OBGY
Subspecialties
Essentials for Postgraduates

OBGY Subspecialties
Essentials for Postgraduates

Editors

Deepti Goswami MD, FRCOG
Director-Professor
Department of Obstetrics and Gynecology
Maulana Azad Medical College
New Delhi

Sangeeta Bhasin MD
Chief Medical Officer (NFSG)
Department of Obstetrics and Gynecology
Lok Nayak Hospital
New Delhi

Anjali Tempe MD
Director-Professor and Head
Department of Obstetrics and Gynecology
Director, IVF Centre
Maulana Azad Medical College
New Delhi

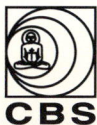

CBS

CBS Publishers & Distributors Pvt Ltd

New Delhi • Bengaluru • Chennai • Kochi • Kolkata • Mumbai

Bhopal • Bhubaneswar • Hyderabad • Jharkhand • Nagpur • Patna • Pune • Uttarakhand • Dhaka (Bangladesh)

OBGY
Subspecialties
Essentials for Postgraduates

ISBN: 978-93-88178-96-9

Copyright © Authors and Publisher

First Edition: 2019

Published by Satish Kumar Jain and produced by Varun Jain for

CBS Publishers & Distributors Pvt Ltd
4819/XI Prahlad Street, 24 Ansari Road, Daryaganj, New Delhi 110 002, India.
Ph: 23289259, 23266861, 23266867   Fax: 011-23243014   Website: www.cbspd.com
e-mail: delhi@cbspd.com; cbspubs@airtelmail.in.

Corporate Office: 204 FIE, Industrial Area, Patparganj, Delhi 110 092
Ph: 4934 4934   Fax: 4934 4935   e-mail: publishing@cbspd.com; publicity@cbspd.com

Branches

- **Bengaluru:** Seema House 2975, 17th Cross, K.R. Road,
  Banasankari 2nd Stage, Bengaluru 560 070, Karnataka
  Ph: +91-80-26771678/79   Fax: +91-80-26771680   e-mail: bangalore@cbspd.com
- **Chennai:** 7, Subbaraya Street, Shenoy Nagar, Chennai 600 030, Tamil Nadu
  Ph: +91-44-26680620, 26681266   Fax: +91-44-42032115   e-mail: chennai@cbspd.com
- **Kochi:** 42/1325, 1326, Power House Road, Opp KSEB Power House,
  Ernakulam 682 018, Kochi, Kerala
  Ph: +91-484-4059061-65   Fax: +91-484-4059065   e-mail: kochi@cbspd.com
- **Kolkata:** 6/B, Ground Floor, Rameswar Shaw Road, Kolkata-700 014, West Bengal
  Ph: +91-33-22891126, 22891127, 22891128   e-mail: kolkata@cbspd.com
- **Mumbai:** 83-C, Dr E Moses Road, Worli, Mumbai-400018, Maharashtra
  Ph: +91-22-24902340/41   Fax: +91-22-24902342   e-mail: mumbai@cbspd.com

Representatives

• Bhopal	0-8319310552	• Bhubaneswar	0-9911037372	• Hyderabad	0-9885175004
• Jharkhand	0-9811541605	• Nagpur	0-9021734563	• Patna	0-9334159340
• Pune	0-9623451994	• Uttarakhand	0-9716462459	• Dhaka (Bangladesh)	01912-003485

Printed at: HT Media Ltd., Greater Noida, UP India

Contributors

Aastha Raheja
Resident
Department of Obstetrics and
Gynecology, Maulana Azad Medical
College, New Delhi

Aditi Aggarwal
Senior Research Associate
Department of Radiotherapy
Lok Nayak Hospital
New Delhi

Amee Prapanna
Senior Resident
Department of Obstetrics and
Gynecology, Lok Nayak Hospital
New Delhi

Anjali Tempe
Director-Professor and Head
Department of Obstetrics and
Gynecology, Maulana Azad Medical
College, New Delhi

Anubhuti Rana
Senior Resident
Department of Obstetrics and
Gynecology, Lok Nayak Hospital
New Delhi

Arun Kumar Rathi
Director-Professor
Department of Radiotherapy
Maulana Azad Medical College
New Delhi

Ashima Aron
Resident
Department of Obstetrics and
Gynecology, Maulana Azad Medical
College, New Delhi

Ashok Kumar
Director-Professor
Department of Obstetrics and
Gynecology, Maulana Azad Medical
College, New Delhi

Asmita M Rathore
Director-Professor
Department of Obstetrics and
Gynecology, Maulana Azad Medical
College, New Delhi

Bidhisha Singha
Specialist
Department of Obstetrics and
Gynecology, Lok Nayak Hospital
New Delhi

Chetna A Sethi
Specialist
Department of Obstetrics and
Gynecology, Lok Nayak Hospital
New Delhi

Deepali Dhingra
Fellow, Reproductive Medicine
Department of Obstetrics and
Gynecology, Maulana Azad Medical
College, New Delhi

Deepti Goswami
Director-Professor
Department of Obstetrics and
Gynecology, Maulana Azad Medical
College, New Delhi

Devender Kumar
Professor
Department of Obstetrics and
Gynecology, Maulana Azad Medical
College, New Delhi

Divya KV
Resident
Department of Obstetrics and
Gynecology, Maulana Azad Medical
College, New Delhi

Garima Sharma
Fellow, Reproductive Medicine
Department of Obstetrics and
Gynecology, Maulana Azad Medical
College, New Delhi

Garima Singh
Resident
Department of Obstetrics and
Gynecology, Maulana Azad Medical
College, New Delhi

Gauri Gandhi
Director-Professor
Department of Obstetrics and
Gynecology, Maulana Azad Medical
College, New Delhi

Gazala Parveen
Fellow, High risk pregnancy and
Neonatology, Department of
Obstetrics and Gynecology, Maulana
Azad Medical College, New Delhi

Hemlata Garg
Clinical Associate
Department of Obstetrics and
Gynecology, B.L. Kapoor Hospital
New Delhi

Kanika Gupta
Resident
Department of Obstetrics and
Gynecology, Maulana Azad Medical
College, New Delhi

Karishma Gupta
Senior Resident
Department of Obstetrics and Gyneco-
logy, Lok Nayak Hospital New Delhi

Kashika Kathuria
Fellow, Reproductive Medicine
Department of Obstetrics and
Gynecology, Maulana Azad Medical
College, New Delhi

Khushboo Tong
Resident
Department of Obstetrics and
Gynecology, Maulana Azad Medical
College, New Delhi

Kishore Singh
Director-Professor and Head
Department of Radiotherapy, Maulana
Azad Medical College, New Delhi

Komal Rastogi
Senior Resident
Department of Obstetrics and
Gynecology, Lok Nayak Hospital
New Delhi

Krishna Agarwal
Professor
Department of Obstetrics and
Gynecology, Maulana Azad Medical
College, New Delhi

Latika Sahu
Director-Professor
Department of Obstetrics and
Gynecology, Maulana Azad Medical
College, New Delhi

Madhavi M Gupta
Professor
Department of Obstetrics and
Gynecology, Maulana Azad Medical
College, New Delhi

Muthyala Tanuja
Assistant Professor
Department of Obstetrics and
Gynecology, Maulana Azad Medical
College, New Delhi

Narayan Adhikari
Senior Resident
Department of Radiotherapy
Lok Nayak Hospital, New Delhi

Niharika Dhiman
Assistant Professor
Department of Obstetrics and
Gynecology, Maulana Azad Medical
College, New Delhi

Nilanchali Singh
Assistant Professor
Department of Obstetrics and
Gynecology, Maulana Azad Medical
College, New Delhi

Poonam Kashyap
Assistant Professor
Department of Obstetrics and
Gynecology, Maulana Azad Medical
College, New Delhi

Poonam Sachdeva
Senior Specialist
Department of Obstetrics and
Gynecology, Lok Nayak Hospital
New Delhi

Preeti Singh
Associate Professor
Department of Obstetrics and
Gynecology, Maulana Azad Medical
College, New Delhi

Priyanka Khandey
Senior Resident
Department of Obstetrics and
Gynecology, Lok Nayak Hospital
New Delhi

Pushpa Mishra
Senior Medical Officer
Department of Obstetrics and
Gynecology, Lok Nayak Hospital
New Delhi

Rachna Sharma
Senior Specialist
Department of Obstetrics and
Gynecology, Lok Nayak Hospital
New Delhi

Rashmi Pillania
Fellow, Reproductive Medicine
Department of Obstetrics and
Gynecology, Maulana Azad Medical
College, New Delhi

Reetu Yadav
Resident
Department of Obstetrics and
Gynecology, Maulana Azad Medical
College, New Delhi

Renu Tanwar
Professor
Department of Obstetrics and
Gynecology, Maulana Azad Medical
College, New Delhi

Rini Pachori
Resident
Department of Obstetrics and
Gynecology, Maulana Azad Medical
College, New Delhi

Rubee Khattar
Consultant
Department of Obstetrics and
Gynecology, Alshifa Hospital
New Delhi

Ruchi Gupta
Fellow, High Risk Pregnancy and
Neonatology, Department of
Obstetrics and Gynecology
Maulana Azad Medical College
New Delhi

Sana Tiwari
Resident
Department of Obstetrics and
Gynecology, Vardhman Mahavir
Medical College, New Delhi

Sangeeta Bhasin
Chief Medical Officer (NFSG)
Department of Obstetrics and
Gynecology, Lok Nayak Hospital
New Delhi

Sangeeta Gupta
Director-Professor
Department of Obstetrics and
Gynecology, Maulana Azad Medical
College, New Delhi

Saumya Prasad
Senior Resident
Reproductive Medicine
Department of Obstetrics and
Gynecology, Lok Nayak Hospital
New Delhi

Savita Arora
Assistant Professor
Department of Radiotherapy
Maulana Azad Medical College
New Delhi

Shakun Tyagi
Associate Professor
Department of Obstetrics and
Gynecology, Maulana Azad Medical
College, New Delhi

Shivangini Rana
Resident
Department of Obstetrics and
Gynecology, Maulana Azad Medical
College, New Delhi

Sneha Mishra
Resident
Department of Obstetrics and
Gynecology, Maulana Azada Medical
College, New Delhi

Sneha Sharma
Senior Resident
Department of Obstetrics and
Gynecology, Lok Nayak Hospital
New Delhi

Snigdha Pathak
Senior Resident
Department of Obstetrics and
Gynecology, Lok Nayak Hospital
New Delhi

Sudha Prasad
Director-Professor
Department of Obstetrics and
Gynecology, Maulana Azad Medical
College, New Delhi

Swati Rai
Senior Resident
Department of Obstetrics and
Gynecology, Lok Nayak Hospital
New Delhi

Tarang Preet Kaur
Resident
Department of Obstetrics and
Gynecology, Maulana Azad Medical
College, New Delhi

Vijay Zutshi
Professor and Consultant
Department of Obstetrics and
Gynecology, Vardhman Mahavir
Medical College, New Delhi

YM Mala
Director-Professor
Department of Obstetrics and
Gynecology, Maulana Azad Medical
College, New Delhi

Foreword

The medical science has seen an explosion of knowledge and technology during the last few decades resulting in evolution of subspecialties in different fields. The specialty of obstetrics and gynecology has been no exception and the subspecialties in the form of maternal-fetal medicine, reproductive medicine, gynecologic oncology and urogynecology have emerged and established themselves. As the dean of prestigious Maulana Azad Medical College, I have been a witness to the growth and development of some of these subspecialties in the college. Therefore, I am particularly pleased to write the Foreword.

The concomitant dissemination of information to the common man via internet has resulted in everincreasing patient demands that have had a positive impact by way of clinicians striving to achieve optimal outcomes with the ultimate aim of achieving patient satisfaction. This has put additional responsibility on the generalists to be aware of the evolving science so that the deserving patients are referred to appropriate specialists. The Department of Obstetrics and Gynecology, Maulana Azad Medical College and associated Lok Nayak Hospital has shouldered this challenging responsibility by bringing out this book *OBGY Subspecialties: Essentials for Postgraduates*. The book is divided into five sections covering specialties of Maternal-fetal Medicine, Reproductive Endocrinology, Infertility and Assisted Reproductive Technology, Gynecologic Oncology, Urogynecology and a General section, which addresses the important issues related to sexual violence. All the Authors are renowned professionals with expertise in their respective fields and are also familiar with working in limited resource settings. The Editors have marvelously performed the difficult task of making the text simple and lucid so that the postgraduates find it easy to comprehend.

In my opinion, the Editors and the Authors have succeeded in providing a comprehensive overview of Obstetrics and Gynecology subspecialties, which will be useful not only to the postgraduates in preparation of their examinations, but also to general obstetricians and gynecologists to update themselves and counsel the patients appropriately when in need of a subspecialty care. The team deserves to be congratulated for their commendable efforts.

Dr Deepak K Tempe
Director-Professor
Department of Anesthesiology and
Intensive Care
GB Pant Institute of Postgraduate Medical
Education and Research
Former Dean
Maulana Azad Medical College, New Delhi

Preface

In this world of specializations, it becomes difficult sometimes, for doctors, to render speciality care to patients unless they themselves have a basic working knowledge of different subspecialties in their subjects. To bridge this loophole in knowledge, an endeavor is being made to provide a ready reckoner in speciality care for both students and practitioners of obstetrics and gynecology.

The Department of Obstetrics and Gynecology, MAMC, has been running speciality clinics in infertility and assisted reproductive technology (ART), reproductive endocrinology, gynecologic oncology, fetal medicine and high risk obstetrics for the past many years. Likewise, this book titled *OBGY Subspecialties: Essentials for Postgraduates*, has been divided into different sections.

The first section on Maternal-fetal Medicine deals with patients requiring aneuploidy screening, patients having fetal growth restriction, patients at risk of preterm labor and those having fetal hydrops, from the perspective of a fetal medicine specialist. The second section on Reproductive Endocrinology dwells on commonly encountered endocrine disorders like amenorrhea, hyperprolactinemia and polycystic ovarian syndrome. The third section on Infertility and Assisted Reproductive Technology deals with intrauterine insemination, *in vitro* fertilization protocols that are commonly prescribed and state of the art subjects like cryopreservation, fertility preservation in cancer and uterine transplantation. The fourth section on Gynecologic Oncology which includes both preventive and therapeutic aspects of management of different gynecological cancers. Fifth section on Urogynecology and Sixth section on General dealing with the important topics of contraception and clinical and medicolegal aspects of care of a survivor of sexual violence has also been included.

The book has been written in an 'easy to read' and 'easy to understand' problem-based format. Common case scenarios (as they present in the outpatient department) are followed by questions and answers.

The authors are all experts in their own right and the editors are grateful to them for their clinical and intellectual inputs.

We hope that our efforts in providing this ready access to information are appreciated and enjoyed by all, particularly the postgraduate students.

Happy reading!

Deepti Goswami
Sangeeta Bhasin
Anjali Tempe

Contents

Section I MATERNAL-FETAL MEDICINE

Section 2 REPRODUCTIVE ENDOCRINOLOGY

Section 5 UROGYNECOLOGY

Section 6 GENERAL

Aneuploidy Screening

Sangeeta Gupta

Aneuploidy screening during pregnancy is the standard of obstetric care. It has evolved from taking maternal age of 35 years as cut off for invasive testing to the most recent addition of NIPT to its armamentarium. The following case discussions will highlight the principles of aneuploidy screening.

Case 1

A 26 years primigravida visits the antenatal clinic at 13 weeks pregnancy. Her friend has recently delivered a baby boy with Down's syndrome. She is very anxious and is aware that testing in early pregnancy can help detection of this disorder in fetus.

Q1. What will you advise her?

- The patient is explained about combined first trimester screening (cFTS) with ultrasound and serum markers. A thorough pre-test counselling is done to explain that it is a screening test with false-positive and false-negative results. A positive result would warrant a confirmatory test, that is, invasive testing and options of termination of pregnancy in case of affected fetus.
- The essential criteria for optimal performance of screening tests are
  - Parameters like maternal age (MA), weight, ethnicity, insulin dependent diabetes, smoking, number of fetus and IVF pregnancy (self or donor), should be addressed
  - Accurate gestational age (GA) determination, confirmed by ultrasound

  - Accredited sonographers for measurement of crown rump length (CRL), nuchal translucency (NT) and nasal bone (NB).
  - Accredited laboratory and proper standardisation for analysing serum markers
- The first step is to perform a first trimester ultrasonography (USG) to confirm gestational age by measuring the CRL, number of fetuses, measure NT and NB.

Q2. What criteria should be fulfilled during USG examination?

- The scan should be done between 11 weeks and 13 weeks + 6 days gestational age and the fetal CRL should be between 45 and 84 mm.
- The image to measure crown rump length should be captured in the perfect mid-sagittal section and fetus should be horizontal. The fetus should be in neutral position. For NT and NB measurement, the image is magnified so that the head and upper thorax occupy the whole screen.[1]

Q3. Patient follows the next day with the following USG: Single intrauterine pregnancy, cardiac activity present, CRL 68.3 mm, GA corresponds to 13 weeks, NT 1.7 mm and nasal bone is seen. What would you do now?

Since her CRL is 68.3 mm maternal serum sample is collected for analysis of PAPP-A and free β-hCG.

Q4. **The report of cFTS is as follows (Fig. 1.1). What would you explain to her?**

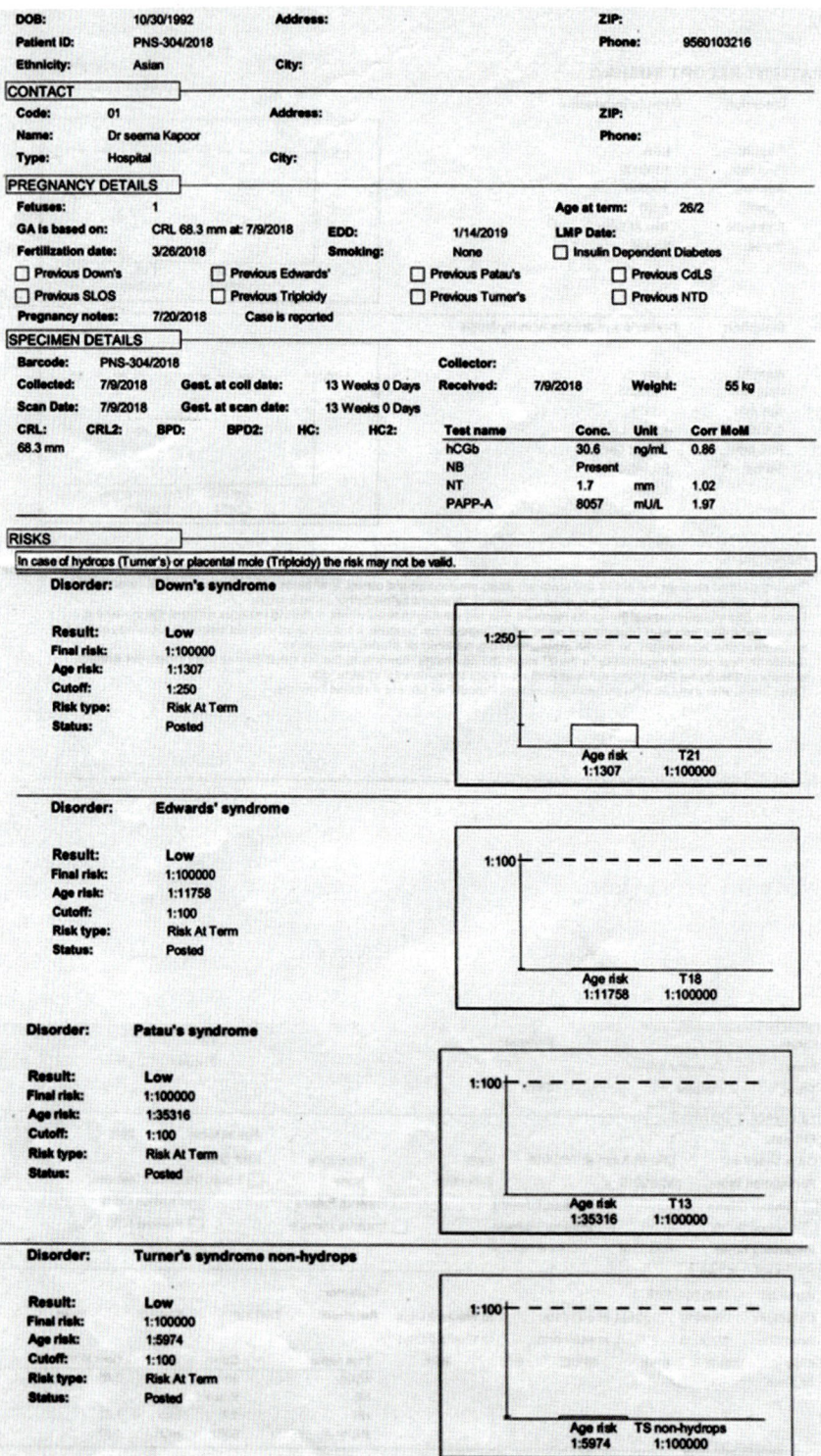

Fig. 1.1: cFTS report of Case 1

As the results are low risk, the couple needs no further testing.

Q5. What if results are high risk, for example, 1 in 86? What are the options available in such a case?

The patient can be offered NIPS or invasive testing (Further discussion will be similar as in Case 4).

Q6. In a similar case scenario if the results are 1 in 350, what are the options?

The following options can be considered:
- No further testing
- However, some fetal medicine specialists classify the risk in three categories of high risk (more than 1 in 100), intermediate risk (1 in 100 to 1 in 1000) and low risk (less than 1 in 1000) (Fig. 1.2).

In the above case risk can be reassigned by the contingent method, to reduce the invasive procedure rate. If after using the contingent method, patient has high risk result, invasive testing is done. If she has a low risk, she needs no further testing. The contingent method increases specificity, does not decrease sensitivity and lowers fasle positive rates (FPR) thus reduces number of invasive tests.[2]

Case 2

A 32 years G2P1L1 comes for her first antenatal check-up at 16 weeks GA.

Q1. What options are available for aneuploidy screening?

She can be offered triple or Quad test which includes maternal serum markers (listed in Table 1.1). The correct GA determination is

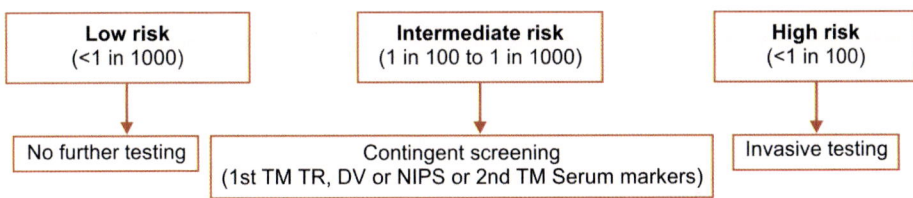

Fig. 1.2: Flow diagram depicting risk categorisation and strategy

Table 1.1: Aneuploidy screening tests			
Screening test	*Components*	*Period of performance*	*DR@5% FPR*
First trimester Serum screening: "double marker test"	Free beta hCG and PAPP-A	GA 10–3+6 weeks or CRL 33–84 mm	60%
Nuchal scan	Nuchal translucency (NT)	GA 11–13+6 weeks or CRL 45–84 mm	75–80%
Combined screening test	NT, Free β-hCG, PAPP-A	GA 11–13+6 weeks or CRL 45–84 mm	90%
Triple screening test	AFP, β-hCG, uE3	GA 15–22 weeks or BPD 32–52 mm	65–70%
Quadruple screening test (QST)	AFP, β-hCG, dimeric inhibin A (DIA), uE3	GA 15-22 weeks or BPD 32–52 mm	80%
Integrated test	NT, PAPP-A at first trimester, β-hCG, AFP, DIA, uE3 at second trimester	As per each visit	94%

essential for optimal performance of these tests, hence scan for accurate dating is essential by CRL in first trimester or BPD in second trimester. The permissible BPD range for performing the above two tests is 32–52 mm or GA between 15 and 22 weeks. The triple test is not recommended anymore due to low DR (65–70%) and hence increased number of invasive tests. At minimum, any prenatal screen offered should have a detection rate of 75% with no more than a 5% false-positive rate. Therefore, offering maternal age or triple test should be avoided. Table 1.1 enlists various screening tests[3].

Case 3

A 29 years G2P1L1 comes at 19 weeks GA with second trimester ultrasound done for anomalies. In the scan two soft markers, echogenic intracardiac focus and short femur are seen. Other soft markers are not seen.

Q1. Patient has come for further work up. What should be done?

For estimation of risk for trisomy 21 based on second trimester ultrasound findings, two important figures are the apriori risk and the likelihood ratio (LR). The apriori risk would be the maternal age (in case of no previous screening) or second trimester serum bio-chemical testing or cFTS. The positive and negative likelihood ratios for each soft marker are derived by study by Agathokleous (Table 1.2). For final risk, the apriori risk (MA or cFTS or second trimester biochemical screening) is multiplied by positive LR of each marker found to be present and the negative LR of each marker looked for but not found.[4]

First or second trimester screening results were not available for the patient. As the patient is 19 weeks, Quadruple test was advised. The results were 1 in 482. Hence, the apriori risk was taken as 1 in 482. The soft markers LR were filled in excel spreadsheet allowing automated calculations (Table 1.3). The combined LR was 6.21 thus after multiplying by 1/482, the final risk is 1 in 78. Thus, now patient falls in high risk zone and was offered amniocentesis.

Non-invasive Prenatal Screening

Non-invasive Prenatal Screening (NIPS) uses cell free fetal DNA (cffDNA) in maternal blood and has potential to screen for fetal aneuploidies. cffDNA is derived from breakdown of fetal cells of placental origin mostly. cffDNA clears from maternal system quickly and is undetectable within hours after delivery, hence representative of current fetus only. About 3–13% DNA in maternal serum is of fetal origin after 10 weeks of gestation. It is diagnostic for

Table 1.2: Positive and negative likelihood ratios of sonographic markers for trisomy 21 and LR of individual isolated markers

Marker	LR (+)	LR (–)	Isolated marker LR
Echogenic intracardiac focus	5.83	0.80	0.95
Ventriculomegaly	27.52	0.94	3.81
Increased nuchal fold	23.30	0.80	3.79
Echogenic bowel	11.44	0.90	1.65
Mild hydronephrosis	7.63	0.92	1.08
Short humerus	4.81	0.74	0.78
Short femur	3.72	0.80	0.61
ARSA	21.48	0.71	3.94
Absent or hypoplastic nasal bone	23.27	0.46	6.58

Table 1.3: Soft markers LR of case 3 in excel sheet with automated calculations

Marker	Present/absent (choose from drop-down)	LR
Intracardiac echogenic focus	Present	5.83
Mild hydronephrosis	Absent	0.92
Short femur	Present	3.72
Echogenic bowel	Absent	0.90
Increased nuchal fold	Absent	0.80
Aberrant right sub-clavian artery	Not known	1.00
Absent or hypoplastic nasal bone	Normal size	0.46
Ventriculomegaly	Absent	0.94
LR for combination:		**6.21**

fetal sex, Rh negative status and paternally derived mutation. For screening for aneuploidies, the quantitative analysis of DNA fragments from different chromosomes is done. The detection rate is 99% at FPR of 0.5%.[5]

Case 4

- A 37 years primigravida who has conceived by IVF (no donor oocytes) presents at 12+ weeks pregnancy.
- USG: Single live fetus, CRL 54 mm, GA corresponds to 12 weeks, NT 1.7 mm
- cFTS: Risk I in 57

Q1. What are her options for further testing?
The options for further testing offered are invasive testing versus NIPS—thorough counselling about advantages and disadvantages of all options was done (Table 1.4).

The couple opted for NIPS. The following report followed suggestive of high risk of trisomy 21 (Fig. 1.3).

When we interpret the reports of NIPS, we must check the *fetal fraction*. The minimum fetal fraction on which results are interpreted is 4%. Results of NIPS are available in 7–14 days.[6]

Couple underwent chorionic villus sampling, fetus was diagnosed with trisomy 21 (karyotype) and termination of pregnancy was done as desired by the couple.

Advantages of NIPS
- No risk to the pregnancy
- Highly sensitive screening test for Down syndrome, which means that a normal result would be very reassuring in this setting
- High detection rates so less number of invasive procedures

Disadvantages of NIPS
- A *positive result requires confirmation by invasive testing* before action is taken
- A small proportion of women have a failed NIPS result, usually on the basis of a low fetal fraction—*should have invasive testing*
- *False negative results*: There have been several reports of false negative results, rates in the range of 0–1.4%

Messages[7,8]
- Whom to offer NIPS—High risk cases and **not recommended as primary screening tool** in general population.
- Pretest counselling: **The use of NIPS in clinical practice should be an informed patient choice.**

	NIPT (Screening)	cFTS (Screening)	Chorionic villus sampling/ amniocentesis (Diagnostic)
Risk to pregnancy	No	No	Yes, 0.5–1%
Detection rate for Down syndrome	High (sensitivity, or true positive ≥99.5% or higher)	Moderately high	Diagnostic test (≥99.9%)
False-positive rate	Low (specificity, or true negative ≥99.8%)	Moderate	Diagnostic test (≥99.9%)
Ability to detect other chromosomal abnormalities	Currently 13, 18, 21 (+/– and Y). These account for ~70% of the major chromosomal abnormalities	Targeted to screen for trisomy 13, 18, 21	Yes • Plain karyotype: All chromosomes to a resolution visible on microscopy (5–10 million DNA base pairs) • Chromosome microarray: All chromosomes to a relatively high submicaroscopic resolution (generally less than 250,000 DNA base pairs)

Table 1.4: Comparison of NIPT, cFTS and invasive tests

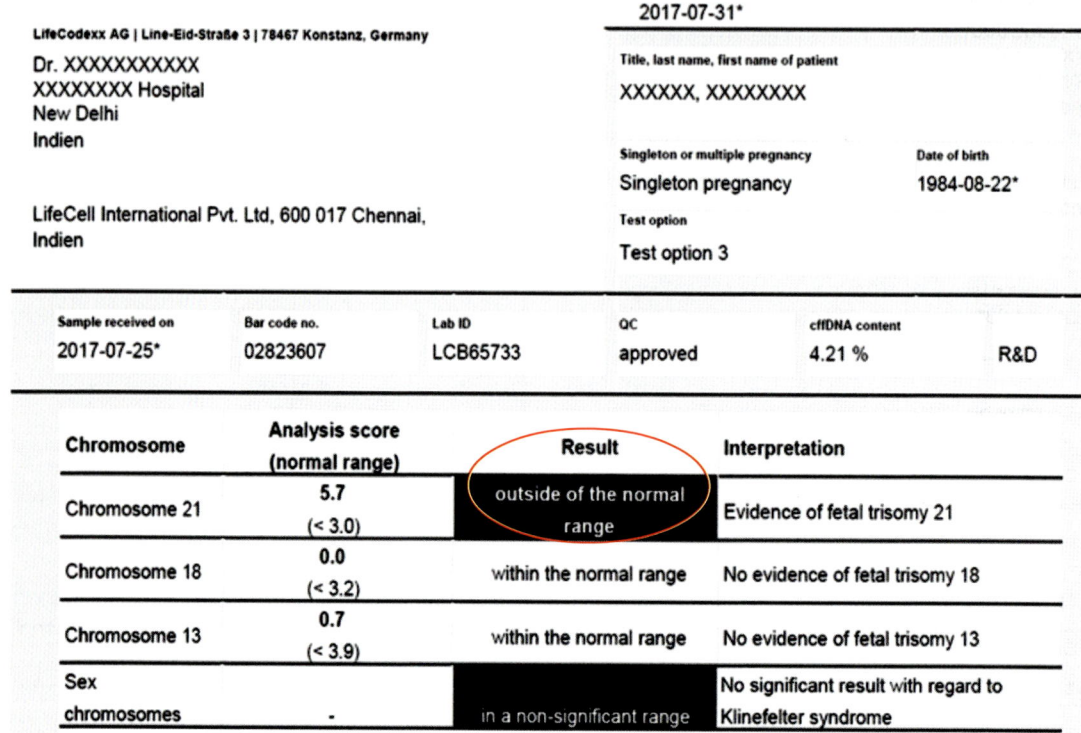

Fig. 1.3: NIPS report of Case 4

- **Abnormal NIPS to be confirmed by diagnostic test:** CVS/Amniocentesis. No irrevocable obstetrical decision should be made in pregnancies with a positive noninvasive prenatal testing result without confirmatory invasive diagnostic testing.

Case 5

A 34-year-old lady, G2P1L1, POG 10 weeks had previous baby with Down's syndrome. She seeks help for early detection in this pregnancy but is concerned about risk of miscarriage with invasive testing.

Q1. The couple enquires if NIPS is an option.

Yes it is. But patient would still require a first trimester scan for dating and NT.

Figure 1.4 shows the NIPS report of the patient.
- The patient had a low risk in NIPS. She was reassured that the baby is unlikely to be affected with Down's syndrome and

requires no further testing. The patient delivered a normal baby at 38 weeks of gestation.
- Indications of NIPS [7]
  - Women >35 years or older
  - Positive first/second trimester screening result
  - USG findings indicative of aneuploidy
  - History of trisomy offspring
  - Parent carrying balanced translocation with increased risk of trisomy 21/13.

Case 6

Case A
- 28 years G2P1L1 with 13+ weeks pregnancy
- USG: Single IUP, CA+, CRL 70 mm, GA corresponds to 13 weeks 1 d, **NT 1.8 mm (50th percentile)**
- PAPP-A: 0.25 MoMs/β-HCG: 1.8 MoMs
- cFTS: Risk I in 57

LifeCodexx AG	Line-Eid-Straße 3	78467 Konstanz, Germany Dr. XXXXXXXXXXX XXXXXXXX Hospital New Delhi Indien LifeCell International Pvt. Ltd, 600 017 Chennai, Indien	Title, last name, first name of patient XXXXXXX, XXXXXX

| | | | Singleton or multiple pregnancy
Singleton pregnancy | Date of birth
1977-12-04* |
| | | | Test option
Test option 3 | |

Sample received on 2017-11-23*	Bar code no. 02827216	Lab ID LCB75405	QC approved	cffDNA content 14.23 %

Chromosome	Analysis score (normal range)	Result	Interpretation
Chromosome 21	-0.1 (< 3.0)	within the normal range	No evidence of fetal trisomy 21
Chromosome 18	0.9 (< 3.2)	within the normal range	No evidence of fetal trisomy 18
Chromosome 13	-0.1 (< 3.9)	within the normal range	No evidence of fetal trisomy 13
Sex chromosomes	-	within the normal range	No evidence of Turner, Triple-X, Klinefelter or XYY syndrome

Fig. 1.4: NIPS report of Case 5

Case B

- 28 years G2P1L1 13+ weeks pregnancy
- USG: Single intrauterine pregnancy, CA+, CRL 70 mm, GA corresponds to 13 weeks 1 d, **NT 2.8 mm (96th percentile)**
- PAPP-A: 0.63 MoMs/β-hCG: 1.02 MoMs
- cFTS: Risk I in 57

Q1. In the above two cases which patient can be offered NIPS?

Though the cFTS risk in both cases is same, Case A can be offered NIPS, however in Case B CVS should be offered as NT is increased (>90th percentile). An increased NT is associated with other abnormalities besides aneuploidy.

Case 7

Case A

- 32 years G3P1L1A1, 17 weeks
- Anomaly scan: Two soft markers—echogenic intracardiac focus and dilated pelvi calyceal system.

Case B

- 30 years G2P1L1, 17 weeks
- Anomaly scan: Isolated omphalocele

Q1. What test would you offer to the above two cases?

In case A, the patient can be offered NIPS but in case B as a major malformation is seen, direct invasive testing, that is, amniocentesis should be done.

Messages [7,8]

- If associated ultrasound abnormality is present, offer invasive testing and not NIPS. However, for ultrasound markers, NIPS is an option.
- NT measurement should always be done even if NIPS taken as first line screening modality.

Case 8

- 30 years Primi, BMI 31 kg/m², POG: 13 weeks

- USG: Single live fetus, CRL 66 mm, GA 12 weeks 6 days, NT 1.1 mm
- cFTS: 1 in 127
- NIPS: **Low fetal fraction (2%),** no call
- Repeat NIPS: Failed
- POG 16 weeks—amniocentesis: Normal karyotype
- USG: Normal

Q1. What do you understand by this report?

This is a case of *Low fetal fraction (<4%)/No call/ Failed NIPS*[7]

- Incidence is 1–8%
- Causes
  - Obesity
  - GA <10 weeks
  - Aneuploidy (T13, T18, Monosomy X, triploidy)
- Repeat sample may give result in 50–60% patients

Messages
- Must do invasive test in these patients as low fetal fraction is associated with aneuploidy
- Confirmation of GA by USG must before giving sample for NIPS

False positive result[7]
- Confined placental mosaicism
- Vanishing twin
- Maternal chromosomal abnormalities (mosaicism)
- Maternal malignancies

Message: Invasive testing is must in positive NIPS.

Limitations of NIPS (versus conventional screening)[7]
- Does not screen for open neural tube defects.
- Does not replace first trimester USG—accurate dating, NT, multiple pregnancy, placental abnormalities and CMF.
- Not used in higher-order pregnancies.
- No role in predicting late-pregnancy complications like pre-eclampsia.

Limitations of NIPS (versus Invasive testing)[7,8]
- Chromosomal abnormalities such as unbalanced translocations, deletions, and duplications will not be detected by NIPS. With fetal anomalies, invasive diagnostic testing and CGH array are more likely to detect chromosomal imbalances—better testing option
- NIPS cannot distinguish Down syndrome is trisomy 21, a Robertsonian translocation or mosaicism
- NIPS does not screen for single-gene mutations.

 Key Points

- Pre-test and post-test counselling are an integral part of any screening test.
- Strict quality control for ultrasound examination and laboratory assays is essential for optimal performance of the screening method.
- NIPS
  - 'Super (?)' screening test—not diagnostic, reduces invasive testing but cannot replace it
  - To be done at more than 10 weeks
  - USG mandatory before NIPS
  - No role if abnormal USG findings
  - Not to be done in low risk population-—use as a contingent method but not as primary screening modality
  - Confirm with invasive testing in 'High risk' and 'No call'.

REFERENCES

1. https://fetalmedicine.org/education/the-11-13-weeks-scan.
2. Kagan KO, Wright D, Nicolaides KH. First-trimester contingent screening for trisomies 21, 18 and 13 by fetal nuchal translucency and ductus venosus flow and maternal blood cell-free DNA testing. Ultrasound Obstet Gynecol 2015;45: 42–7.
3. Practice bulletin No. 163: screening for fetal aneuploidy. Obstet Gynecol 2016;127:e123–37.
4. Agathokleous M, Chaveeva P, Poon LC, Kosinski P, Nicolaides KH. Meta-analysis of second-trimester markers for trisomy 21. Ultrasound Obstet Gynecol 2013;41:247–61.

5. Kinnings SL, Geis JA, Almasri E, Wang H, Guan X, McCullough RM, et al. Factors affecting levels of circulating cell-free fetal DNA in maternal plasma and their implications for noninvasive prenatal testing. Prenat Diagn 2015;35:816–22.

6. Carlson LM, Vora NL. Prenatal diagnosis: Screening and diagnostic tools. Obstet Gynecol Clin North Am 2017;44:245–56.

7. Committee opinion No. 640: cell-free DNA screening for fetal aneuploidy. Obstet Gynecol 2015;126:e31–7.

8. Gregg AR, Gross SJ, Best RG, Monaghan KG, Bajaj K, Skotko BG, et al. ACMG statement on noninvasive prenatal screening for fetal aneuploidy. Genet Med 2013;15:395–8.

Hydrops Fetalis

Asmita M Rathore, Ruchi Gupta, Gazala Shahnaz

Hydrops fetalis (HF) is defined as the abnormal accumulation of fluid in fetal soft tissues and/ or serous cavities. The USG finding of fetal hydrops is a clinical entity with wide spectrum of causes and associations2 and thus warrants thorough search for underlying cause.

Hydrops fetalis is broadly categorised as (a) immune (10–20%) mainly due to maternal Rh D alloimmunization and (b) nonimmune hydrops fetalis (NIHF) (80–90%) due to variety of other causes like infections, aneuploidies, etc. With the introduction of widespread immunoprophylaxis for RhD alloimmunization and the use of intrauterine blood transfusions (IUBT) for immune hydrops therapy, NIHF accounts for almost 90% of hydrops cases and prevalence ranges from 1/1500 to 1/4000 birth in developed world.[1] In India, exact figures are not available but it is not unusual to see cases of hydrops due to Rh alloimmunization as the uptake and quality antenatal care is not universal.

DIAGNOSIS

Hydrops fetalis is essentially an ultrasonographic diagnosis and is defined as effusions in at least two spaces—peritoneal, pleural, pericardial or subcutaneous edema. Fluid in any one of these spaces may be an early finding and such fetuses should undergo follow-up to ensure that hydrops is not developing. The degree of severity of hydrops is generally subjective. Polyhydramnios or placental thickening is often associated.

a. *Fetal ascites:* Appears as an echolucent rim of varying size in the fetal abdomen in USG. It should be visible all the way around the abdomen in the transverse plane (Fig. 2.1).
b. *Pleural effusion:* Appear as small rim of fluid outlining the pleural space and diaphragm. It may be unilateral or bilateral; commonly they are large and compress the lungs (Fig. 2.2).

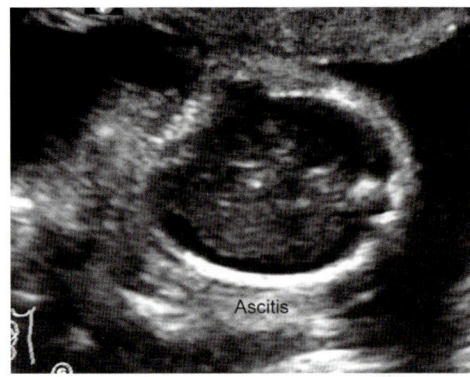

Fig. 2.1: Fetal ascites

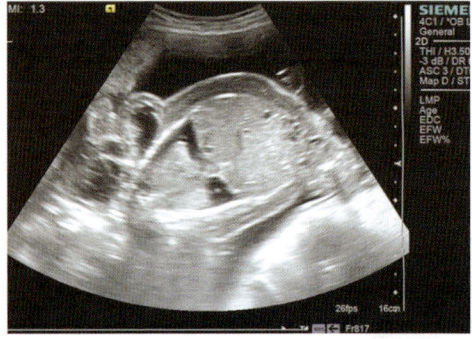

Fig. 2.2: Fetal pleural effusion (*Courtesy:* Dr Anju Garg, Head, Department of Radiodiagnosis, MAMC)

c. *Pericardial effusion:* Pericardial effusion indicates cardiac decompensation and is the earliest sign of hydrops in fetuses with cardiac lesions. It is usually smaller in volume and more difficult to see (Fig. 2.3).

d. *Skin edema (>5 mm of subcutaneous tissue)* is a generalized process. It is easiest to see with USG over the chest wall or scalp (Fig. 2.4).

e. *Placental thickening:* Thickness greater than 4 cm in second trimester and 6 cm in third trimester.

f. *Polyhydramnios:* Usually present in 40 to 75% of cases of hydrops. However, in some cases, oligoamnios is present, and is considered as an ominous or late sign.

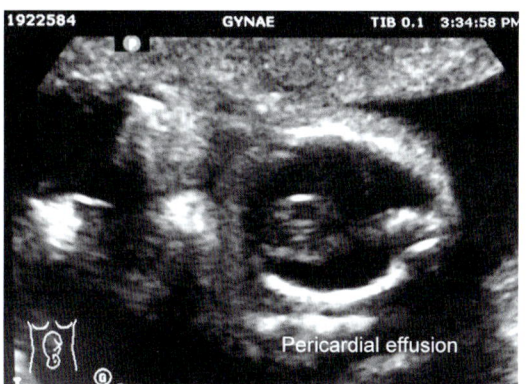

Fig. 2.3: Fetal pericardial effusion

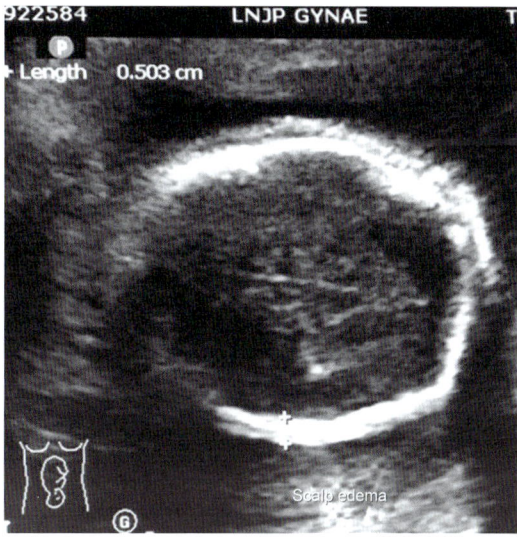

Fig. 2.4: Scalp edema

IMMUNE HYDROPS FETALIS

The commonest cause of immune hydrops is blood group Rh incompatibility, seen mostly with RhD antigen, constituting 97% of cases in pregnancy. The other rare antibodies associated with fetal or neonatal hydrops are Rh non D (E, e, C, c), Kell, Kidd , Duffy, MNSs.

Pathophysiology

When mother is Rh negative and fetus is Rh positive, fetal red cells in maternal circulation elicit an immune response leading to auto-antibody generation. On subsequent exposure to Rh-positive red cells, these antibodies are formed more rapidly and destroy fetal RBCs causing anaemia and high output cardiac failure with resultant hydrops.

Case 1

A 31-year-old G5P1L1A3 was referred at 28 weeks of pregnancy from a secondary care hospital in view of Rh negative pregnancy and positive indirect Coombs test with titre 1:32.

Obstetric History

First pregnancy: Spontaneous abortion at two months gestation, injection anti D not received.

Second pregnancy: Full term vaginal home delivery, injection anti D not received.

Third and fourth pregnancy: Spontaneous abortion at two months gestation, injection anti D not received.

Past and family history: Unremarkable.

General systemic examination: Unremarkable.

Abdominal examination: Uterus 26–28 weeks, cephalic, FHS + regular 130 bpm.

Diagnosis: G5P1L1A3 with POG 32 weeks with Rh alloimmunization.

Q1. How do you diagnose alloimmunisation?

Rh alloimmunisation is diagnosed by indirect Coombs test (ICT) in maternal blood sample, which detects presence of Rh antibodies in maternal serum. Their concentration is determined by double dilution method. The critical titre may vary from lab to lab and is mostly between 1:8 and 1:32.[2] If the titre exceeds the critical dilution or there is significant rise in titre between two consecutive samples even if the upper dilution does not reach the critical level the diagnosis of alloimmunization is made. Once the alloimmunization is diagnosed then further monitoring by antibody titre is not done.

Q2. What are the risk factors for maternal alloimmunization?

- Pregnancy (maternal fetal blood group incompatibility)
- Mismatched blood transfusions
- Abortions—spontaneous, therapeutic, threatened abortion, ectopic pregnancies
- Invasive prenatal procedures—chorionic villus sampling (CVS), amniocentesis, cordocentesis
- Blunt abdominal trauma
- Intrauterine fetal demise in second and third trimesters
- External cephalic version
- Manual removal of placenta

Q3. How will you manage this patient?

Apart from routine antenatal care, the woman needs to be monitored for severity and progression of fetal anemia. If the titre exceeds the critical value, next line of management is assessing the severity of anemia by measuring middle cerebral artery peak systolic velocity (MCA-PCV) and detailed USG to detect fetal hydrops.[3]

Pregnancy is monitored by 1–2 weekly MCA-PSV till 36 weeks of gestation. The MCA PSV value is plotted on nomograms developed by Marie et al. The critical threshold of 1.5 MOMs is used for further intervention. The correct technique of measuring MCA-PSV is important to get accurate result. The sensitivity of MCA-PSV in predicting moderate to severe HDFN is 100% with false positive rate of 12%.[3] Beyond 36 weeks it should be used with caution as sensitivity for detection of fetal anemia

decreases and termination of pregnancy should be considered.

Ultrasound is performed 1–2 weekly to look for early signs of hydrops like cardiomegaly, fluid collection in single cavity. Gross hydrops indicates severe anemia.

If MCA-PSV exceeds 1.5 MoMs or signs of hydrops appear before 34 weeks of gestation then fetal blood sampling to diagnose severity of anemia and intrauterine blood transfusion (IUBT) are required and patient should be referred to fetal medicine specialist.[3]

Follow up of Case 1

The woman was monitored by weekly MCA PSV. The reports were
30 weeks, 32 weeks: 1–1.25 MOM; 34 weeks: 1.25–1.5 MOM.
She was given steroid cover and was delivered at 34 weeks and 5 days gestation.
Baby: Weight: 2.5 kg; Direct Coombs' test (DCT): positive, Hb: 10 g%, serum bilirubin: 6 mg%
Baby was managed with phototherapy, responded well, was discharged on postnatal day 15.

Q4. What are the various manifestations of hemolytic disease in fetus and neonate (HDFN)?

- *Hydrops fetalis:* It is the most severe affection characterised by excessive destruction of red blood cells leading to severe anemia and tissue hypoxemia. Placental hyperplasia occurs in an effort to improve oxygen delivery to fetus. Anoxia damages liver leading to hypoproteinemia causing ascites, hydrothorax and generalised edema. Fetal death ensues after high output cardiac failure.
- *Icterus gravis neonatorum:* It is less severe form of fetal affection where there are no signs of intrauterine affection, but baby develops jaundice after 24 hours of birth. It occurs as the newborn liver is unable to clear bilirubin resulting in neonatal jaundice.
- *Congenital anemia of newborn:* Mildest affection. Anemia develops slowly within first few weeks of life but there is no evidence of jaundice. Usually resolves by 6 weeks.

Q5. How do you monitor neonate after delivery?

After delivery cord blood should be sent for hemogram, DCT, serum bilirubin. Then 1–2 weekly hematocrit and reticulocyte determination is performed till 3 months of age. Infants with Hb <6 g% need top up transfusions.

Q6. What is role of prophylactic anti D to prevent alloimmunization?

The most effective intervention to reduce alloimmunization is use of prophylactic anti D, however, alloimmunization cannot be completely prevented.

Routine anti D prophylaxis[4]

Antenatal:

*   An antibody screen is performed at first antenatal visit, if negative again at 28 week. If still negative, 300 μg of injection anti D should be given. It neutralises fetomaternal hemorrhage of up to 30 mL and reduces risk of isoimmunization from 2% to 0.1%. For women reporting late, the prophylactic anti D can be given later but if she delivers within 3 weeks of antenatal prophylaxis, postnatal dose may be omitted as the effect of anti D persists for about 12 weeks.
*   After CVS, amniocentesis, cordocentesis.
*   After blunt abdominal trauma, antepartum hemorrhage and external cephalic version.

Postnatal: Injection anti D 300 μg is given within 72 hours after birth of an Rh positive infant. It can be given up to 28 days of birth. However, its efficacy gets compromised.

Postabortal: Injection anti D is given in ectopic pregnancies managed either medically or surgically, after induced abortions—medical or surgical, molar pregnancy. There is insufficient evidence regarding anti D administration after spontaneous or threatened miscarriage before 12 weeks of gestation.[5]

Q7. What are the tests available to detect fetomaternal hemorrhage?

The estimation of volume of fetomaternal hemorrhage is important to calculate the neutralising dose of anti D required (approximately 10 μg for 1 mL of fetal blood).

The methods to estimate volume of fetomaternal hemorrhage are:

*   *Kleihauer-Betke test* which is based on the fact that fetal hemoglobin resists denaturation by acid as compared to adult hemoglobin.[6]
*   *Flow cytometry:* It is more precise then Kleihauer-Betke test. It is utilized when large fetomaternal hemorrhage is suspected which requires accurate quantification.
*   *Rosetting method:* This test is used in postpartum Rh-negative mother with Rh-positive fetus within 72 hours. Any positive rosette test needs quantification by Kleihauer-Betke test.

Case 2

A 31-year-old G2P1L1 was referred by radiologist at 30 weeks gestation in view of USG features of fetal hydrops.

Previous pregnancy: Term vaginal home delivery, had postpartum hemorrhage. No anti D given. Male baby 3 years, alive and healthy.

Examination: Uterus 30–32 weeks, cephalic, FHR 134 bpm.

Investigations: Blood group A-negative, husband's blood group A-positive, ICT-1: 128, other investigations were normal.

USG: Single live fetus 28 weeks, no malformations, placenta anterior, amniotic fluid index (AFI)-18, MCA PSV >1.5 MOM.

Diagnosis: Rh Alloimmunization.

Q1. How will you manage this pregnancy further?

The presence of hydrops indicates severe anemia in fetus with Hb deficit of >7 g% for the period of gestation. She should be referred to a fetal medicine unit. The next step is fetal blood sampling to determine fetal hemoglobin and hematocrit to quantify the severity of fetal anemia. Intrauterine transfusion is indicated if fetal Hb <9 g% or hematocrit <30%, at less than 34 weeks of gestation.

Q2. How is IUBT performed?

The IUBT is performed under continuous USG guidance by a team with expertise at a center well equipped to handle such procedures. Appropriate counselling of parents and informed consent is mandatory. The IUBT can be performed by two routes:

- *Intraperitoneal (IPT):* The blood is injected into peritoneal cavity from where RBCs are absorbed in fetal circulation via lymphatics. In hydropic fetuses, presence of ascites reduces its efficacy and may cause fetal bradycardia due to increased intraperitoneal pressure compromising venous return. Intraperitoneal route is used in nonhydropic fetuses when IVT is technically not possible.
- *Intravascular (IVT):* The blood is transfused into the umbilical vein generally in the placental end of cord but free cord loop or intrahepatic portion can also be used. It is the preferred route as it is associated with better survival and reduced rate of neonatal exchange transfusion.
- *Combined IPT and IVT:* Reduces the total volume of blood to be transfused intra-vascularly to achieve target hematocrit thus reducing its complications.

The donor blood used in IUBT should be O Rh-negative or ABO identical with the fetus (if known), compatible with mother, should not be more than 5 days old with citrate phosphate dextrose as anticoagulant, CMV negative, irradiated, with hematocrit of 70–80%. After irradiation blood should be transfused within 24-hours.[3] K-negative blood is recommended to decrease the risk of alloimmunization.

Q3. How do you calculate the amount of blood to be transfused during IUBT?

The blood volume to be transfused (V) depends on the route of transfusion and is calculated by following formula:

Intraperitoneal route:

V= [gestation in weeks – 20] × 10 mL

Intravenous route[7]:

V= fetoplacental volume [initial] × [target hematocrit – initial hematocrit]/hematocrit of transfused blood

Fetoplacental volume (FP) is based on estimated fetal weight and nomograms for FP volume.[8] Target should be achieving hematocrit of 50% for nonhydropic foetuses. Hydropic foetuses have myocardial dysfunction and may not tolerate calculated infusion volume.[9] So their target hematocrit after first transfusion is 25% and second transfusion can be repeated earlier (as early as after 24 hours).

Q4. What are the complications of IUBT?

IUBT is a highly specialised procedure requiring close collaboration between fetal medicine specialist, hematologist, neonatologist and even in most expert hands carries a risk of fetal death of 1–3% per procedure. The other acute complications include fetal distress during or after procedure (due to cord accidents), volume overload, chorioamnionitis, premature rupture of membranes and preterm labour. Long term complications include fetal anemia due to suppression of erythropoiesis, transmission of viral infections, fetomaternal hemorrhage and further sensitisation with worsening of hemolytic disease in fetus and newborn.

Q5. How do you monitor woman after IUBT?

Monitoring with MCA PSV after IUBT is less reliable especially after two transfusions due to changes in circulatory hemodynamics and usually second IUBT is given after 2 weeks. The decline in fetal hemoglobin is at the rate of 0.3 g% per day and subsequent transfusions can be timed accordingly from post-transfusion hematocrit.[2] Weekly USG is performed to look for signs of hydrops.

Q6. When and how to deliver?

The pregnancy is continued till 34–36 weeks, after which risk of procedure outweighs benefit and termination of pregnancy is recommended after steroid cover. Mode of delivery is as per obstetric indication.

NONIMMUNE HYDROPS FETALIS (NIH)

NIH comprises the subgroup of cases not caused by red cell alloimmunization. It has causal relationship with many etiologies through a variety of mechanisms.

Common causes of nonimmune hydrops:[10]

- Cardiovascular (cardiac anomalies, arrhythmia): 17–35%.
- Chromosomal: 7–16%
- Hematologic (anemia, alpha thalassemia): 4–12%
- Infections (CMV, parvovirus, toxoplasmosis): 5–7%
- Twin-twin transfusion: 3–10%
- Lymphatic dysplasia: 5–6%
- Structural abnormalities:
  - Thoracic: 6%
  - GIT, urinary anomalies: 2.5–7%
  - Skeletal dysplasia: 3–4%
  - Tumors: 2–3%
- Syndromic: 3–4%
- Inborn errors of metabolism: 1–2%
- Miscellaneous: 3–15%
- Unknown: 15–25%

Pathophysiology of NIH

The pathophysiology of NIH varies according to etiology and it is clearly understood only in a few conditions. But the basic mechanism is an imbalance of interstitial fluid production and the lymphatic return. More than one mechanism may be responsible for hydropic changes in a fetus.

The possible mechanisms are:

- Increased central venous/lymphatic pressure, inadequate diastolic ventricular filling, e.g. cardiac anomalies, arrhythmias.
- Lymphatic dysplasia, e.g. Turner syndrome, Down syndrome, other aneuploidies.
- Anaemia, high output cardiac failure, hypoxia, e.g. alpha thalassemia, parvovirus infection, G6PD deficiency, hemangiomas, sacrococcygeal teratomas.
- Endothelial cell damage and increased capillary permeability, e.g. fetal infections—CMV, parvovirus, toxoplasma, syphilis.
- Vena caval obstruction, increased intrathoracic pressure, impaired venous return, e.g. intrathoracic masses (congenital pulmonary airway malformation), diaphragmatic hernia.

Case 3

A 24–year-old G3P2A0L0 presented at 24 weeks gestation with USG report of hydrops fetalis. She had previous two preterm macerated stillbirths at 8 months gestation. No structural anomalies were identified in the babies. Her routine antenatal screening was normal. She and her husband, both had B positive blood group. Indirect Coombs test was negative.

Q1. How will you evaluate this case?

With advancement in USG, identification of the case of hydrops is not difficult. Main challenge in nonimmune hydrops is to make an etiological diagnosis for potentially treatable conditions and determine the appropriate therapy (if available) and timing of delivery. Figure 2.5 shows flowchart for evaluation of NIH.

Immediate evaluation includes:

a. *Clinical evaluation*
  - Three generation pedigree
  - *Maternal history*: Age, consanguinity, recent infection/illness, anemia, or medication, hereditary diseases.

b. *Fetal imaging* in a tertiary care centre
  - Detailed obstetrical ultrasound
  - Doppler (MCA, venous, arterial)
  - Fetal echocardiogram

c. *Maternal blood testing*
  - Complete blood count, ABO blood group, Rh typing, indirect Coombs test
  - *Infection screen*: VDRL, syphilis, TORCH, parvovirus
  - *Autoimmune antibodies:* Anti RO, anti LA
  - *Selectively:* Hemoglobin electrophoresis, G6PD deficiency screen.

Q2. What is role invasive prenatal testing in NIH?

All women with NIH after preliminary maternal evaluation should be referred to specialised fetal medicine unit for genetic counselling and testing. Invasive fetal testing with amniocentesis or fetal blood sampling may be needed to diagnose treatable conditions

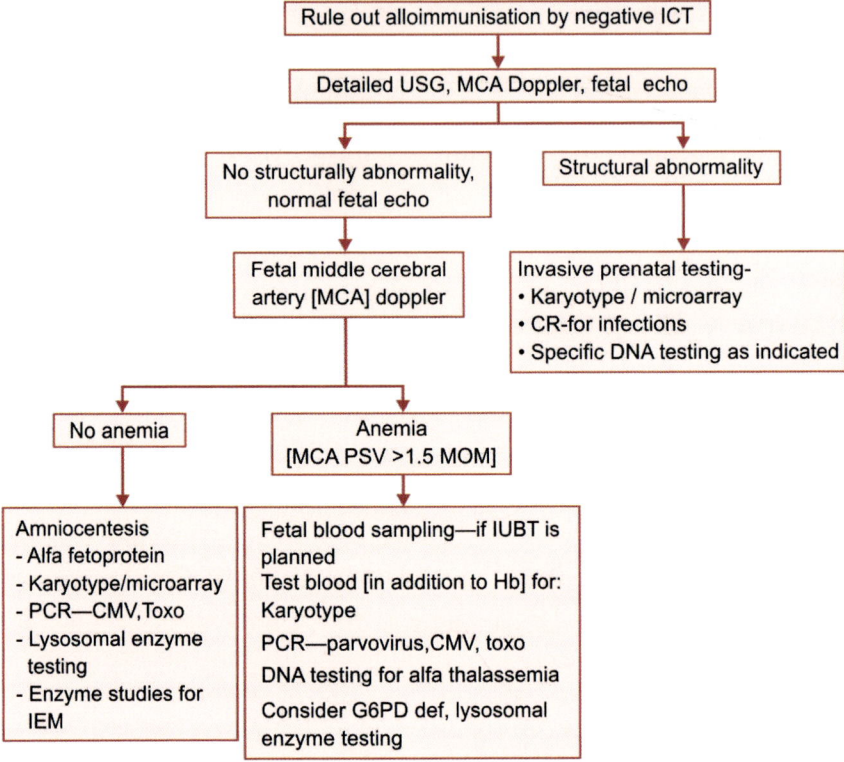

Fig. 2.5: Flowchart for evaluation of NIH

like fetal infections and genetic disorders. Following tests can be considered:

a. *Amniotic fluid*

- FISH or QF-PCR followed by karyotype or microarray analysis
- PCR for CMV, parvovirus-B19, toxoplasmosis
- Keep the amniotic cells and supernatant for future studies
- DNA extraction—if alpha-thalassemia suspected

b. *Fetal blood sampling*

- Complete blood count, reticulocyte count, platelets, direct Coombs test, blood group and type
- Karyotype/genetic microarray
- TORCH/viral serologies
- Metabolic testing (in selected cases)
- Hemoglobin electrophoresis (depending on ethnicity).

Q3. How will you prognosticate a case of NIH?

Presence of hydrops is generally an ominous sign of underlying pathology and prognosis mainly depends on etiology and period of gestation at diagnosis.

The etiology generally fall into three categories:

a. **Those amenable to fetal therapy**, e.g. arrhythmia, fetal infections—referral to a specialized centre, urgent treatment, corticosteroid therapy and antepartum surveillance may improve outcome.

b. **Those with a lethal prognosis**, e.g. aneuploidy—pregnancy termination or comfort care is the only option.

c. **Idiopathic:** Prognosis, though uncertain, is likely to be poor.

Neonatal survival is often less than 50%, even in absence of aneuploidy.[2] Overall prognosis is poor and pregnancy termination should be offered if NIH is diagnosed prior to 20 weeks of pregnancy.

Q4. This patient was evaluated, cordocentesis was performed after genetic counselling and cord blood sent for karyotyping, hematocrit, DCT, PCR for parvovirus and TORCH but no cause could be identified. How will you manage this case?

A specific cause for NIH is found only in 50–60% cases.[11] Since this case falls into idiopathic category and onset of hydrops was in early pregnancy she should be counselled about guarded prognosis and advised weekly follow up. It is also important to counsel about possibility of maternal complications with expectant management including mirror syndrome and serial evaluation of maternal blood pressure is therefore recommended.

Q5. At 26 weeks of pregnancy, she reported with loss of fetal movements and USG confirmed diagnosis of intrauteine fetal demise. How will you manage now?

The woman can be offered termination of pregnancy and timing and suitable method can be decided after discussion with family. After delivery detailed evaluation of the fetus and placenta should be done:

- Clinical pictures
- Skeletal survey
- Cord blood karyotype/microarray if not done antenatally
- Bank fetal DNA, fetal cells culture (if indicated)
- Placental pathology
- Autopsy

Follow up of Case 3
Patient delivered macerated stillborn baby weighing 800 gms.
Examination of fetus—soft cystic swelling of 3 × 2 cm in posterolateral part of fetal neck with generalized edema. Infantogram was normal. No other gross structural fetal anomaly was identified. Patient refused autopsy.

Case 4

A 29-year-old lady G3P1L1A1 was referred at 28 weeks gestation with USG report of fetal bradycardia (fetal heart rate 60 bpm) with cardiomegaly.

Her routine antenatal investigations were normal.

Anomaly scan, performed at 20 weeks was normal and fetal heart rate was 132 bpm.

She was a known case of hypothyroidism. There was no history of systemic lupus erythematous or diabetes mellitus.

Fetal echocardiography diagnosed sinus bradycardia, cardiomegaly and minimal pericardial effusion but there was no associated structural anomaly.

Anti Ro/La test was negative.

Q1. What are the causes of fetal bradycardia and how will you manage this case?

The common causes of fetal bradycardia include fetal distress, sinus bradycardia, congenital heart block due to structural heart disease or autoimmune antibodies. Fetal sinus bradycardia due to sinus node dysfunction generally does not need specific therapy antenatally. Very low ventricular rate of <55 bpm is associated increased risk of hydrops, neonatal cardiac failure and need for pacing. The parents were counselled about the condition, need for monitoring by multidisciplinary team of obstetrician, cardiologist and neonatologists and delivery at tertiary care hospital. She was monitored with weekly USG with Doppler studies and fetal echocardiography.

Q2. How you will decide mode and time of delivery?

There is no evidence that elective preterm delivery will improve the fetal outcome. In the absence of clinical deterioration or other indications for earlier intervention, delivery by 37–38 weeks should be considered. Cesarean section may be the preferred mode of delivery (a) to avoid soft tissue dystocia due to edema if severe hydrops is present and (b) to avoid difficulty in intrapartum monitoring due to fetal bradyarrhythmia.

Q3. Which causes of NIH are amenable to antenatal fetal therapy?

Only about 20–30% fetuses with NIH may be amenable to fetal therapy even in best centres. Fetal interventions should be considered after counselling of parents when gestational age is remote from term and maternal contraindications to therapy are ruled out.

Hydrops associated with only certain conditions may benefit with therapy (Table 2.1).

Follow up of Case 4

Repeat scan was performed weekly, pleural effusion and polyhydramnios were noticed at 34 weeks scan. FHR remained between 50–80 bpm. Steroid cover was given, baby was delivered by elective caesarean section and was referred to cardiologist for cardiac pacing.

Table 2.1: Antenatal therapy for nonimmune hydrops

Etiology	Therapy and recommendation
Cardiac tachyarrhythmia	Maternal transplacental administration of *antiarrhythmic medication(s).*
Fetal anemia	Fetal blood sampling followed by *intrauterine transfusion* (IUT)
Fetal hydrothorax	*Fetal needle drainage of effusion* or placement of *thoracoamniotic shunt*; if gestational age is advanced, needle drainage prior to delivery in selected cases
Fetal congenital pulmonary airway malformation (CPAM)	**Macrocystic type:** *Fetal needle drainage of effusion or placement of thoracoamniotic shunt;* **Microcystic type**: Maternal administration of *corticosteroids*
Twin-to-Twin Transfusion Syndrome (TTTS) and Twin Anemia Polycythemia Sequence (TAPS)	*Laser ablation* of placental anastomoses or selective termination (if NIH < 26 weeks)
Twin-reversed arterial perfusion sequence	*Percutaneous radiofrequency ablation*

🧠 Key Points

- Hydrops fetalis is an ultrasonographic diagnosis and is defined as effusions in at least two spaces: peritoneal, pleural, pericardial or subcutaneous edema.
- Hydrops fetalis could be immune (10–20%) or nonimmune (80–90%)
- The risk factors for maternal alloimmunisation include pregnancy, mismatched blood transfusions, abortions, invasive prenatal procedures, external cephalic version, manual removal of placenta.
- The Rh alloimmunisation is diagnosed by indirect Coombs test in maternal blood sample and the critical titre is mostly between 1:8 and 1:32.
- MCA PSV is mainstay of diagnosis and monitoring of fetal anemia after the ICT titre exceeds the critical value.

- Fetal blood sampling and IUBT are indicated when MCA-PSV exceeds 1.5 MoM or if signs of hydrops appear before 34 weeks of gestation.
- Anti-D prophylaxis is the most effective intervention to reduce Rh alloimmunisation. 300 µg of anti D immunoglobulin is given to non-immunised Rh-negative women at 28 weeks of pregnancy and within 72 hours after delivery.
- The common causes of nonimmune hydrops include cardiac anomalies, arrhythmia, chromosomal abnormalities, fetal infections, structural abnormalities and inborn errors of metabolism.
- Only about 20–30% fetuses with NIH may be amenable to fetal therapy and these include fetal tachyarrhythmia, fetal anemia, isolated fetal hydrothorax, CPAM and TTTS.
- Overall prognosis is poor if NIH is diagnosed prior to 20 weeks POG.
- In cases of fetal death, detailed evaluation of fetus and placenta is done after delivery.

REFERENCES

1. Okeke TC, Egbugara MN, Ezenyeaku CC, Ikeako LC. Non-immune hydrops fetalis. Niger J Med 2013;22:266–73.

2. Satoskar P, Agrawal S. Intrauterine transfusion. In: Sahetya R, Malhotra J, Purandarey H,eds. Principles and Practice of Fetal Medicine. 1st ed. Jaypee Brothers Medical Publishers. New Delhi India. 2017:238–244.

3. RCOG, green top guidelines 65. The management of women with red cell antibodies during pregnancy; 2014.

4. Bernstein PS, Cole DS. Rh alloimmunisation . Medscape Ob/Gyn 2002; 7(2).

5. Karanth L, Jaafar SH, Kanagasabai S, Nair NS, Barua A. Anti-D administration after spontaneous miscarriage for preventing Rhesus alloimmunisation. Cochrane database syst Rev 2013;(3): CD009617.

6. Kim YA, Makar RS. Detection of fetomaternal hemorrhage. Am J Hematol 2012;87:417–23.

7. Rodeck CH, Nicolaides KH, Warsof SL, Fysh WJ, Gamsu HR, Kemp JR. The management of severe rhesus isoimmunization by fetoscopic intravascular transfusions. Am J Obstet Gynecol 1984; 150:769–74.

8. Nicolaides KH, Clewell WH, Rodeck CH. Measurement of human fetoplacental blood volume in erythroblastosis fetalis. Am J Obstet Gynecol 1987; 157:50–3.

9. Weiner CP, Pelzer GD, Heilskov J, Wenstrom KD, Williamson RA. The effect of intravascular transfusion on umbilical venous pressure in anemicfetuses with and without hydrops. Am J Obstet Gynecol 1989; 161:1498–501.

10. Society for Maternal-Fetal Medicine (SMFM), Norton ME, Chauhan SP, Dashe JS. Society for maternal-fetal medicine (SMFM) clinical guideline no. 7: nonimmune hydrops fetalis. Am J Obstet Gynecol 2015 ;212:127–39.

11. Acharya A. Nonimmune hydrops. In: Deka D, Malhotra N, eds. An introduction to Genetics and Fetal medicine. 2nd ed. FOGSI JAYPEE Publication. New Delhi. 2010:227–33.

Screening and Prediction of Preterm Labor

Karishma Bhatia, Kanika Gupta, Preeti Singh

Preterm labor is the onset of regular uterine contractions with cervical effacement or dilation anytime before 37 completed weeks of pregnancy. India, being a developing country, bears the brunt of 3.5 million preterm births every year.[1] India is the 5th country worldwide with respect to the number of preterm births.[2] Preterm birth and its complications are the leading cause of death among children under 5 years of age. Three-quarters of these deaths could be prevented if preterm labor is diagnosed early and managed appropriately.

Case 1

A 26-year-old lady G2P1L1 with 17 weeks of period of gestation came to the antenatal OPD for routine check up. On eliciting a detailed history, it was found that her previous pregnancy resulted in a preterm vaginal delivery at 35 weeks of gestation.

Obstetric history: Married for 4 years, non-consanguineous marriage.

First pregnancy spontaneous conception, 2 years back, delivered a preterm male child weighing 1.6 kg at 35 weeks of gestation vaginally.

Baby was kept in neonatal ICU for 16 days and discharged at a weight of 1.75 kg.

On examination: General condition fair, pulse: 84/min, blood pressure: 120/80 mmHg.

Per abdomen—uterus corresponds to 18 weeks size. Per speculum examination—os closed, cervical length appeared <2.5 cm, no discharge or bleeding observed.

Her antenatal investigations are normal. Dual test and a level I ultrasound were done at 12 weeks which were normal.

Q1. How will you manage this patient ?

The patient has a history of previous preterm birth. She does not have any complaints at present. She should be counselled about the risk of preterm labor in the current pregnancy. A transvaginal scan should be done for early detection and prediction of preterm labor. If the scan shows cervical length >25 mm, serial measurements (every 1 to 2 weeks) should be done till 24 weeks. If the scan shows a short cervical length <25 mm, the patient should be offered prophylactic cerclage. If a patient has cervical length <25 mm and no history of previous preterm birth then she is advised vaginal progesterone.[2]

Cervical length >25 mm	Repeat weekly till 24 weeks
Short cervical length + history of preterm labor	Prophylactic cerclage
Short cervical length, No history of preterm labor	Vaginal progesterone

Q2. What are the factors predisposing to preterm labor in this case?

In this case, previous preterm birth is a predisposing factor to preterm labor. Other factors include:

Maternal:
- Short inter-conception period
- Multiple pregnancy

- Polyhydramnios
- Preeclampsia, eclampsia
- Antepartum hemorrhage
- Asymptomatic bacteriuria
- Infections
- Idiopathic
- Recurrent second trimester abortions

Utero-cervical
- Cervical incompetence
- Cervical conization and amputation
- Congenital uterine anomalies

Socioeconomic
- Low pre-pregnancy body mass index (BMI)
- Smoking
- Alcohol and substance abuse
- Malnutrition
- Extremes of age
- Trauma

Q3. What are the various modalities available for prediction of preterm labor?

Preterm labor can be predicted by:

a. *Transvaginal ultrasound:* A short cervical length measurement from 16–24 weeks is a very accurate predictor for spontaneous preterm labor (Level B).[3] Transvaginal ultrasound is the best method to measure cervical length as unlike transabdominal scan, it is not affected by obesity, shadowing from fetal parts and cervical position.[4,5] Funnelling can be seen in ultrasound, which is an indicator of cervical incompetence. It is not indicated before 16 weeks as before that, the lower uterine segment is not well formed, making it difficult to distinguish between endocervical canal and lower uterine segment.[6] Its clinical significance after 24 weeks decreases significantly as most interventions that are done in case of short cervical length are studied only until 24 weeks and after it even if short cervical length is found, the benefit of any intervention is controversial.[7–10]

b. *Fetal fibronectin screening:* Fetal fibronectin is a glycoprotein that is present in high concentration in the amniotic fluid. It is normally present in cervical and vaginal secretions before 24 weeks and after 35 weeks. Its presence in cervico-vaginal secretions between 24 and 35 weeks reflects mechanical or inflammatory damage to the membranes and placental separation and is a marker for imminent onset of labor within the next 1–2 weeks. High fFN (>50 ng/mL) has a low positive predictive value and a negative predictive value of more than 95%, thus making it useful in ruling out the onset of labor within the next 2 weeks.[11]

Sexual activity in the past 24 hours, recent cervical examination or cervical bleeding produce a false positive test. It is present as either a bedside rapid test or as an enzyme immunoassay. To collect the sample, a swab stick is inserted into the posterior fornix and rotated for 10 seconds and the sample is sent to laboratory for testing.[11]

c. *IGFBP-1 or the actim partus test:* This is another test used to detect cervical ripening and for prediction of imminent labor. The phosphorylated isoforms of insulin like growth factor binding protein-1 is detected in cervical secretions of women with preterm labor. This test is available as a bedside kit. It has a high negative predictive value, i.e. a negative test indicates patient will not go into preterm labor in the next 7 days.[12]

d. *Risk scoring is not recommended:* It includes systematic, objective measures like age, marital status, threatened miscarriage, smoking, previous low birth weight baby, maternal weight, height, socioeconomic factors.

Its use entails a few ethical issues like the use of an intervention with its potential morbidity in a patient with no proven benefit of the intervention. This is therefore, not recommended (Level B).[13]

e. *Home uterine activity monitoring:* This ambulatory uterine activity monitoring may result in fewer neonatal intensive care unit admissions, but is associated with more unscheduled antenatal visits and unnecessary tocolytic therapy administration and is thus, not recommended (Level A).[13]

f. *Salivary estriol:* Maternal serum estradiol and salivary estriol rise 3–5 weeks before the onset of spontaneous labor. Its value shows a diurnal variation, peaking at night and is suppressed by beta methasone administration. It has a high false positive rate and therefore its clinical implication is low (Level A).[13]

g. *Bacterial vaginosis screening:* Bacterial vaginosis is associated with preterm labor independent of other risk factors. Screening and treatment of bacterial vaginosis has failed to show any impact on the prevention of preterm birth in various trials (Level A).[13]

Q4. How is cervical length measured?

As described by the Society of Maternal Fetal Medicine, cervical length should be measured carefully as follows:

Method of proper cervical length measurement:

- Ask the patient to empty her bladder
- Under aseptic precautions, gently insert the probe into the patient's vagina
- Advance the probe into the anterior fornix
- Gently withdraw the probe until a clear image is obtained without undue pressure.
- Both the internal and external os should be visible clearly.
- Enlarge the image so that the cervix occupies 2/3rd of the screen
- Measure the cervical length along the endocervical canal, between the internal and external os, taking three measurements.
- Use the shortest best measurement.

Serial (1–2 weekly) cervical length measurement is recommended for women with short cervical length and a high risk for preterm birth (previous history of spontaneous preterm birth). Routine cervical length measurement is not indicated in:

- Multiple gestation
- Preterm premature rupture of membranes

- Women with no history of previous preterm birth

Q5. Are there any interventions which may prevent onset of preterm labor?

In a woman with high risk of preterm birth, transvaginal ultrasound guided cervical length measurement is done at 16 weeks. If her cervical length is found to be less than 25 mm, two treatment modalities can be offered:

- *Prophylactic progesterone:* Progesterone acts by inhibiting myometrial contractility. In women with history of preterm labor and cervical length more than 25 mm—It can be given as either weekly intramuscular injections of 17-alpha-hydroxy caproate or intravaginal progesterone (progesterone gel 90 mg daily or micronised progesterone 200 mg daily). Both routes are equally efficacious with fewer systemic side effects with vaginal use.[13] Prophylactic intramuscular progesterone is offered to women with transvaginal ultrasound guided cervical length of >30 mm and a prior history of spontaneous preterm birth or mid-trimester loss.[14] It is started between 16 and 20 weeks and continued till 37 weeks or delivery, whichever occurs first.[14] In women with short cervix vaginal progesterone is preferred.[13]

- *Prophylactic cervical cerclage:* Prophylactic cervical cerclage is offered to women with short cervical length of <25 mm on transvaginal ultrasound and a prior history of preterm birth before 34 weeks, mid-trimester loss, preterm premature rupture of membranes (PPROM) in previous pregnancy or a history of cervical trauma. It involves placement of a stitch at the cervico-uterine junction.[2] It may be done transabdominally or transvaginally. Haemorrhage is more with transabdominal route and therefore, it is reserved generally for cases with failed transvaginal cerclage or at those with hypoplastic cervix.

Cerclage is done between 16 and 24 weeks and removal is done between 36 and 37 weeks,

Prophylactic cerclage	Therapeutic cerclage	Rescue cerclage
It is when cerclage is done based only on the basis of history of previous preterm birth	This is when cerclage is done based on transvaginal ultrasound guided short cervical length	Cerclage done when the patient is in labour with painless dilation of cervix and bulging of intact membranes is rescue cerclage

or at onset of labor, whichever is earlier.[2] Tocolysis either before or after cerclage is not indicated.

Q6. What are the different routes for performing cervical cerclage?

Cervical cerclage may be performed by transvaginal or transabdominal route.

Transvaginal route

a. *McDonald's stitch application:* In this method a purse string suture is applied on the cervix as high as possible near the cervical os using a permanent suture. The knot is tied anteriorly and is cut when the patient goes into labor or at 36 weeks.

b. *Shirodkar's method:* In this technique the vaginal mucosa is dissected and the bladder and rectum are retracted to expose the cervix at the cervical os. This method has more blood loss compared to McDonald's method.

Transabdominal route: This route is useful for patients in whom transvaginal cerclage cannot be performed due to hypoplastic cervix or congenitally malformed cervix or in cases with a previously failed transvaginal cerclage. The advantages are that in this approach the stitch can be placed high up on the cervix near the internal os and can be performed where vaginal approach fails.

The disadvantages are that the patient ends up needing two laparotomies; one for the cerclage and another for caesarean section later. Also if the patient goes into preterm labor prior to viability or patient has an intrauterine death a hysterotomy would still have to be done to deliver the baby.[15]

Q7. What are the indications for performing cervical cerclage?

- Short cervical length on transvaginal ultrasound

- History of recurrent midtrimester losses with cervical insufficiency
- Rescue cerclage in women in preterm labor

Q8. What are the sonographic appearance of short cervix?

The relationship of lower uterine segment to cervical canal is 'T' shaped in normal pregnancy. In cervical incompetence, the relation appears as a 'Y', denoting early cervical dilation. This progresses to 'V' and then 'U' as the pregnancy advances.

Q9. How is cervical incompetence diagnosed?

It is diagnosed by history and examination along with ultrasound features:

- *History:* Recurrent midtrimester losses
- *Examination*
  - Easy passage of Hegar's cervical dilator no.8 (this method is seldom used now)
  - Dilation of cervix with herniation of membranes on per speculum examination
- *Ultrasound*
  - Funneling of internal os
  - Cervical length <25 mm

Q9. What are the possible complications of a cerclage procedure?

Complications of cerclage operations

- Sepsis
- Hemorrhage
- Premature rupture of membranes
- Onset of uterine contractions
- Cervical fibrosis leading to dystocia in the future thus increasing chances of caesarean section.

Q10. What is the post operative advice for the patient?

- Bedrest
- Avoid constipation
- Avoid sexual intercourse

- Prophylactic antibiotics or tocolysis is not recommended
- Patient is counselled to return as soon as she goes into labor or at 36 weeks, whichever is earlier.

Case 2

A 23-year-old G3P2L2 with 31 weeks of gestation came to the gynae emergency with complaints of pain abdomen. She was a booked case at our hospital with regular antenatal visits and was sure of dates. Pain was starting in the back and radiating to groin, occurring at regular intervals with increasing frequency.

Obstetric history

- P1–5 years back, male child delivered at term by normal vaginal delivery at hospital, weighed 2.6 kg at birth, alive and healthy, no antenatal or postnatal complications.
- P2–2 years back, female child delivered at term by normal vaginal delivery at hospital, weighed 2.2 kg at birth, alive and healthy, no antenatal or postnatal complications.

On examination

- Per abdomen—uterus corresponds to 30 weeks of gestation, head engaged, mild contractions present, FHS regular at 130 beats/min
- Per speculum—os closed, cervix length appears less than 1 cm.

Q1. How will you diagnose whether this woman is in preterm labor?

This patient is in suspected preterm labor. First we will perform diagnostic tests to confirm preterm labor.

Suspected preterm labor: It is when a woman who complains of labor symptoms has clinical assessment findings (cervical dilatation and effacement) consistent with labor but not with established preterm labor.[2]

Diagnosed preterm labor: When she is in suspected preterm labor and has had a positive diagnostic test for preterm labor.[2]

Established preterm labor: When a women with suspected preterm labor has progressive cervical dilatation from 4 cm with regular contractions.[2]

To diagnose preterm labor, transvaginal scan for cervical length should be performed as described above. If it is less than 15 mm then patient is said to be in diagnosed preterm labor. If it is more than 15 mm then patient is not in preterm labor and should be reassured and offered to return home.[2]

If transvaginal scan is not available, fetal fibronectin testing should be done. If its value is more than 50 ng/mL the test is said to be positive and woman is in diagnosed preterm labor.

If transvaginal scan or fetal fibronectin testing both are not available then patient should be treated as diagnosed preterm labor.[2]

If either of these tests are negative then patient is not in preterm labor. And may go home and is advised to return to emergency in case of pain abdomen. Performing both the tests in not advisable.[2]

Q2. How does one manage patient with diagnosed preterm labor?

If patient has been diagnosed with preterm labor she should be admitted in labor room. Patient should be counselled regarding the risks associated with preterm delivery.

Management involves the following interventions:

a. Antenatal corticosteroids—for fetal lung maturity
b. Maternal tocolytic therapy—till steroid cover is complete
c. Group B Streptococcus (GBS) prophy-laxis—antibiotics
d. Magnesium sulphate for neuroprotection
e. Delivery at a facility with appropriate neonatal facility.

The patient is kept on conservative manage-ment till fetal lung maturity is attained or till 36 weeks is reached.

Q3. In which condition is conservative management contraindicated?

Conservative management is contraindicated in:

- Non reactive non stress test
- Oligohydramnios
- Absent or reversed end diastolic flow on umbilical artery Doppler
- Repetitive severe variable decelerations
- Abruption
- Fetal demise
- Chorioamnionitis
- Pregnancy >34 weeks of gestation.

Q4. Discuss the role of tocolytics in preterm labor ?

Tocolytic agents act by decreasing uterine contractions and causing uterine relaxation. They do not prevent preterm labor, but act only as a method to prolong pregnancy and delay labor for the next 48 hours, which is the time required for steroids to act (Level A evidence).[14] All the contraindications to conservative management are a contraindication to tocolytic use as well. The various tocolytics that can be used are:

a. *Nifedipine:* It is a calcium channel blocker and acts by blocking the cell membrane calcium channels, thus reducing intracellular calcium. It is associated with statistically and clinically better outcomes and fewer side effects and is therefore the first line agent according to RCOG.[2] It is given in a loading dose of 20 mg, followed by 3 additional doses of 20 mg each if contractions continue. Maintenance dose is 20–40 mg every 4 hourly for 48 hours. It is contraindicated in heart disease patients as it causes hypotension, tachycardia, hypoglycemia, headache, dizziness and facial flushing.

b. *Atosiban:* It is a modified form of oxytocin which acts as a competitive inhibitor of oxytocin receptors. It is given as an initial loading dose of 6.75 mg in 0.9 mL IV over one minute followed by a continuous infusion of 24 mL/hr for 3 hours, after which the rate of infusion is reduced to 8 mL/hr for 45 hours. It is sold by the brand name of Tosiban in India at ₹ 1500/6.75 mg, which makes it a very expensive tocolytic agent. It is used in cases where nifedipine is contraindicated.

Side effects include headache, dizziness, hot flashes, tachycardia, hypotension, hyperglycemia, vomiting and rarely, post-partum haemorrhage.

c. β-mimetics-like ritodrine, terbutaline, isoxsuprine were used earlier but are no longer in use due to serious side effects like palpitations.

Q5. What is the role of steroids? When and how to give steroid course?

Steroids are given for fetal lung maturity. They reduce the incidence of respiratory distress syndrome, transient tachypnoea of newborn, intraventricular haemorrhage and necrotising enterocolitis. A single course of steroids is offered to women between 26 to 33 + 6 weeks if they are in established preterm labor or if labor is anticipated within the next 48 hours.

One should consider steroid cover at 24 to 25 + 6 weeks and at 34 to 35 + 6 weeks.[16–20]

Steroid course may be repeated (rescue dose) once when the pregnancy is less than 34 weeks and previous steroid course was given more than 14 days back and delivery is imminent within the next 7 days[21] (Level B evidence).

Both dexamethasone and betamethasone are equally efficacious. The maximum effect is seen within 2–7 days. Even a single dose confers some protective effect and thus should be given even if it seems that delivery will occur before the next dose.[16]

Betamethasone—12 mg intramuscular 24 hours apart × 2 doses.

Dexamethasone—6 mg intramuscular 12 hourly × 4 doses.

Q6. What is the role of magnesium sulphate?

Women who are more than 24 weeks but less than 32 weeks and are in preterm labor, benefit by administration of low dose magnesium sulphate. It acts as a neuroprotective agent for the fetal brain and reduces the long term risk of cerebral palsy (Level A evidence).[22]

It is given as a bolus dose of 4 g IV over 15 minutes, followed by 1 g/hr IV infusion for 24 hrs or till delivery occurs, whichever is earlier.

The signs of magnesium toxicity need to be watched for by measuring the pulse, BP, respiratory rate and deep tendon reflexes every 4 hours and checking hourly urine output.

Q7. Is there any role of giving antibiotics in this case?

RCOG recommends universal administration of Group B streptococcal (GBS) prophylaxis to all women in preterm labor (irrespective of membrane status) and less than 37 weeks of gestation to prevent neonatal GBS infection as GBS is one of the leading causes of early (<7 days) infection in neonates. The prophylaxis should be continued for a minimum of 72 hours.[23]

Q8. What is the preferred mode of delivery?

Mode of delivery depends on various factors such as the gestational age, viability, any congenital anomalies, presentation of the baby.

In cephalic presentation, vaginal mode of delivery is preferred as cesarean section is associated with increased incidence of intraventricular hemorrhage. Also, caesarean section is technically more difficult due to poor formation of the lower uterine segment. Vacuum delivery is avoided in fetus less than 34 weeks due to increased risk of intraventricular haemorrhage and cephalhematoma and thus, forceps are preferred. In case of breech presentation, cesarean section is preferable for a viable fetus with no congenital anomalies.

Q9. What are the neonatal complications of preterm delivery?

- Short term complications
  - Respiratory distress syndrome
  - Necrotising enterocolitis
  - Intraventricular haemorrhage
  - Retinopathy of prematurity
  - Hypoglycemia
  - Hypothermia
  - Hypotension
  - Patent ductus arteriosus
  - Infection
- Long term complications
  - Neurodevelopmental delay
  - Cerebral palsy
  - Visual impairment
  - Hearing defect
  - Growth impairment

Case 3

Mrs A presented to casualty with complaint of leaking per vaginum. She gives history of soakage of clothes. She is 30 weeks pregnant and this is her first pregnancy.

Pulse: 90/min, afebrile, blood pressure 120/88 mmHg.

Per abdomen examination: Uterus 28 to 30 weeks size, non-tense, non-tender, FHS 140/min.

Per speculum: os closed, leaking not observed.

Q1. How should this patient be managed?

Since leaking is not observed further tests are required to confirm premature preterm rupture of membranes. If available, insulin-like growth factor binding protein-1 test or placental alpha-microglobulin-1 test of vaginal fluid is done. If negative then it is unlikely that patient has PPROM. If positive then treat the patient as a case of PROM.[2] An ultrasound is done for amniotic fluid index to confirm premature rupture of membranes. History of soakage of clothes and a reduced amniotic fluid index confirm PPROM in this case.

Q2. How does one monitor for signs of chorioamnionitis?

Clinically pulse rate and temperature charting should be done. On per abdomen examination uterus should not be tense or tender. On per

Code	Quality of evidence	Definition
A	High	Several high-quality studies with consistent results In special cases: one large, high-quality multi-centre trial
B	Moderate	One high-quality study Several studies with some limitations
C	Low	One or more studies with severe limitations
D	Very low	Expert opinion No direct research evidence One or more studies with very severe limitations

speculum examination one should watch out for any foul smelling discharge.

Investigations: Total leucocyte counts should be done on alternate days, C reactive protein once a week and fetal heart rate tocography are done to monitor for signs of chorio-amnionitis. One must consider termination if there is any suspicion of chorioamnionitis or at 34 weeks whichever is earlier.[2]

Q3. What antibiotics should be prescribed to her?

Tablet erythromycin 250 mg QID for 10 days or till the woman goes into established labor whichever is earlier. Co-amoxyclav (augmentin) should not be given as it increases the risk of necrotising enterocolitis in the baby.[24]

 Key Points

- Early detection and management of preterm labor can reduce perinatal mortality and morbidity.
- In women with history of previous preterm labor screening with transvaginal ultrasound for cervical length is recommended from 16 to 24 weeks.
- History of preterm labor with cervical length less than 25 mm—cervical cerclage should be done.
- If there is no history of preterm labor but cervical length is less than 25 mm—vaginal progesterone is recommended.
- Fetal fibronectin and IGFBP-1 are bedside tests to detect preterm labor with high negative predictive value.
- Management of preterm labor involves administration of steroid cover, tocolysis till steroid cover is completed and transfer to a suitable facility with NICU facilities.

- Magnesium sulphate for neuroprotection should be considered at 24 to 32 weeks gestation if delivery is imminent or planned in the next 24 hours.

REFERENCES

1. Blencowe H, Cousens S, Oestergaard MZ, Chou D, Moller AB, Narwal R et al. National, regional, and worldwide estimates of preterm birth rates in the year 2010 with time trends since 1990 for selected countries: a systematic analysis and implications. Lancet 2012;379:2162–72.
2. NICE. Preterm Labor and birth NG25. National Institute for Health and Clinical Excellence, London. 2015.
3. Sonek JD, Iams JD, Blumenfeld M, Johnson F, Landon M, Gabbe S. Measurement of cervical length in pregnancy: comparison between vaginal ultrasonography and digital examination. Obstet Gynecol 1990;76:172–5.
4. Doyle NM, Monga M. Role of ultrasound in screening patients at risk for preterm delivery. Obstet Gynecol Clin North Am 2004;31:125–39.
5. Leitich H, Brunbauer M, Kaider A, Egarter C, Husslein P. Cervical length and dilatation of internal cervical os detected by ultrasonography as markers for preterm delivery:a systematic review. Am J Obstet Gynecol 1999;181:1465–72.
6. Mella MT, Berghella V. Prediction of preterm birth: cervical sonography. Semin Perinatol 2009; 33:317–24.
7. Greco E, Gupta R, Syngelaki A, Poon LC, Nicolaides KH. First-trimester screening for spontaneous preterm delivery with maternal characteristics and cervical length. Fetal Diagn Ther 2012;31:154–61.
8. Berghella V, Talucci M, Desai A. Does transvaginal sonographic measurement of cervical length before 14 weeks predict preterm delivery in high risk pregnancies? Ultrasound Obstet Gynecol 2003;21:140–4.

9. Antsaklis P, Daskalakis G, Pilalis A, et al. The role of cervical length measurement at 11–14 weeks for the prediction of preterm delivery. J Matern Fetal Neonatal Med 2011; 24:465–70.

10. Berghella V, Roman A, Daskalakis C, Ness A, Baxter JK. Gestational age at cervical length measurement and incidence of preterm birth. Obstet Gynecol 2007;110:311–7.

11. Deshpande SN, Van Asselt AD, Tomini F, Armstrong N, Allen A, Noake C, et al. Rapid fetal fibronectin testing to predict preterm birth in women with symptoms of premature labour: A systematic review and cost analysis. Health Technology Assessment 2013;17:1–138.

12. Ballic D, Latifagic A, Hudic I. Insulin-like growth factor-binding protein-1 (IGFBP-1) in cervical secretions as a predictor of preterm delivery. J Matern Fetal Neonatal Med 2008;21:297–300.

13. Farine D, Mundle W, Dodd J. The use of progesterone for prevention of preterm labour. J Obstet Gynaecol Can 2008;30:67–71.

14. ACOG. Prediction and Prevention of Preterm Birth Practice Bulletin 130. The American College of Obstetrics and Gynecologists 2012;120:964–73.

15. Novy MJ. Transabdominal cervicoisthmic cerclage: A reappraisal 25 years after its introduction. Am J Obstet Gynecol 1991;164:1635–41.

16. Periviable birth. Obstetric Care Consensus No.4. American College of Obstetricians and Gynaecologists. Obstet Gynecol 2016;127:e157–69.

17. Iams JD, Goldenberg RL, Meis PJ, Mercer BM, Moawad A, Das A, et al. The length of cervix and the risk of spontaneous premature delivery. National Institute of Child Health and Human Development Maternal Fetal Medicine Unit Network. N Engl J Med 1996;334:567–72.

18. Owen J, Iams JD. What we have learned about cervical ultrasound. National Institute of Child Health and Human Development Maternal Fetal Medicine Units Network.Semin Perinatol 2003;27:194–203.

19. Management of preterm labor. Practice Bulletin No.171. American College of Obstetricians and Gynaecologists. Obstet Gynecol 2016;128: e155–64.

20. Antenatal corticosteroids revisited:repeat courses. NIH Consens Statement 2000;17:1–18.

21. Garite TJ, Kurtzman J, Maurel K, Clark R. Impact of a 'rescue course' of antenatal corticosteroids:a multicenter randomized placebo-controlled trial. Obstetrix Collaborative Research Network [published erratum appears in Am J Obstet Gynecol 2009;201:428. Am J Obstet Gynecol 2009; 200:248.e1–9.

22. Nelson KB, Grether JK. Can magnesium sulfate reduce the risk of cerebral palsy in very low birth-weight infants? Pediatrics 1995; 95:263–269.

23. Hughes RG, Brocklehurst P, Steer PJ, Heath P, Stenson BM. Prevention of early-onset neonatal group B streptococcal disease. Green-top Guideline No. 36. BJOG 2017;124:e280–e305.

24. Kenyon S, Boulvain M, Neilson JP. Antibiotics for preterm rupture of membranes. Cochrane Database Syst Rev 2013;(12):CD001058.

Intrauterine Fetal Growth Restriction

Krishna Agarwal, Sneha Mishra, Aastha Raheja

BACKGROUND

Size of the fetus follows a normal distribution pattern. Normally, ultrasonographically estimated fetal weight (EFW) or abdominal circumference (AC) is measured to estimate the fetal size. When the fetal EFW or AC is between 10th and 90th centile for the gestation, the fetus is labeled as appropriate for gestational age (AGA).[1] Fetus with EFW or AC less than 10th centile for the gestational age is called as small for gestational age (SGA) and fetus with EFW or AC more than 90th centile is termed as large for gestational age (LGA).[1] Fetal growth restriction (FGR) is defined as a condition where fetus is unable to achieve its genetic growth potential due to underlying pathological condition.[2]

A growth restricted fetus is at a higher risk of adverse outcomes which include higher risk of intrauterine demise, intrapartum asphyxia and preterm delivery.[2] There are no well defined physical criteria to identify a growth restricted fetus and it is difficult to identify a fetus who has not achieved its genetic growth potential. Therefore, all SGA fetuses are considered to be suspected FGR. However, all SGA fetuses are not growth restricted and all growth restricted fetuses are not SGA.

70% of SGA fetuses are constitutionally small and 30% are FGR. Studies have shown that SGA fetuses with EFW or AC between 3rd to 10th centile are mostly constitutionally small and they show linear growth pattern with normal Doppler studies and normal liquor. Mostly, the SGA fetuses <3rd centile are pathologically growth restricted.[3]

Case 1

- Mrs X, G2P1L1, with 34 weeks period of gestation
- Referred in view of fundal height smaller by 6 weeks than the period of gestation
- She is sure of dates with good dates and POG is corresponding with BPD on second trimester scan
- On fetal biometry, AC is <10th centile for the gestational age on Intergrowth curve and pregnancy is labeled as SGA.

Q1. What are the causes of pregnancy with SGA fetus?

Almost 70% of SGA fetuses are constitutionally small.[3] These babies are small and healthy and there is no pathological growth restriction. On growth monitoring they show linear growth pattern, normal fetal Doppler studies and amniotic fluid volume.

The second main cause of SGA fetus is uteroplacental insufficiency.

Rest of the causes for SGA fetus are various maternal and fetal causes. The maternal causes include pre-eclampsia, pre-gestational diabetes, autoimmune disorders, heart diseases, etc. The fetal causes include multiple pregnancy, congenital anomalies like gastroschisis, heart diseases, aneuploidies and fetal infections like cytomegalovirus, varicella, toxoplasma, syphilis, malaria, etc.[4]

Q2. What do you understand by uteroplacental insufficiency?

In normal pregnancy, development of placenta is marked by trophoblastic migration and invasion of muscular layer of the spiral arterioles in the myometrium which turns the high resistance vessels to low resistance vessels. However, when this trophoblastic invasion fails, there is high resistance in the spiral arterioles leading to reduced blood flow to placenta and decreased nutritional supply. This condition of uteroplacental insufficiency leads to fetal growth restriction and sometimes pre-eclampsia.

Q3. How will you differentiate between FGR and constitutionally small fetuses?

For answer *see* Table 4.1

Q4. What are the risk factors for FGR?

History of previous SGA or previous still birth is a significant risk factor. History of medical disorders in the mother like hypertensive disorders of pregnancy, pre-gestational diabetes and autoimmune disorders make her high risk for FGR. Smoking and age >40 years are also significant risk factors.[4]

Q5. How do you screen for FGR?

The medical and the obstetric history should be reviewed for the presence of risk factors.

Serial fundal height measurements will be done from 24 weeks onwards. If the fundal height lags by 3 weeks or if fundal height is <10th centile for the gestation on fundal height growth chart (intergrowth 21 chart),[5] then the fetus may be SGA and growth restricted.

If the fundal height lags for the gestational age and the risk factors for FGR are present, diagnosis of suspected FGR will be made.

Q6. When do you label a fetus as growth restricted?

When FGR is suspected, ultrasonography will be done for fetal biometry which includes biparietal diameter (BPD), head circumference (HC), abdominal circumference (AC) and femur length (FL).

The fetal growth parameters would be plotted on the fetal growth curves. There are customized growth curve and intergrowth curves available.[5] Though there are no recommendations regarding which curves should be used, the intergrowth curves may be used because standardized criteria were used for creating these curves and charts.

So, a fetus having <10th centile AC on intergrowth curve would be labeled as SGA. Serial

Table 4.1		
Parameter	*Small and healthy fetus (maternal and fetal causes for SGA ruled out)*	*Placental insufficiency*
Growth pattern	Symmetrically small; all parameters BPD, HC, AC and FL are <10th centile	Asymmetrical; BPD and FL are normal, AC and EFW are <10th centile
Abdominal circumference/EFW curve	Growth centile maintained	The growth centile progressively falls
1st trimester aneuploidy screen	Low	Low
PAPP-A	Normal	Low
Liquor	Normal	May be reduced
Doppler studies	Normal	May be abnormal

fetal biometry will be measured at 2–3 weeks interval and plotted on the curve. A fetus with AC <3rd centile or flattening of growth curve will point towards FGR.

Q7. What specific investigations for FGR would you like to do?

A detailed anomaly scan would be done to rule out any congenital anomaly. Genetic sonogram including soft markers for aneuploidy would be performed.

Oral glucose tolerance test would be done to rule out gestational diabetes and regular blood pressure monitoring would be done.

Though no clear evidence is available about when to start fetal surveillance, it can be started at 30–32 weeks. Fetal surveillance is done by fetal growth monitoring, feto-placental Doppler studies, and biophysical profile (BPP). The optimal interval is not established but weekly Doppler studies and BPP should be done. Fetal growth monitoring by serial fetal biometry every 2–3 weeks should be continued.

Q8. How does Doppler study help you in management of pregnancy with FGR?

Following vessels provide useful information for fetal monitoring in pregnancy with FGR.

A. Umbilical artery

The most important vessel in management of pregnancy with FGR is umbilical artery. Doppler flow velocity in umbilical artery reflects the placental function. It is reported that Umbilical artery pulsatility index (PI) >95th centile for the gestation suggests more than 50% placental insufficiency whereas absent end diastolic flow may be present when placental insufficiency is >70% and reversal of flow in umbilical artery suggests >90% placental insufficiency.

One can measure systolic diastolic ratio (SD ratio), pulsatility index (PI) or the resistive index (RI) in the umbilical artery.

The most important Doppler parameter which correlates with placental insufficiency is considered to be PI and the reference tables for PI with 5th centile, mean and 95th centile are

available. PI is calculated as (peak systolic velocity-end diastolic velocity)/mean velocity (area under curve).

B. Uterine artery

Another important artery is uterine artery which reflects development of the placenta. The reference table for uterine artery PI from 14 to 41 weeks of gestation is available. Though, abnormal uterine artery Doppler may point towards placental insufficiency, we do not depend upon uterine artery Doppler for management of FGR pregnancy.

C. Middle cerebral artery

Other two important vessels are middle cerebral artery and ductus venosus which reflect how the FGR fetus is coping with the placental insufficiency. In FGR, there is compensatory increased flow to brain during systole due to brain sparing effect. Therefore, the PI in MCA reduces and MCA PI <5th centile for the gestation is considered to be associated with neonatal acidosis and is an indication for delivery.

D. Ductus venosus

This is another vessel which is considered important in deciding the time of delivery in SGA fetuses. Ductus venosus reflects the pressure and volume changes in right atrium. When there is hypoxia and metabolic acidosis due to placental insufficiency, it causes cardiac compromise and there is absent "a" wave in ductus venosus ("a" wave represents atrial filling in diastole). On further worsening, there may be reversal of "a" wave which is considered ominous and warrants immediate delivery of SGA pregnancy.

Q9. How do you decide timing of delivery of growth restricted fetus?

There are two studies GRIT (growth restriction intervention trial) and DIGITAT (disproportionate intrauterine growth intervention trail at term) which have looked at the timing of delivery in pregnancy with FGR.[6,7]

GRIT study looked at the timing of delivery in FGR fetus <34 weeks of pregnancy. No difference was found in short term or long term neonatal survival in early delivery versus expectant management groups.

DIGITAT study compared delivery versus expectant management in FGR fetus >36 weeks gestation. No difference in terms of neonatal survival was found in the two groups.

ACOG (2013) suggested the following criteria for delivery in FGR:[8]

1. If fetal Doppler study and BPP is normal, then delivery may be considered between 38-0/7 to 39-6/7 weeks of POG.
2. If there is decreased liquor or abnormal Doppler study then delivery is to be considered between 34-0/7 to 37-6/7 weeks

Antenatal corticosteroids are to be given if delivery is considered before 34 weeks and magnesium sulfate for neonatal neuroprotection if delivery is considered before 32 weeks.

Q10. What is the dose of magnesium sulfate for neuro-protection?

For women with imminent preterm birth between 24 and 34 weeks of gestation who are expected to deliver within 24 hours, Injection magnesium sulphate 4 gm of 20% solution intravenous loading dose is given over 20–30 minutes to the mother followed by 1 gm/hr maintenance infusion till birth or for a maximum of 24 hours. It is found to be neuroprotective in premature neonates.[9]

Key Points

- Fetal growth restriction is defined as a condition where fetus is unable to achieve its genetic growth potential due to underlying pathological condition.
- Fetus with EFW or AC less than 10th centile for the gestational age is called as small for gestational age.
- 70% of SGA fetuses are constitutionally small and 30% are FGR.
- Intrinsic fetal conditions as well as maternal and environmental factors lead to development of FGR
- Screening is done by serial fundal height measurements which is further confirmed by ultrasound findings
- Suspected pregnancies are followed up with tests for fetal well being like biophysical profile and Doppler velocimetry studies.

- The timing and mode of delivery is usually individualized where the consequences of prematurity and operative interferences are weighed against the risk of IUD .
- ACOG 2013 suggested the following for delivery in FGR:
  - If fetal Doppler study and BPP is normal, then delivery may be considered are 38-0/7 to 39-6/7 weeks of POG
  - If there is decreased liquor or abnormal Doppler study then delivery is to be considered between 34-0/7 to 37-6/7 weeks

REFERENCES

1. Rad S, Beauchamp S, Morales C, Mirocha J, Esakoff TF. Defining fetal growth restriction: abdominal circumference as an alternative criterion. J Matern Fetal Neonatal Med 2017;17:1–6.
2. Galan HL. Timing of delivery of growth restricted fetus. Semin perinatol 2011;35:262–9.
3. Ott WJ. The diagnosis of altered fetal growth. Obstet Gynecol Clin North Am 1988;15:237–63.
4. Royal college of obstetricians and gynaecologists. The investigation and management of the small for gestational age fetus. Green-top guidelines No. 31, London: RCOG 2013.
5. Villar J, Altman DG, Purwar M, Noble JA, Knight HE, Ruyan; International Fetal and Newborn Growth Consortium for the 21st Century. The objectives, design and implementation of the intergrowth-21st Project. BJOG 2013;120 (Suppl 2):9–26.
6. Walker DM, Marlow N, Upstone L, Gross H, Hornbuckle J, Vail A, et al. The Growth Restriction Intervention Trial: long-term outcomes in a randomized trial of timing of delivery in fetal growth restriction. Am J Obstet Gynecol 2011; 204:34.e1–9.
7. Boers KE, Vijgen SM, BIjlenga D, van der Post JA, Bekedam DJ, Kwee A, et al; DIGITAT study group. Induction versus expectant monitoring for intrauterine growth restriction at term: randomized equivanlence trial (DIGITAT). BMJ 2010;341: c7087.
8. American college of obstetricians and gynecologists. ACOG Practice bulletin no. 134: fetal growth restriction. Obstet Gynecol 2013;121:1122–33.
9. Royal college of obstetricians and gynaecologists. Magnesium sulphate to prevent cerebral palsy following preterm birth. Green-top Guidelines No. 29, London: RCOG; 2011.

Recurrent Pregnancy Loss

Chetna Arvind Sethi, Shivangini Rana

Pregnancy loss is defined as spontaneous fetal demise before it reaches viability. Recurrent pregnancy loss (RPL) is historically defined as three or more pregnancy losses which may or may not be consecutive. According to ESHRE, two or more pregnancy losses could be considered as RPL.[1] American Society for Reproductive Medicine also uses term RPL for two or more failed clinical pregnancies.[2]

The prevalence of RPL is 2–5%, making it an important health issue and a cause for grief for many a couple.[2] The incidence of RPL varies widely because of the differences in population, lifestyle and criteria for diagnosis.

Recent data suggests that the risk of adverse pregnancy outcomes in subsequent pregnancies is 30 and 33% respectively after two and three pregnancy losses. Hence the workup of RPL should be considered after two rather than three pregnancy losses.

The concerned pregnancies in RPL should have been confirmed by an ultrasound or histopathology, molar and ectopic pregnancies should be excluded.

The RPL is termed primary RPL if there is no previous viable pregnancy. When RPL occurs after one or more pregnancies progressing beyond viability it is termed secondary RPL. Tertiary RPL is considered when multiple pregnancy losses occur between normal pregnancies.

Q1.   What are the causes of RPL?

The cause of RPL can be established in only up to 50% of the cases (Table 5.1)[3]

Table 5.1: Causes of RPL	
Cause	*Incidence (%)*
Unexplained Including Non-APS Thrombophilias	40–50
Autoimmune	20
Endocrine factors	17–20
Anatomic factors	10–15
Genetic factors	2–5
Infections	0.5–5

The various established causes of RPL are:
- Increased maternal age
- Genetic
- Endocrine
- Autoimmune—antiphospholipid antibody (APLA) syndrome
- Anatomic—congenital uterine anomalies.

The controversial causes being:
- Anatomic (acquired)—intrauterine adhesions, fibroids, polyps.
- Infections
- Immunological causes
- Various lifestyle factors including stress

Q2.   What are the risk factors of RPL?

a. *Maternal age:* It plays an important role in RPL. There is an increase in the risk of clinical miscarriages with the rise in maternal age. Relatively the risk is low below 30 years of age. The risk of RPL increases sharply after the age of 35 years and more so after 40 years.

b. *Previous pregnancy losses:* The risk of RPL increases with the increasing number of previous miscarriages.

c. *Smoking:* It increases the risk of RPL in a dose dependent manner. This is mainly due to the vaso-constrictive and anti-metabolic role of some of the agents present in cigarette smoke.

d. *Alcohol:* The risk of RPL is almost double with increased consumption of alcohol (more than two drinks per day, the risk is almost double).

e. *Caffeine:* High caffeine consumption (more than 3 cups per day) is associated with high risk of RPL.

f. *Obesity:* A BMI >25 kg/m^2 is associated increased with risk of miscarriages.

g. *Stress:* Many studies suggest that increased stress level is associated with adverse pregnancy outcomes but it is unclear whether stress causes RPL or vice versa. [4]

Case 1

A 32-year-old lady, G4A3 came to antenatal clinic with history of 3 spontaneous miscarriages, all around 6 weeks in the past 2 years, now presenting with 5 weeks amenorrhoea. She has a consanguineous marriage.

Q1. What further points in history and examination would you like to elicit in a case of RPL?

A detailed history and examination play an important part along with investigations in such a case scenario. Apart from maternal age, number and sequence of pregnancy outcomes and consanguinity, the history should include the following points:

- Details of previous pregnancy losses including
  - Gestational age at which previous pregnancy losses occurred
  - Whether the ultrasound was done in the previous pregnancies and if yes, whether cardiac activity was confirmed
  - Whether products of conception were analysed by karyotyping
- History of diabetes, thyroid disorder, hypertension
- History of substance abuse
- History of any curettage or cervical surgical procedure
- History of any genital infections
- Detailed menstrual history
- Family history including history of thrombophilias.

Examination should include the following:
- General physical examination with body mass index (BMI), blood pressure and thyroid examination.
- Per speculum examination for any discharge, bleeding and cervical abnormality.
- Per vaginal examination for any uterine abnormality.

Q2. Describe the genetic factors involved in RPL in such a clinical setting.

Genetic cause of RPL should be considered in this case, in view of history of consanguineous marriage and all previous pregnancy losses occurring early, at 6 weeks of gestation.

The vast majority of early pregnancy losses (50–60%) are the consequence of chromosomal abnormalities, either in the embryo from parents with normal chromosomes or arising in the embryo with abnormal parental chromosomes.

The most common cause of early pregnancy loss is embryonic aneuploidy. The most commonly found abnormalities are numeric chromosome errors, such as trisomy, polyploidy and monosomy X. The risk of aneuploidy increases with increasing maternal age, making it one of the risk factors for RPL.

The most common parental abnormalities are balanced translocations, found in 2–4% of cases of RPL. [5] These can be detected by karyotyping in parents. Balanced translocations can be reciprocal or Robertsonian.

In a reciprocal translocation, there is exchange of genetic material between the two chromosomes. A Robertsonian translocation involves sharing of centrosome by the long arms of two acrocentric chromosomes.

RPL is rarely associated with single gene defects like cystic fibrosis or sickle cell anemia.

Q3. How will you work up this case to confirm the genetic causes of RPL and what are the treatment options?

Couples with suspected genetic causes for RPL need to undergo genetic counselling and should be explained the need and outcomes of further investigations.

Investigations

a. Karyotyping of both partners, to rule out balanced translocations.
b. Analysis of the products of conception by conventional karyotyping, fluorescence *in situ* hybridization (FISH), or array-based comparative genomic hybridization (array-CGH).

FISH does not necessarily detect all chromosomal causes of miscarriage as it uses probes only for certain chromosomes. Array CGH is the currently preferred technique, as it scans all the chromosomes and so the limitations associated with conventional karyotyping and FISH are avoided.[6] New techniques such as next generation sequencing (NGS) may prove to be useful in the future but are yet to be extensively studied in the genetic analysis of conceptus.[7]

The analysis of the products of conception is done if miscarriage occurs the second time and as the presence of abnormality in the analysis does not rule out other causes of RPL, they still need to be investigated.

Treatment

- *In vitro* fertilisation (IVF) with pre-implantation genetic diagnosis (PGD) should be considered (regardless of maternal age) in pregnancies suspected with genetic factors.
- In women carrying balanced translocations, option of IVF with donor oocytes should also be given.

Q4. What do you understand by pre-implantation genetic diagnosis and how is it different from pre-implantation genetic screening?

The process of pre-implantation genetic testing involves controlled ovarian hyper-stimulation cycle and retrieval of mature oocyte followed by IVF with sperm from the partner. The embryos thus formed are biopsied and a blastomere is removed at either the eight cell cleavage state or tropho-ectoderm cells are obtained at the blastocyst stage. The DNA obtained from the embryos is then tested for genetic abnormalities. The term pre-implantation genetic diagnosis (PGD) is used if the genetic defect is already known like in cases with a diagnosed balanced translocation in parents. When there is no chromosomal defect identified in the parents, the process of pre-implantation DNA testing of the embryo is termed pre-implantation genetic screening (PGS).

Q5. What is Antiphospholipid Antibody Syndrome (APS)? How is it implicated in RPL?

Antiphospholipid Syndrome is a possibly treatable cause of RPL. It is an autoimmune disorder in which the auto antibodies are directed towards the phospholipids binding plasma proteins most commonly β2 glyco-protein.[1] It is associated with pregnancy complications like recurrent pregnancy loss, pre-eclampsia, thrombosis, foetal growth restriction and autoimmune thrombocyto-penia.

In APS, the antibodies directed towards the platelets, promote platelet adhesion and those directed towards the vascular endothelium, cause vasoconstriction. This leads to thrombosis in uteroplacental circulation and associated adverse feto-maternal outcomes. There is recent evidence which also points towards abnormal trophoblastic invasion as one of the mechanisms causing early as well as late pregnancy loss. Antiphospholipid antibodies may cause inhibition of trophoblastic invasion or may directly cause damage to trophoblasts leading to pregnancy loss.

Q6. How will you diagnose a case of APS?

Diagnosis of APS requires presence of one clinical criteria and one laboratory criteria.

Clinical Criteria

a. Vascular thrombosis

b. Pregnancy morbidity

    i. One or more losses after the 10th week of a morphologically normal foetus.

    ii. One or more premature births of a normal neonate before the 34th week, because of preeclampsia or eclampsia or placental insufficiency.

    iii. Three or more unexplained consecutive early miscarriages.

Laboratory Tests

a. Lupus anticoagulant (LAC)

b. Anticardiolipin antibody (aCLA: IgG or IgM)

c. Anti β2 glycoprotein 1 antibody (IgG or IgM)

All these antibodies must be present on 2 or more occasions at least 12 weeks apart. The test is done at least six weeks after a pregnancy loss in the inter conceptional period.

Q7. How do you manage APS?

Treatment for APS includes:

a. Aspirin (anti platelet agent)

b. Heparin (anticoagulant)

Many studies suggest that a combined treatment with aspirin and heparin is superior to either of the two alone. Aspirin (75–100 mg/day) should be started when the woman plans to conceive. Heparin should begin with the first indication of live pregnancy.

Low molecular weight heparin (LMWH) is preferred over unfractionated heparin. It has an increased anti thrombotic ratio, lesser incidence of osteopenia and thrombocytopenia and also longer half life, permitting less frequent dosages in comparison to unfractionated heparin.

Prednisone and IV immunoglobulin have a doubtful role in APS. The risks of prednisone like diabetes and hypertension outweigh its benefits.

Q8. What is the role of immunological screening in RPL?

Maternal immunological recognition of conceptus and responses to it are known to have important role in a normal pregnancy and abnormalities of the same may be responsible for recurrent pregnancy loss. Still available investigations like Human Leukocyte Antigen testing, screening for presence of specific HLA allele, cytokines testing or natural killer cell testing are not recommended as a routine. Further the immune therapies in the form of intravenous immunoglobulin or paternal leukocyte immunization cannot be advocated as treatment options as they have not proven to improve outcomes in RPL.

According to European Society of Human Reproduction and Embryology (ESHRE), antinuclear antibody (ANA) testing could be considered in RPL for explanatory purpose since the majority of case-control studies document an association with RPL.[1]

Case 2

A lady visits the antenatal clinic with history of 2 consecutive pregnancy losses at 14 weeks and 16 weeks, now again pregnant at 8 weeks seeking medical advice.

Q1. What is the most common cause of RPL at the above mentioned periods of gestation and what investigations and treatment can be offered to this lady?

Since the lady has recurrent mid trimester pregnancy loss, uterine structural abnormalities should be considered as a cause of RPL. As the patient has reported during pregnancy she can be offered a transvaginal sonography (TVS), 3-D ultrasound (USG) and if not available an magnetic resonance imaging (MRI). Other invasive modalities like hysterosalpingography (HSG), saline infusion salpingography (SIS), laparoscopy and hysteroscopy cannot be done. The scope of treatment in the antenatal period is also limited. If serial ultrasounds reveal cervical incompetence, she must be advised to undergo a cervical cerclage.

However, if such a patient with a history of mid trimester losses reports to us in the inter conception period, she should be thoroughly investigated to rule out anatomic causes of RPL.

Anatomic causes implicated in second trimester losses include congenital uterine abnormalities, intrauterine adhesions, fibroids and polyps, mainly because they lead to abnormal placentation.

Uterine septum is the anomaly most commonly implicated as a cause of RPL. Others being bicornuate, unicornuate and didelphic uterus. All these uterine anomalies are usually linked with urinary tract anomalies except septate uterus, hence women need screening for the same.

Intrauterine adhesions or synechiae occur due to curettage, uterine surgery or infections when the basal layer of endometrium is destroyed, therefore affecting placentation.

Intramural fibroids greater than 5 cm and submucosal fibroids can cause RPL via mechanical and molecular mechanisms.

Cervical incompetence, caused by either surgical trauma to the cervix or associated with congenital factors is an important cause of RPL in the second trimester.

Q2. How will you investigate this lady in inter conceptional period for uterine structural anomalies?

The various modalities available for diagnosing uterine structural abnormalities are ultrasound (TVS /3D), HSG, SIS / SHS, laparoscopy and hysteroscopy and MRI. In the review by Saravelos, combined hysteroscopy and laparoscopy are considered as gold standard for diagnoses of malformations of the uterus, as they allow a direct visualization of the internal and external uterine contour.[8]

Sonohysterography (or hysterosonography) (SHG) is a safe procedure providing more information about uterine abnormalities as compared to HSG or ultrasound alone.[8] TVS and HSG are suboptimal in diagnosing malformations of the uterus because of poor accuracy and limited potential in classifying malformations, especially when used in isolation.[9]

Three-dimensional US is non invasive, with high sensitivity and specificity. The internal as well as external contour of the uterus can be visualised with precision.

MRI is not recommended as a first line option due to high cost and absence of additional diagnostic advantage compared to 3D USG. It is may be used where 3D USG is not available or in cases where a surgery is planned.

Q3. How do you treat the anatomic causes of RPL?

For a septate uterus, hysteroscopic metroplasty has become the indicated treatment of choice.[10] According to the available data surgical treatment is not recommended in unicornuate, arcuate or uterus didelphys and should be used as the last resort in bicornuate uterus. Unification process in a case of uterus didelphys if done, unifies the two fundi and leaves the two cervices intact. Hysteroscopic resection of uterine adhesions should be done. When myomas do not encroach or distort the uterine cavity, surgery is not indicated in the absence of other symptoms attributable to myomas that need to be treated. Myomectomy is recommended for submucous and intramural fibroids greater than 5 cm.

Cervical cerclage is reserved for women with previous second trimester pregnancy losses or cervical shortening. A recent review states that benefit of cerclage is limited to women with three prior adverse events, and those with a short cervix (<25 mm) who have had a prior preterm birth.[11] According to recent guidelines women with recurrent second-trimester pregnancy losses with suspected cervical weakness should be offered serial sonography for cervical surveillance and those with a singleton pregnancy and second-trimester RPL attributable to cervical weakness, could be considered for cerclage. There is still a lack of evidence that this intervention improves perinatal outcome.

Case 3

An obese hypothyroid woman with history of three recurrent early pregnancy losses, presents to the outpatient department for preconception counselling.

Q1. How does overt hypothyroidism affect pregnancy? What are the other endocrine and metabolic causes of RPL?

Overt hypothyroidism impacts pregnancy in many ways. It causes fetal death, miscarriages, lower childhood IQs, preterm deliveries, abruption and gestational hypertension. Hence, it needs to be treated with levothyroxine. Many studies in recent times also link subclinical hypothyroidism with miscarriages.[12–14]

Polycystic ovarian syndrome (PCOS), hyper-prolactinemia, diabetes mellitus and luteal phase defect (LPD) are among the other endocrine and metabolic causes implicated in RPL.

Hypothyroidism, both overt and subclinical is found to be associated with RPL and screening for thyroid disorders with serum thyroid-stimulating hormone (TSH) and Anti-TPO antibodies is recommended. The treatment is with levothyroxine. In previously diagnosed hypothyroid women, the levothyroxine dose should be increased by 30% as soon as the pregnancy is diagnosed. Treatment with levothyroxine in euthyroid women with anti thyroid antibodies is under evaluation.

A number of studies have shown the correlation between PCOS and recurrent pregnancy loss. The various reasons being hyper secretion of luteinizing hormone (LH), hyper insulinemia, hyper androgenemia and high levels of plasminogen activator inhibitor-1. The treatment includes lifestyle modification, clomiphene citrate (ovulation induction) and metformin (insulin sensitising). The combined treatment with clomiphene and metformin has not been found to be superior to clomiphene alone.

Diabetic women with uncontrolled sugar levels in the first trimester are more likely to suffer pregnancy losses, hence need a good glycaemic control in the peri conceptional period.

Hyperprolactinemia is associated with infertility and miscarriages because it alters the hypothalamic-pituitary-ovarian axis, leading to impaired folliculogenesis and anovulation. Testing for serum prolactin is not indicated in absence of symptoms of hyperprolactinemia. Normalising prolactin levels with dopamine agonist improves pregnancy outcomes in patients with RPL.

LPD is due to insufficient production of progesterone by the corpus luteum and the endometrium not being mature enough for placentation. LPD is diagnosed when there is a lag of greater than two days between the day of the menstrual cycle and the histology of the endometrium. The true prevalence of LPD as a cause of RPL is still unknown but is probably low.

The various methods used to diagnose LPD are serum progesterone concentrations, endometrial biopsy and short luteal phase duration (less than 13 days). The various treatment modalities are treatment of the underlying cause (increased prolactin or thyroid), ovulation induction and supplementation with progesterone, estrogen and HCG. LPD can be viewed as a form of ovulation dysfunction, so ovulation induction is a logical choice. Exogenous progesterone is usually started 2 to 3 days after ovulation, but it can delay menses further causing anxiety.

Vitamin D deficiency is also associated with adverse pregnancy outcomes, therefore, it can be supplemented up to a dose of 4000 IU per day during pregnancy and can be given prophylactically when a woman comes for preconception counselling.

The routine assessment of homocysteine levels is not recommended in a case of RPL as its association is still unclear.

Q2. What is the role of infections in patients with RPL?

Ureaplasma urealyticum, Mycoplasma hominis, Chlamydia, *Listeria monocytogenes, Toxoplasma gondii,* rubella, cytomegalovirus, herpesvirus and other less known pathogens have been identified in women with sporadic miscarriages. However, there is no convincing data that infections cause RPL so these

Table 5.2: RPL—etiology, diagnosis and treatment options		
Etiology	*Tests for diagnosis*	*Treatment options*
Genetic	Karyotype of product of conception Parental karyotype	Genetic counseling Preimplantation genetic diagnosis for balanced translocation
Uterine factor	3D ultrasonography, sonohysterography, HSG, hysteroscopy, MRI	Hysteroscopic resection of septum, myomectomy, hysteroscopic removal of polyps, adhesiolysis
Antiphospholipid syndrome	aCLA, Anti-β2GP1, lupus anticoagulant	Heparin + aspirin
Endocrine abnormality	– TSH, Anti -TPO antibodies – Prolactin – Fasting glucose or HbA1c – Mid-luteal progesterone, endometrial biopsy (LPD)	– Levothyroxine – Bromocriptine – Diabetes control (weight loss, nutrition, metformin) – Progesterone supplementation, ovulation induction
Environmental factors	Screen for smoking, drug use, excessive alcohol and caffeine intake	Eliminate environmental toxins
Psychological		Psychological support in a specialized setting
Chronic endometritis	Endometrial biopsy	Antibiotic treatment
Other infections	Cultures	Appropriate treatment
Unexplained		Progesterone supplementation (no consensus) immunomodulating treaments (no consensus) Preimplantation genetic screening (no consensus)

organisms are not routinely tested for in patients of RPL.

Q3. What do you understand by unexplained RPL?

In almost half of the cases of RPL no definitive cause can be identified. This is termed as unexplained RPL. The management of unexplained RPL is a challenge as the etiology is unclear. Various treatment modalities have been evaluated including lymphocyte immunization therapy (LIT) with paternal or third party donor lymphocytes, intravenous immunoglobulins, glucocorticoids, anticoagulants (asprin or heparin) but are not recommended in clinical practice due to lack of proven benefits and associated adverse effects. Folic acid supplementation is given for prevention of neural tube defects but its role in prevention of RPL is not proven. Other modalities like G-CSF, endometrial scratching are still under evaluation.

Progesterone supplementation by vaginal or oral route has been used empirically by many practitioners. Vaginally administered progesterone supplementation in early pregnancy has shown no proven benefit for women experiencing unexplained RPL.[15] There is some evidence that oral dydrogesterone started after documentation of fetal cardiac activity may prove beneficial.[16] Progesterone is important during implantation of the embryo, hence supplementation with progesterone starting from the luteal phase, rather than after pregnancy confirmation may prove beneficial. More trials are needed to evaluate role of oral progesterone in unexplained RPL.

Key Points
- The causes of RPL could be genetic, anatomic, autoimmune or endocrinological.
- No definite cause is identified in nearly half of the cases.

- Careful history and examination may suggest the possible cause.
- Specific investigations are needed to diagnose autoimmune and endocrinological causes.
- Imaging helps in diagnosing structural defects causing RPL.
- Treatment depends on the underlying cause.

REFERENCES

1. ESHRE guideline: Recurrent pregnancy loss. The ESHRE Guideline Group on RPL: Atik RB, Christiansen OB, Janine Elson Elson J, Kolte AM, Lewis S, et al. Human Reproduction Open. 2018; 2:hoy004https://doi.org/10.1093/hropen/hoy004.

2. Practice Committee of the American Society for Reproductive Medicine. Evaluation and treatment of recurrent pregnancy loss: a committee opinion. Fertil Steril 2012;98:1103–11.

3. Jaslow CR, Carney JL, Kutteh WH. Diagnostic factors identified in 1020 women with two versus three or more recurrent pregnancy losses. Fertil Steril 2010;93:1234–43.

4. Li W, Newell-Price J, Jones GL, Ledger WL, Li TC. Relationship between psychological stress and recurrent miscarriage. Reprod Biomed Online 2012;25:180–9.

5. De Braekeleer M, Dao TN. Cytogenetic studies in couples experiencing repeated pregnancy losses. Hum Reprod 1990;5:519–28.

6. Mathur N, Triplett L, Stephenson MD. Miscarriage chromosome testing: utility of comparative genomic hybridization with reflex microsatellite analysis in preserved miscarriage tissue. Fertil Steril 2014;101:1349–52.

7. Shamseldin HE, Swaid A, Alkuraya FS. Lifting the lid on unborn lethal Mendelian phenotypes through exome sequencing. Genet Med 2013;15: 307–9.

8. Saravelos SH, Cocksedge KA, Li TC. Prevalence and diagnosis of congenital uterine anomalies in women with reproductive failure: a critical appraisal. Hum Reprod Update 2008;14:415–29.

9. Tur-Kaspa I, Gal M, Hartman M, Hartman J, Hartman A. A prospective evaluation of uterine abnormalities by saline infusion sonohysterography in 1,009 women with infertility or abnormal uterine bleeding. Fertil Steril 2006;86: 1731–35.

10. Valle RF, Ekpo GE. Hysteroscopic metroplasty for the septate uterus: review and meta-analysis. J Minim Invasive Gynecol 2013;20:22–42.

11. Story L, Shennan A. Cervical cerclage: an established intervention with neglected potential? Eur J Obstet Gynecol Reprod Biol 2014;176:17–19.

12. Schneuer FJ, Nassar N, Tasevski V, Morris JM, Roberts CL. Association and predictive accuracy of high TSH serum levels in first trimester and adverse pregnancy outcomes. J Clin Endocrinol Metab 2012;97:3115–22.

13. Benhadi N, Wiersinga WM, Reitsma JB, Vrijkotte TG, Bonsel GJ. Higher maternal TSH levels in pregnancy are associated with increased risk for miscarriage, fetal or neonatal death. Eur J Endocrinol 2009;160:985–91.

14. Negro R, Schwartz A, Gismondi R, Tinelli A, Mangieri T, Stagnaro-Green. Increased pregnancy loss rate in thyroid antibody negative women with TSH levels between 2.5 and 5.0 in the first trimester of pregnancy. J Clin Endocrinol Metab 2010;95:E44–48.

15. Coomarasamy A, Williams H, Truchanowicz E, Seed PT, Small R, Quenby S, Gupta P, Dawood F, Koot YE, Bender Atik R et al. A Randomized Trial of Progesterone in Women with Recurrent Miscarriages. N Engl J Med 2015;373:2141–48.

16. Kumar A, Begum N, Prasad S, Aggarwal S, Sharma S. Oral dydrogesterone treatment during early pregnancy to prevent recurrent pregnancy loss and its role in modulation of cytokine production: a double-blind, randomized, parallel, placebo-controlled trial. Fertil Steril 2014;102: 1357–63.

Hypertension in Pregnancy

Ashok Kumar, Khushboo Tong

INTRODUCTION

Hypertensive disorders complicates 5–10% of all pregnancies and contribute significantly to maternal and perinatal morbidity and mortality. According to the World Health Organization (WHO), hypertensive disorders account for 16% of maternal death in developed countries.

Case 1

A 34-year-old at 32 weeks of gestation in her first pregnancy presented to antenatal clinic for an routine check up, she was found to have blood pressure of 150/100 mm Hg. Blood pressure remained same when checked after 4 hours.

Q1. What will be the important points to be noted while taking history of this patient?

- Age-young and nulliparous women are vulnerable to developing pre-eclampsia (3–0%). Chronic hypertension with superimposed pre-eclampsia are more common in older women. The incidence of pre-eclampsia in multipara ranges from 1.4–4%[1].
- Any complaint of headache, blurring of vision, epigastric pain, right upper quadrant pain and decreased urine output.
- Any complaint of easy fatigability, dyspnea, orthopnea (signs of CHF).
- Any complaint of pain abdomen, leaking per vaginum, bleeding per vaginum and decreased fetal movements.

Obstetric History

- Parity—nulliparous women are at a greater risk of developing pre-eclampsia.
- Present pregnancy related risk factors: The incidence of gestational hypertension is 13% in twin gestation as compared to 6% in singletons. Hydatiform mole and hydrops fetalis are also associated with increased risk of hypertension in pregnancy.
- History of hypertension in previous pregnancy—women with history of hypertensive disorder of pregnancy in previous pregnancy have 16–47% risk of developing the same in subsequent pregnancy.[1]
- Longer interval between pregnancies (more than 10 years) is also one of the risk factors for pre-eclampsia.

Past History

Presence of underlying disorders: Diabetes, autoimmune diseases such as systemic lupus erythematosus (SLE) or antiphospholipid antibody syndrome, collagen vascular disease, factor V Leiden mutation, protein C and protein S deficiency, sickle cell and other haemoglobinopathies, polycystic ovarian syndrome (PCOS), chronic kidney disease, maternal hyperhomocystinemia, metabolic syndrome are also the risk factors associated with pre-eclampsia.

Family History

Family history of hypertension: There is two to four fold increase in risk of pre-eclampsia in patients having first degree relative with medical history of the disorder.

Personal History

Smoking reduces the risk of hypertension during pregnancy because it upregulates placental adrenomedullin expression, which regulates volume homeostasis.

Q2. What are the important points in examination?

General physical examination
- Vital parameters like pulse, blood pressure, temperature, respiratory rate.
- Pallor, icterus, pedal edema.
- Any thyroid enlargement should be noted and investigated.
- Respiratory system, cardiovascular system and central nervous system examination.
- Look for signs of congestive heart failure like dyspnea, basal crepitations, tachypnea, raised jugular venous pressure (JVP).

Fundus examination

Check patellar reflex

Abdominal examination

Symphysiofundal height and abdominal girth to monitor fetal growth. Fetal growth restriction is commonly seen with hypertensive disorders in pregnancy. Fundal height more than period of gestation is suggestive of molar pregnancy, twins and hydraminos, these conditions can also be associated with hypertension in pregnancy.

Q3. How will you classify hypertensive disorders of pregnancy?

The classification of hypertensive disorders of pregnancy—according to task force of the American College of Obstetricians and Gynecologists (ACOG), 2013.[2]
a. Gestational hypertension
b. pre-eclampsia and eclampsia syndrome
c. Chronic hypertension
d. pre-eclampsia superimposed on chronic hypertension

Gestational Hypertension

Gestational hypertension is defined as new hypertension (systolic blood pressure ≥140 mmHg or diastolic blood pressure ≥90 mmHg or both) presenting at or after 20 weeks gestation without proteinuria or other features of pre-eclampsia and hypertension resolves by 12 weeks postpartum. Around 50% of them later on develop pre-eclampsia syndrome.

Pre-eclampsia and Eclampsia Syndrome

Pre-eclampsia is pregnancy-specific syndrome which can involve every organ system.

Pre-eclampsia is defined as hypertension with significant proteinuria or gestational hypertension with new onset proteinuria (Table 6.1). Pre-eclampsia can occur without proteinuria, with hepatic, hematopoietic, or other manifestations. Edema is no longer a specific diagnostic criterion for pre-eclampsia. Pregnant women with hypertensive disorder of pregnancy with other adverse features but no proteinuria should have further evaluation for pre-eclampsia.[2]

Eclampsia

Eclampsia is defined as new onset generalized seizures in women with pre-eclampsia. Some women presenting with eclampsia do not have diagnosed pre-eclampsia, and some women may present with eclampsia in the post-partum period.

Other causes of seizures:
- Bleeding arteriovenous malformation
- Ruptured aneurysm
- Idiopathic seizure disorder

Chronic Hypertension

Chronic underlying hypertension is diagnosed in women with documented blood pressures >140/90 mm Hg before pregnancy or before 20 weeks gestation, or both.

Chronic Hypertension with Superimposed pre-eclampsia

It is defined as new-onset or worsening base-line hypertension associated with new-onset

Table 6.1: Diagnosis of pre-eclampsia

- Blood pressure ≥140/90 mmHg after 20 weeks of gestation in a woman with previously normal blood pressure, 2 readings at least 4 hours apart.
- Proteinuria ≥300 mg/24 hours.
- Protein/creatinine ratio 0.3
- Urine albumin by dipstick >1+
  In patients without proteinuria, any new onset hypertension with any of the following
  - Thrombocytopenia (Platelet count < 1 lac/µL)
  - Serum creatinine ≥ 1.1 mg/dL
  - Liver function test—ALT and AST twice normal concentration.
  - Cerebral and visual disturbances
  - Pulmonary edema

proteinuria or other findings as discussed above. Superimposed pre-eclampsia commonly develops earlier in pregnancy. It also tends to be more severe and is more often accompanied by fetal growth restriction.

Q4. What are the severe features of pre-eclampsia?

These are summarized in Table 6.2.

Q5. What investigations are required in this case?

The investigations include:

a. Complete blood count including platelet count.

b. Urine albumin—an automated reagent strip can be used to detect proteinuria and if a result of 1+ or more is obtained, proteinuria should be quantified using a spot urinary protein: creatinine ratio or 24 hours urine collection.

c. If urine protein: Creatinine ratio is greater than 30 mg/mmol or a 24-hour urine collection shows greater than 300 mg protein significant proteinuria is diagnosed.

d. Liver function test including enzymes aspartate transaminase (AST) and alanine transaminase (ALT) levels.

e. Lactate dehydrogenase (LDH)—LDH levels may be elevated in women with pre-eclampsia and eclampsia. Higher LDH level has significant correlation with high blood pressure as well as poor maternal and perinatal outcome. LDH level of >800 IU/L in pre-eclamptic women shows significant association with pre-eclampsia related complication like abruption, eclampsia and others.[3]

f. Fundus examination—the retinal changes (hypertensive retinopathy) are graded according to Keith Wagener classification into:

   Grade I: Mild generalized arterial attenuation, particularly of small branches

   Grade II: More severe Grade I + focal arteriolar attenuation

   Grade III: Grade II + hemorrhages, hard exudates, cotton wool spots

   Grade IV: Grade III = optic disc swelling (papilledema)

g. Prothrombin time international normalised ratio, if platelet count is abnormal.

Table 6.2: Severe features of pre-eclampsia

- Blood pressure ≥160 mm Hg systolic and a diastolic blood pressure ≥110 mmHg.
- Proteinuria ≥300 mg/24 hours.
- Protein/creatinine ratio ≥ 0.3
- Urine albumin dipstick >1+
- Thrombocytopenia (Platelet count < 1 lac/µL)
- Serum creatinine ≥ 1.1 mg/dL
- Liver function tests—ALT and AST twice normal concentration.
- Cerebral and visual disturbances
- Pulmonary edema

Q6. How will you manage this patient?

This patient should be investigated for the presence of end organ dysfunction and quantification of proteinuria needs to be done. A diagnosis of gestational hypertension is made when there is no proteinuria or any feature suggestive of end organ dysfunction. Hospitalisation is advisable at least initially for 48 hours to rule out severe hypertension. During this period investigations and four hourly blood pressure measurements are performed. Patients with controlled blood pressure and normal investigations can be managed on outpatient basis. She should follow weekly in antenatal clinic and should be explained about the importance of daily BP measurement at home and symptoms suggestive of end organ damage (blurring of vision, headache, epigastric pain) in which case they should immediately report to hospital. The management of gestational hypertension is summarized in Table 6.3.

Q7. What is DELTA hypertension?

Delta hypertension is defined as a sudden rise in mean arterial pressure later in pregnancy. It signifies pre-eclampsia even if blood pressure is <140/90 mmHg. These women will develop HELLP syndrome while still normotensive.

Q8. What is white coat hypertension?

White coat syndrome is a phenomenon in which patients shows a blood pressure level above the normal range, in a clinical setting, although they do not exhibit it in other settings. It is believed that the phenomenon is due to anxiety experienced during a clinic visit.

Case 2

A 30-year-old lady gravida 2 Para1 with 35+ 2 weeks period of gestation comes to antenatal clinic with complaint of epigastric pain and blurring of vision. BP is 170/110 mm Hg and urine albumin on dipstick is 2+.

Q1. What is the diagnosis and what additional points should be noted in history and examination?

The diagnosis is pre-eclampsia with severe features. If patient is a known case of hypertension or gives history of hypertension before 20 weeks of gestation, then it is chronic hypertension with superimposed pre-eclampsia.

Additional point to be noted
History
- Ask about headache, epigastric pain or right upper quadrant pain
- Ask history of excessive weight gain
- History of decrease urine output.

Table 6.3: Management of gestational hypertension in pregnancy	
Management of gestational hypertension in pregnancy	
Antihypertensive treatment	Start oral labetalol as first line drug if BP >150/100 mm Hg Aim is to keep diastolic BP between 80–100 mm Hg and systolic BP <150 mm Hg
BP measurement	At least twice daily
Dipstick or Urinary protein:creatinine ratio	At least twice daily
Blood investigations	Weekly complete blood count, kidney function test, electrolytes, serum bilirubin, transaminase
Fetal monitoring	Daily fetal movement count Non stress test weekly Fundal height measurement at each visit Ultrasound for fetal growth and amniotic fluid index and Umbilical artery Doppler velocimetry every 3 weeks.

- History of convulsions
- Any history of chest pain, breathlessness suggestive of pulmonary edema/impending cardiac features.

Examination
- *Reflexes:* Brisk deep tendon reflexes occur as a result of nervous system irritability. In some cases, twitching of digits and clonus may also occur.
- *Fundus:* Segmental vasospasm and increase vein to artery ratio are common finding in severe pre-eclampsia. Presence of hemorrhage, exudates suggest chronic hypertension.

Q2. What is the role of expectant management in severe pre-eclampsia? What are the indications for delivery in a patient with pre-eclampsia with severe features receiving expectant management?

Definitive treatment of severe pre-eclampsia is the delivery of the fetus, however, expectant management has been tried in a women remote from term without compromising maternal condition for better fetal outcome. It is useful between 28 and 34 weeks of gestation in a tertiary care hospital with intensive fetal and maternal monitoring. Antihypertensive agents are given for blood pressure control and a course of antenatal corticosteroids is given for fetal lung maturity. Prophylactic anticonvulsant therapy with magnesium sulphate may be required. Prompt delivery is indicated in the conditions enlisted in Table 6.4.

Q3. What are the different antihypertensive drugs used in pregnancy?

The role of antihypertensive therapy in mild to moderate hypertension is controversial. Antihypertensive therapy may decrease progression to severe hypertension. The benefit is mainly maternal to prevent cerebrovascular accidents.

The drugs used to control BP, their doses and side effects are summarized in Table 6.5.

Q4. What is the mechanism of action of magnesium sulphate and what are the different regimens for prevention and treatment of seizure activity in patients of severe pre-eclampsia?

Its action is mediated via following ways:
- Reducing presynaptic release of neurotransmitter glutamate
- Blocking glutaminergic N-methyl-D-aspartate receptors
- Increased mitochondrial calcium buffering and blockage of calcium entry through voltage gated channel
- Enhancement of adenosine action

Table 6.4: Indications for delivery	
Maternal indication	**Fetal indications**
• Persistent severe headache or visual changes	• Severe fetal growth restriction (estimated fetal weight <5th percentiles)
• Uncontrolled hypertension despite maximum dose of two antihypertensive drugs	• Persistent oligohydraminos (maximum vertical pocket <2 cm)
• Progressive renal insufficiency (serum creatinine >1.1 mg/dL or doubling of serum creatinine absence of other renal disease)	• Reversed or absent umbilical artery end-diastolic flow
• Elevated liver enzymes with persistent severe epigastric pain or right upper quadrant pain	• Biophysical profile <4 on at least two occasions 6 hours apart.
• Persistent thrombocytopenia or HELLP syndrome	• Recurrent variable or late decelerations during nonstress test (NST)
• Eclampsia	
• Pulmonary edema	
• Abruptio placentae	

Various Regimen of Magnesium Sulphate

Pritchard Regimen

Loading dose—$MgSO_4$ 4 gm is given IV slowly over 3 to 4 minutes as 20 mL of 20% solution followed by 5 gm in each buttock intramuscularly as 10 mL 50% solution.

Maintenance dose—$MgSO_4$ 5 gm is given IM in alternate buttock 4 hourly as 10 mL of 50% solution.

Zuspan Regimen

Loading dose 4 gm IV followed by IV infusion of 1gm per hour until 24 hours after delivery.

Sibai Regimen

This has been recommended by ACOG 2013.[2] It gives reliable blood magnesium level and there is no risk of gluteal abscess. Loading dose of 6 gm $MgSO_4$ IV over 15–20 minutes followed by 2 gm per hour IV infusion.

Table 6.5: Antihypertensive drugs used in pregnancy

Labetalol (alpha 1 and nonselective beta blocker)

First line drug for managing hypertension in pregnancy that acts by decreasing peripheral vascular resistance.

- It is given intravenously for hypertensive emergencies: 20 mg initial dose followed by 40–80 mg every 15– 20 minutes until the therapeutic response is achieved. Maximum dose is 220 mg.
- Onset of action—5 minutes
- Peak action—10–20 minutes
- When used orally, the initial dose is 100 mg twice daily which may be increased according to patient's response up to a maximum dose of 2400 mg per day.
- Side effects include maternal hypotension, bradycardia, fatigue, depression, dizziness. It also masks signs of hypoglycaemia in insulin treated diabetic patients.

Methyldopa (centrally acting adrenergic agonist)

- The usual starting dose is 250 mg thrice a day. Maximum dose is 2 gram per day.
- Its maximum response is achived in 4–6 hours and duration of action is 8 hours.
- Side effects include postural hypotension, depression, excessive sedation, dryness of mouth. Positive coombs test (haemolytic anemia) and abnormal liver function test (drug induced hepatitis).

Nifedipine (calcium channel blocker)

An orally administered agent effective in controlling acute pregnancy-related hypertension. Oral nifedipine is now considered as one of the first line therapy options.[4] The ACOG (2017a), the NHBPEP Working Group (2010), and the Royal College of Obstetricians and Gynaecologists (2006) recommend a 10-mg oral dose to be followed in 20–30 minutes with 10–20 mg if necessary.

- Sublingul nifedipine is no longer recommended as it is associated with dangerous side effects.
- Maximum dose: 90 mg per day.
- Facial flushing and headache are common side effects.

Hydralazine (peripheral vasodilator)

It is administered intravenously.

- Initial dose is 5–10 mg followed by 10 mg doses at 15–20 minute intervals until a satisfactory response.
- The ACOG (2017a) recommends labetalol therapy if severe hypertension persists after the second dose.
- Side effects—tachycardia, hypotension, utero-placental insufficiency and fetal heart deceleration due to rapid fall in BP.

Diuretics

- Potent loop diuretics can further compromise placental perfusion. Immediate effects include redistribution of the intravascular volume, which is already reduced in severe pre-eclampsia. Therefore, diuretics are not used to lower blood pressure during pregnancy.
- Diuretics are used in pregnancy only for the management of heart failure and pulmonary edema.

Dhaka Regimen

A loading dose of 4 gm IV slow infusion with 3 gm IM in each buttock along with maintenance dose of 2.5 gm IM in alternate buttock every 4 hours for 24 hours after last fit or delivery, whichever is later. This regimen may be more suitable for use in Indian women with low BMI and in poor resource settings where clinical monitoring is limited. This is used in women with jeoparadised renal function.[5]

The following should be monitored before administration of maintenance dose:

- Deep tendon reflex
- Urine output should be >30 mL per hour
- RR >14 minutes

Therapeutic level of magnesium is 4–7 mEq/ L

- Depression of patellar reflex occur at serum level of 8–10 mEq/L and is the earliest sign of magnesium toxicity
- Respiratory depression occurs at 12–14 mEq/L
- Cardiac arrest occurs at 25–30 mEq/L

If respiratory depression develops stop magnesium sulphate and gives 10 mL of 10% calcium gluconate IV slowly over 3 minutes.

Q5. What is the risk of recurrence of hypertensive disorder?

A woman who had gestational hypertension has 16–47% risk of developing gestational hypertension in future pregnancy and 2–7% risk of developing pre-eclampsia in future.

In women with pre-eclampsia in first pregnancy, the risk of recurrence in next pregnancy is 16%. The risk of recurrence for eclampsia is 1.4%.

Q6. How can you identify a woman at risk of developing pre-eclampsia?

Vascular resistance testing and tests for assessing placental perfusion help in identifying women at risk of developing pre-eclampsia.

Provocative Pressor Test

- Roll over test
- Isometric exercise test
- Angiotensin infusion test

Uterine artery Doppler velocimetry at 22–24 weeks is useful to identify women at risk of early onset pre-eclampsia. It reflects faulty trophoblastic invasion of the spiral arteries. Elevated flow resistance results in an abnormal vessel waveform represented by an exaggerated diastolic notch or pulsatility index above 95th percentile. These pregnancies are associated with six fold increase in risk of pre-eclampsia. Abnormal uterine artery Doppler has a sensitivity of 20–60% for predicting pre-eclampsia.

Fetal-Placental Unit Endocrine Function

Human chorionic gonadotrophin (hCG), alpha fetoprotein, estriol, pregnancy associated plasma protein, inhibin A, activin A, etc.

Renal Function Tests

- Hyperuricemia
- Isolated gestational proteinuria

Endothelial Dysfunction and Oxidant Stress

- Fibronectins are high-molecular weight glycoproteins released from endothelial cells and extracellular matrix following endothelial injury.
- Thrombocytopenia and platelet dysfunction are unique features of pre-eclampsia. Markers of oxidative stress

Other Markers

Cell free DNA—it is released in pre-eclampsia by accelerated apoptosis of cytotrophoblasts.

Q7. What are the angiogenic markers of pre-eclampsia?

Serum levels of vascular endothelial growth factor (VEGF) and placental growth factor (PlGF) fall significantly below normal levels before pre-eclampsia develops. Antiangiogenic factors, such as sFlt-1 and sEng, begin to increase as angiogenic factors fall. Determination of the sFlt-1/PlGF ratio in women admitted near 37 weeks gestation to exclude pre-eclampsia has been found to be useful.[6]

Q8. What is the expectant management of preterm severe pre-eclampsia?

For answer *see* Figure below.

Q9. What are the clinical features of eclampsia?

Eclampsia is development of seizure that cannot be attributed to other causes and unexplained coma during pregnancy or puerperium in a woman with pre-eclampsia.

Impending Eclampsia Signs/Symptoms

- Persistent headache: Frontal or occipital
- Visual disturbances: Blurred vision or photophobia
- Restlessness or agitation
- Right upper quadrant pain/epigastric pain
- Nausea/vomiting

- Oliguria
- Lab evidence of disseminated intravascular coagulation (DIC).

Stages of Eclampsia

- *Premonitory stage:* Patient is unconscious with twitching of muscles of face, tongue or limbs. Eyeball is turned to one side and becomes fixed and it lasts for 30 seconds.
- *Tonic stage:* In this stage whole body goes into tonic spasm, trunk ophisthotonus limbs are flexed, hands are clenched, respiration ceases and tongue protrudes. Cyanosis develops and this stage lasts for 30 seconds.
- *Clonic stage:* All muscles of body undergo contraction and relaxation. Twitching starts in face then involve one side of extremity and whole body is gradually involved in

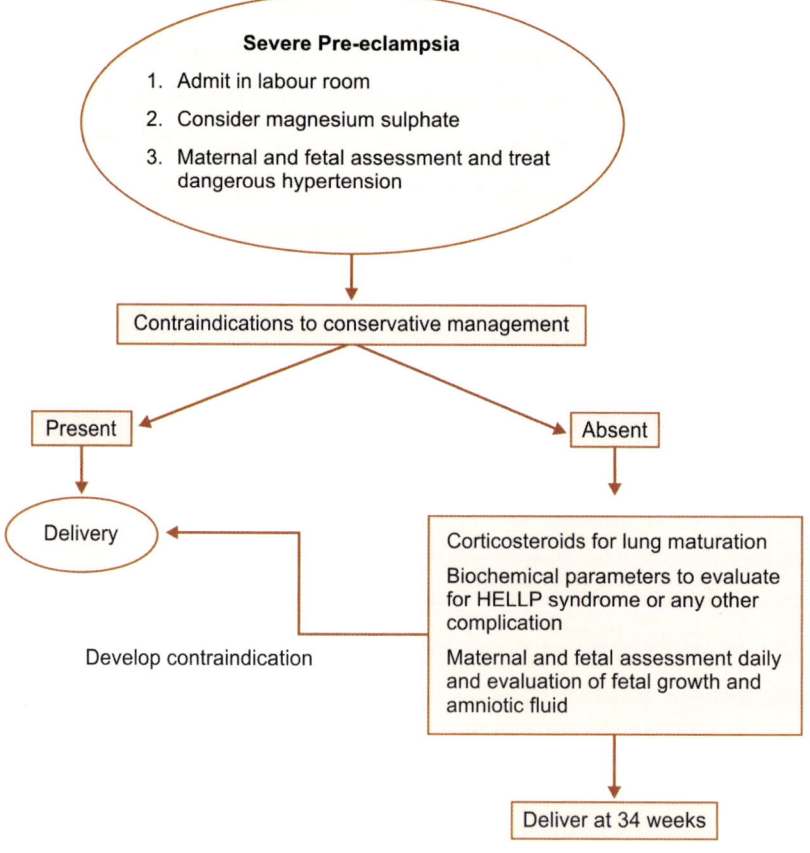

convulsions. Breathing becomes stertorus and bloodstained frothy discharge fills mouth. Tongue bite occurs and cyanosis gradually disappears. This stage lasts for 1–4 minutes.

- *Coma stage:* Patient goes in coma for brief period or coma persists till patient has another convulsion.

Associated Clinical Features

- Diminished urine output or anuria
- Generalized edema
- Hemoglobinuria
- High fever—grave sign indicates cerebral hemorrhage.

Q10. What is the role of aspirin in high risk patients? What is ASPRE Trial and new recommendations for aspirin in pregnancy?

Low-dose aspirin (81 mg/day) prophylaxis is recommended in women at high risk of pre-eclampsia and should be initiated between 12 weeks and 28 weeks of gestation (optimally before 16 weeks) and continued daily until delivery.

Clinical Risk Assessment for pre-eclampsia

High Risk Factors

History of pre-eclampsia, multifetal gestation, chronic hypertension, Type 1 or 2 diabetes, renal disease, autoimmune disease (systemic lupus erythematosus, antiphospholipid syndrome).

Moderate Risk Factors

Nulliparity, obesity (body mass index greater than 30), family history of pre-eclampsia (mother or sister), sociodemographic characteristics (African American race, low socioeconomic status), age 35 years or older, personal factors (e.g. low birthweight or small for gestational age, previous adverse pregnancy outcome, more than 10-year pregnancy interval).[8]

The ASPRE Trial

The ASPRE (combined multi marker screening and randomized patient treatment with aspirin for evidence-based pre-eclampsia prevention) trial was a prospective first-trimester multi-center study on screening for preterm pre-eclampsia in 26 941 singleton pregnancies by means of an algorithm that combines maternal factors, mean arterial pressure (MAP), uterine artery pulsatility index (UtA-PI), and maternal serum pregnancy-associated plasma protein-A (PAPP-A) and placental growth factor (PlGF) at 11-13 weeks' gestation. In the aspirin group, the incidence of preterm pre-eclampsia was reduced by 62%.[7]

New recommendations of ACOG 2018 and SMFM for low dose aspirin are:[8]

The American College of Obstetricians and Gynecologists (ACOG) and the Society for Maternal-Fetal Medicine (SMFM) make the following recommendations:

- Low-dose aspirin (81 mg/day) prophylaxis is recommended in women at high risk of pre-eclampsia and with more than one of the moderate risk factors and should be initiated between 12 weeks and 28 weeks of gestation (optimally before 16 weeks) and continued daily until delivery.
- Low-dose aspirin prophylaxis is not recommended solely for the indication of prior unexplained stillbirth, fetal growth restriction, spontaneous preterm birth and early pregnancy loss in the absence of risk factors for pre-eclampsia.

Q12. What are the complications associated with pre-eclampsia?

Complications include

Fetal

- IUGR
- Fetal bradycardia/distress
- Hypoxic ischemic encephalopathy
- Intrauterine death

Maternal

- Injuries: Tongue bite or fall from bed
- Placental: Abruption
- Pulmonary: Edema, aspiration pneumonitis, adult respiratory distress syndrome (ARDS)
- Status epilepticus
- Visual: Disturbances like blindness due to occipital edema or retinal detachment
- Cardiac: Left ventricular failure and cardiomyopathy
- Renal: Acute renal failure, oliguria and anuria
- Cerebral: Edema, hemorrhage, psychosis
- Others: DIC, sepsis, shock.

Q12. What are the criteria for the diagnosis of HELLP syndrome and what is its management?

The term HELLP syndrome is an acronym of the following presentations: Hemolysis, elevated liver enzymes and low platelet count.

Hemolysis

- Abnormal peripheral blood smear (schistocytes, burr cells)
- Elevated bilirubin >1.2 g/dL
- Low serum haptoglobin
- Raised serum LDH >600 U/L (twice the upper limit of normal).

Elevated Liver Enzymes

Elevated AST, ALT >40 IU/L.

Low Platelet Count

Less than 150,000/mm^3

Mississippi Classification

Categorizes the severity of HELLP syndrome in to three categories according to maternal platelet count.

- **Class 1:** (Severe thrombocytopenia); platelet count <50,000/mm^3, AST or ALT >70 IU/L, LDH >600 IU/L.
- **Class 2:** (Moderate thrombocytopenia); Platelet between 50,000 and 100,000/mm^3. AST or ALT >40 IU/L, LDH >600 IU/L.
- **Class 3:** (Mild thrombocytopenia); platelet count between 1 lakh and 1.5 lakh/mm^3, AST >40 IU/L, LDH > 600 IU/L.

Tennessee Classification

Tennessee classification classifies HELLP syndrome complete if all the three parameters are abnormal and incomplete or partial syndrome if one or two of the three parameters are abnormal.

Differential Diagnosis as HELLP

Idiopathic thrombocytopenia conditions, haemolytic uremic syndrome, viral hepatitis, acute fatty liver of pregnancy, renal disease, gall bladder disease and hyperemesis gravidarum.

Management

HELLP is associated with 1% risk of maternal mortality. Most of these deaths are due to acute renal failure, abruptio placentae, pulmonary edema and disseminated intravascular coagulation. Perinatal morbidity and mortality are also significantly increased due to prematurity, growth restriction and abruptio placentae. The diagnosis of HELLP syndrome is an indicator for immediate delivery after 34 weeks of gestation or at any gestational age if pulmonary edema, renal failure, severe liver dysfunction, placental abruption, nonassuring fetal status or uncontrolled hypertension is present. For women <34 weeks of gestation delivery may be delayed for 24–48 hours to complete a course of corticosteroids for fetal benefit if maternal and fetal conditions remain stable. Platelet transfusion may be required for platelet count less than 50,000/mm^3. Careful monitoring of the input-output, periodic auscultation of lungs and pulse oximetry is necessary for assessment of pulmonary and renal condition. Data on maternal benefit of dexamethasone in patient with HELLP syndrome are conflicting and at present corticosteroids are not recommended for treatment of HELLP syndrome.

Q13. How will you manage acute severe hypertension?

In acute severe hypertension, first line agent should be used expeditiously to reduce the risk of maternal stroke. Intravenous hydralazine and labetalol are considered first line but now as per latest evidence oral immediate release nifedipine can also be used as first line when intravenous access is not available.

Q14. How will you manage eclampsia?

The basic principles of management are:
- Control of convulsions
- Control of hypertension
- Immediate delivery

The first step is to maintain cardiorespiratory function and prevent maternal injury. Bedsides rails should be elevated and patient is placed in lateral decubitus position to prevent aspiration. Padded tongue blade should be inserted between teeth to avoid injury to the tongue and oral secretions should be suctioned out if needed to keep the airway clean. Oxygen should be supplemented by face mask at 8–10 L/min. Magnesium sulphate is the drug of choice for control of convulsions. It should be continued till 24 hours after delivery or 24 hours after the last convulsion.

Antihypertensives should be used for blood pressure control. Labetalol is the first line antihypertensive drug followed by nifedipine. After initial stabilization of the patient, delivery should be planned. After a seizure, labour often ensues spontaneously, progresses fast or can be induced successfully. If cervix is favourable (Bishop's score >6) amniotomy followed by oxytocin is used. If cervix is unfavourable (Bishop's score <6), intracervical PGE$_2$ gel is used. Cesarean section is done for obstetrics indications like transverse lie, placenta previa or in the presence of prolong fetal bradycardia, fetal growth restriction (FGR), unripe cervix, poor progress in labor, and uncontrolled convulsions.

Q15. What are the long term consequences of pre-eclampsia or eclampsia?

These are summarized in Table 6.6.

Table 6.6: Long term consequences of pre-eclampsia or eclampsia				
Cardiovascular	*Neurovascular*	*Metabolic*	*Renal*	*Central nervous system*
• Chronic hypertension • Ischemic heart disease • Atherosclerosis • Coronary artery calcification • Cardiomyopathy • Thromboembolism	• Stroke • Retinal detachment • Diabetic retinopathy	• Type 2 diabetes • Metabolic syndrome • Dyslipidemia • Obesity	• Glomerular dysfunction • Proteinuria	• White-matter lesions • Cognitive dysfunction • Retinopathy

 Key Points

- Hypertension in pregnancy harms mother as well as the fetus.
- Management involves hypertensive therapy, close maternal-fetal monitoring and termination of pregnancy at optimal time.
- Severe features of pre-eclampsia and occurrence of complications like eclampsia and HELLP require prompt termination of pregnancy.
- Expectant management is done only in selected cases.

REFERENCES

1. Fisher SJ. Why is placentation abnormal in preeclampsia? Am J Obstet Gynecol 2015;213: S115–22.
2. American College of Obstetricians and Gynecologists; Task Force on Hypertension in Pregnancy. Hypertension in pregnancy. Report of the American College of Obstetricians and Gynecologists' Task Force on Hypertension in Pregnancy. Obstet Gynecol 2013;122:1122–31.

3. Qublan HS, Ammarin V, Bataineh O, Al-Shraideh Z, Tahat Y, Awamleh I, et al. Lactic dehydrogenase as biochemical marker of adverse pregnancy outcome in severe preclampsia. Med Sci Monit 2005;11:CR393–7.

4. Committee on Obstetric Practice. Committee Opinion No. 692: Emergent Therapy for Acute-Onset, Severe Hypertension During Pregnancy and the Postpartum Period. Obstet Gynecol 2017;129:e90–e95.

5. Begum R, Begum A, Johanson R, Ali MN, Akhter S. A low dose ("Dhaka") magnesium sulphate regime for eclampsia. Acta Obstet Gynecol Scand 2001;80:998–1002.

6. Stepan H, Herraiz I, Schlembach D, Verlohren S, Brennecke S, Chantraine F, et al. Implementation of the sFlt-1/PlGF ratio for prediction and diagnosis of pre-eclampsia in singleton pregnancy: implications for clinical practice. Ultrasound in Obstetrics and Gynecology 2015;45:241–246.

7. Rolnik DL, Wright D, Poon LCY, Syngelaki A, O'Gorman N, de Paco et al. ASPRE trial: performance of screening for preterm pre-eclampsia. Ultrasound Obstet Gynecol 2017;50:492–495.

8. ACOG Committee Opinion No. 743: Low-Dose Aspirin Use During Pregnancy. Obstet Gynecol 2018;132:e44–e52.

CHAPTER 7

Diabetes in Pregnancy

Ashok Kumar, Divya KV

Diabetes is a disorder of carbohydrate metabolism characterised by elevated blood sugar levels secondary to defective insulin secretion or its action. Diabetes in pregnancy causes maternal and fetal complications.

Q1. How do we classify diabetes in pregnancy?

Diabetes is classified based on the underlying etiology for glucose intolerance:[1]

- Insulin dependent or type 1 diabetes
- Insulin independent or type 2 diabetes
- Gestational diabetes mellitus (GDM)

The other classification is the one proposed by Priscilla White which takes into account the duration of disease (Table 7.1), age at onset of the disease and complications. The classification divides diabetes in pregnancy into mainly two types—gestational and pregestational.

Table 7.1: Priscilla White classification

Type A1	Abnormal oral glucose tolerance test (OGTT), with normal fasting and postprandial glucose
Type A2	Abnormal OGTT with abnormal glucose levels during fasting or after meals
Type B	Onset at the age of 20 or older and duration <10 years
Type C	Onset age 10–19 years and duration of 10–19 years
Type D	Onset before age 10 or duration >20 years
Type E	Overt diabetes with calcified pelvic vessels
Type F	Diabetic nephropathy
Type R	Proliferative retinopathy
Type RF	Retinopathy and nephropathy
Type H	Ischemic heart disease
Type T	Prior kidney transplant

Q2. What are the maternal and fetal complications of diabetes?

These are summarized in Table 7.2.

Table 7.2: Maternal and fetal complications of diabetes

Fetal complications	Maternal complications
Spontaneous abortion (15.79%)	Polyhydramnios (18.8%)
Intrauterine death (15.79%)	Pre-eclampsia (9.9%)
Congenital malformation (5.26%)	Prolonged labor
Shoulder dystocia, macrosomia (16–29%)	Obstructed labour
Birth injuries	Uterine atony
Neonatal hypoglycemia (18.42%)	Postpartum haemorrhage
Infant respiratory distress syndrome	Infection (15.79%)

Q3. What are the fetal malformations caused by preexisting diabetes in first trimester?

Ans. Fetal malformations associated with preexisting diabetes are enumerated below:[2]

Central nervous system: Open neural tube defects, holoprosencephaly, absent corpus callosum, Arnold-Chiari malformation, microcephaly, macrocephaly, agenesis of olfactory tracts, hydrocephaly, sacral agenesis, caudal regression syndrome.

Cardiovascular system: Transposition of great vessels, ventricular septal defect (VSD), atrial septal defect, tetralogy of Fallot, coarctation of aorta, single umbilical artery, hypoplastic left ventricle, cardiomegaly.

Gastrointestinal system: Pyloric stenosis, duodenal atresia, microcolon, anorectal atresia, hernias, omphaloenteric cyst.

Urogenital system: Renal agenesis, renal cysts, hydronephrosis, ureterocoele, uterine agenesis, hypoplastic vagina, hypospadiasis, ambiguous genitalia.

Musculoskeletal system: Caudal dysgenesis, craniosynostosis, limb reduction, club foot, contractures, polysyndactyly.

Most common malformation is VSD and the most specific are caudal regression and sacral agenesis.

Q4. What is Pedersen's hypothesis and how does it explain macrosomia in fetus of diabetic mother?

Pedersen's hypothesis states that hyperglycemia in a diabetic mother leads to hyperglycemia in fetus which leads to hyperinsulinemia in fetus and increased utilization of glucose and hence, increased fetal adipose tissue. The combination of hyperinsulinemia and hyperglycemia leads to an increase in protein and fat stores in the fetus, resulting in macrosomia. Recent research has shown the role of lipids in macrosomia especially the triglycerides, free fatty acids which undergo transplacental transfer and increase fat mass in the fetus. This explains macrosomia inspite of good glycemic control in some of the diabetic women.[3]

Q5. How do you screen and diagnose gestational diabetes?

Pregnant women with high risk factors of GDM should be screened as soon as possible, preferably during their first antenatal visit. Retesting is done at 24–28 weeks gestation if the first trimester screen is negative. Screening is done by two approaches, single step and two step method.[4] Screening and diagnostic tests for diabetes in pregnancy are summarized in Table 7.3.

Q6. How is Glucose challenge test used for screening of Gestational diabetes?

Glucose challenge test is done with 50 g of oral glucose regardless to time of day or last meal and blood glucose is measured after an hour. Screening for diabetes should be done in first trimester itself. If negative, test is repeated at around 24–28 weeks and finally around 32–34 weeks. The cut offs are given in Table 7.4. If GCT is positive, diagnostic test with 100 g of glucose load is performed.[5]

Table 7.3: Screening and diagnostic tests for diabetes in pregnancy					
Criteria	Test	Fasting blood glucose (mg/dL)	1 hr postprandial glucose (mg/dL)	2 hr postprandial glucose (mg/dL)	3 hr postprandial glucose (mg/dL)
WHO[5]	75 g OGTT	92–125	180	153–199	—
ACOG	100 g OGTT	≥ 95	≥ 180	≥ 155	≥ 140
IADPSG[6,7]	75 g OGTT	≥ 92	≥ 180	≥ 153	—
DIPSI[7]	75 g OGTT	—	—	≥ 140	—
NICE	75 g OGTT	≥ 95	—	≥ 140	—
ADA	75 g OGTT	≥ 95	≥ 180	≥ 155	—
FIGO[8]	75 g OGTT	≥ 126	—	≥ 200	—

WHO: World Health Organisation.
ACOG: American College of Obstetrics and Gynaecologists
IADPSG: International Association of Diabetes and Pregnancy Study Group
DIPSI: Diabetes in Pregnancy Study group of India
NICE: National Institute for Clinical Excellence
ADA: American Diabetic Association
FIGO: International Federation of Gynaecology and Obstetrics

Table 7.4: Glucose challenge test		
Serum glucose cut off	*Proportion with positive test*	*Sensitivity for GDM*
>140 mg/dL of plasma glucose	14–18%	80%
>130 mg/dL of whole blood glucose	20–25%	90%

Q7. Write a note on universal screening of pregnant women for diabetes?

Selective screening based on known risk factors has poor sensitivity for detection of GDM. Universal screening as advocated by FIGO is particularly relevant to low and middle resource countries as these account for a large number of cases of gestational diabetes and ascertainment of risk factors is poor owing to poor education and lack of awareness. Universal screening for GDM is essential and it is generally accepted that women of Asian origin and especially ethnic Indians, are at a higher risk of developing GDM and subsequent type 2 diabetes.[9]

Q8. What is the role of glycosylated haemoglobin (HbA1c) in diabetes of pregnancy?

HbA1c is a product of nonenzymatic glycosylation of haemoglobin. HbA1c levels before 14 weeks of pregnancy reflect the quality of blood sugar control over the previous three months. HbA1c value less than 6% indicates good glycemic control. Higher the HbA1c, greater is the risk of congenital malformation. Chance of major congenital malformation is about 8% and 23% when HbA1c values are 9.5 and 10 respectively. However, glycosylated haemoglobin is inadequate as a diagnostic tool, because of underestimation of the average glucose level in pregnant women due to their high physiological turnover of erythrocytes.[5]

Q9. What is the role of diet in a diabetic mother?

Medical nutritional therapy is considered as the first line of treatment in diabetic pregnant women. The total calorie intake should consist of approximately 45% carbohydrate, 30% protein and 25% fat (mainly unsaturated fats). Saturated fat intake should be restricted to <10% of total calories. Total calories need to be spread over the day as three small meals and two–three snacks. Large meals should be avoided to prevent hyperglycemia. Protein requirement is increased in pregnancy. Therefore at least three servings of protein rich foods are required. High fibre diet is added as it helps to control blood sugar by delaying gastric emptying, retarding glucose entry into blood and reduces postprandial blood glucose. Exercise improves glycemic control by increasing sensitivity of peripheral tissues to insulin. Excessive maternal weight gain is associated with fetal macrosomia.[1]

Q10. Write a note on oral hypoglycemics used in GDM?

Oral hypoglycemic agents offer the advantage of oral intake over injections. Metformin and Glyburide are the two oral hypoglycaemics used in pregnancy. Other oral hypoglycaemics are not recommended due to concerns about potential teratogenicity or prolonged neonatal hypoglycaemia. Metformin is a biguanide and it acts by reducing hepatic gluconeogenesis, increases peripheral glucose uptake in skeletal muscle and adipocytes. Metformin freely crosses the placenta.[5]

The Metformin in Gestational diabetes (MIG) trial showed that use of metformin in GDM patients reduces insulin dose and weight gain in pregnancy. NICE guidelines also recommend use of metformin for gestational diabetes. Glyburide is an oral hypoglycemic that primarily enhances insulin secretion by the pancreas.[1]

Q11. How is blood sugar monitored in women with diabetes in pregnancy?

Blood sugar self-monitoring is recommended for pregnant women with diabetes. Postprandial glucose levels are preferable to fasting glucose levels, because they are more strongly associated with macrosomia.[10]

The American Diabetic Association recommends following target blood sugar levels[5]
- Fasting blood sugar < 95 mg/dL
- 1 hour post meal blood sugar <140 mg/dL
- 2 hour post meal blood sugar <120 mg/dL

The risk of macrosomia cannot be excluded despite achieving the target levels. At the same time too tight control may result in small for gestational age babies. Initially blood sugar testing may be required seven times a day which may subsequently be reduced to three times. Usual practice is to check fasting blood glucose, pre-meal and 2 hour post-meal blood glucose on alternate days. Glucose may be checked at 2 AM to document nocturnal hypoglycemia which may occur due to excess bed time insulin and cause fasting hyperglycemia (Somogyi phenomenon).[1]

Q12. Role of Insulin therapy in a diabetic mother?

Insulin therapy is recommended if medical nutrition therapy fails to achieve glycemic control. Insulin does not cross the placenta. Insulin is started initially at 0.7–1 unit/kg/day given in divided doses. Short acting regular insulin has onset of action in 30 min lasting for 6–8 hours. Intermediate acting NPH insulin has onset of action in 1 hour that lasts for 10–14 hours. Ultra short acting insulin like insulin Lispro and Aspart have action beginning in 15 min and are helpful for postprandial glucose management. Glargine (lantus) is not recommended for use in pregnancy due to its mitogenic action and risk of increased fetal growth.[1]

A commonly used plan for insulin therapy: Total insulin dose required is calculated according to the blood sugar profile. Two-thirds of total insulin dose is given in the morning and one-third in the night. The morning dose of insulin is further given as two third NPH and one-third short acting insulin. The night dose of insulin is split as half NPH and half short acting insulin.

Patient should be explained about the symptoms of hypoglycemia. Insulin dose needs to be adjusted in emergency cases like diabetic ketoacidosis, during labour, post-operative period and in patients receiving steroids for fetal lung maturity. NICE guidelines suggest daily testing of urine ketones by dipstick method for patients on insulin therapy.[1]

Q13. What are the advantages of fetal echocardiography in a diabetic mother?

The best tool for prenatal diagnosis of congenital heart defects is fetal echocardiography. Ultrasonic energy can be applied safely in a developing fetus. Maternal hyperglycemia during third trimester and subsequent fetal hyperinsulinemia, lead to neonatal cardiac hypertrophy. Fetus of diabetic mother may have myocardial hypertrophy and diastolic dysfunction along with progressive increase in fetal cardiac wall and septal thickness.[11]

Q14. How is fetal monitoring done in a woman with diabetes in pregnancy?

Antepartum fetal surveillance is done by
- Daily nonstress test
- Biweekly biophysical profile
- Clinical estimation of fetal weight, maternal assessment of fetal activity and measurement of amniotic fluid volume are other parameters monitored in antenatal period.[12]
- Umbilical artery Doppler is not useful in routine cases of gestational diabetes but is required in those affected by vasculopathy or intrauterine growth restriction.

Q15. How will you decide the timing and mode of delivery in a diabetic pregnant woman?

Although most associations recommend delivery after 38 completed weeks of gestation in a diabetic woman, some state that uncomplicated cases of gestational diabetes may be allowed to continue pregnancy up to 40 weeks of gestation with adequate fetal surveillance.

According to *NICE 2015* guidelines, one can wait for spontaneous onset of labour up to 38 week + 6 days.

ACOG (2013)[13]:

- For women with well controlled diabetes, whether pregestational or gestational, delivery before 39 completed weeks is not indicated.
- An early term or term delivery at 38 to 39 weeks + 6 days is suggested if vascular complications are present in women with pregestational diabetes.
- In patients with well controlled diabetes and reassuring fetal conditions, an expectant management is allowed, but generally not beyond the estimated due date.

Government of India (2018):[14]

- Pregnant women with GDM with well controlled blood sugar should be induced at 39 weeks.
- Pregnant women with poorly controlled blood sugar, those with risk factors like hypertensive disorder of pregnancy, previous stillbirth and other complications should be delivered earlier.
- Vaginal delivery should be preferred and caesarean should be done only for obstetric indications.
- In case of fetal macrosomia (estimated birth weight >4 kg) consider a primary caesarean section at 39 weeks to avoid shoulder dystocia.

The main concern with vaginal delivery is the risk of shoulder dystocia due to macrosomia. The ACOG and NICE guidelines suggest that vaginal delivery is not contraindicated for suspected macrosomia unless the estimated fetal weight is >4.5 kg. Indian women with GDM and their babies are small and vaginal delivery should be allowed only after a proper assessment of pelvic adequacy. One study has suggested a cutoff of 3.4 kg for macrosomia for Indian women.[15]

Q16. Discuss the intrapartum monitoring of diabetic mother?

On the evening prior to induction, insulin dose and meal are taken by the patient.

- Morning dose of insulin is omitted and fasting blood glucose is checked. Further blood sugar monitoring is done every two hours with the aim to keep blood sugar level between 70–110 mg/dL.
- IV infusion with normal saline is started and regular insulin is added according to blood sugar level as shown in Table 7.5.

Table 7.5: Government of India guidelines 2018 for insulin administration during labor[14]		
Blood sugar level	Insulin to be added in 500 ml NS	Rate of NS infusion
90–120 mg/dL	0	100 mL/hour (16 drops/min)
120–140 mg/dL	4U	100 mL/hour (16 drops/min)
140–180 mg/dL	6U	100 mL/hour (16 drops/min)
>180 mg/dL	8U	100 mL/hour (16 drops/min)

- If blood glucose level is not maintained then dextrose-insulin neutralizing drip is started.
- It is important to monitor vital signs, fluid intake, urine output, urinary ketones and blood glucose level 1–2 hourly.
- Fetal heart is monitored closely.
- Labour progress is monitored closely.
- Both traumatic and atonic postpartum haemorrhage must be watched for.[1]

Insulin sensitivity increases with the delivery of the placenta and returns to pre-pregnant levels over the following 1–2 weeks. Insulin requirement may decrease in breast feeding women.

Q17. Discuss the important aspects of management of Diabetic Ketoacidosis?

Diabetic ketoacidosis (DKA) is most commonly seen in women with type 1 diabetes. Keto-acidosis can precipitate in conditions like excessive stress, diarrhoea, infection and preterm labour. Management of DKA is done under the guidance of an endocrinologist or a physician.

Diagnosis of DKA is made when

- Blood glucose >250 mg/dL. It may occur at lower glucose level also during pregnancy.
- Presence of ketone bodies in blood and urine.
- Arterial pH <7.3.
- Serum bicarbonate level <15 mEq/L.

Management

Fluid replacement is given. Severe dehydration may result in a large fluid deficit as much as 6–7 litres.

- The estimated fluid deficit must be replaced over 12–24 hours.
- Insulin therapy is started as 0.2 U/kg IV bolus followed by 0.1 U/kg/hr normal saline. Once glucose level is between 200–250 mg/dL, normal saline is replaced with 5% dextrose.
- Hypokalemia is common with DKA. If serum potassium level is <4 mEq/L, correction is needed.
- Bicarbonate replacement is required if pH falls to <6.8
- Antibiotics are also started.
- Periodic monitoring of pulse, blood pressure, input and output, blood glucose, urine ketones and blood arterial gases.
- Fetal heart monitoring is also needed.

The underlying cause that precipitated DKA is treated simultaneously.[1]

Q18. What are the postpartum contraceptive options for women with diabetes in pregnancy?

Women with diabetes have the same contraception options as those without diabetes.

- Barrier methods are ideal (MEC category 1).
- Progesterone only pills can be used (MEC category 2 if <6 week postpartum and MEC category 1 if >6 weeks postpartum).
- Combined oral contraceptive pills are avoided, especially when diabetes is of longer duration because they have adverse effect on carbohydrate and lipid metabolism (MEC category 3).
- Intrauterine contraceptive device is another option (MEC category 1).
- Tubal sterilization and vasectomy are other options.[16]

Q19. How do you follow up these women in the postpartum period?

All women with diabetes in pregnancy should be tested postpartum for impaired glucose tolerance.

ADA (2018): Test at 4–12 weeks postpartum with a 75 g OGTT.[17]

NICE (2015): Test at 6–13 weeks postpartum using fasting blood glucose or glycosylated haemoglobin.

Diabetes Care (2018): Women should also be tested every 1–3 years thereafter if the 4–12 week 75 g OGTT is normal, with frequency depending on other risk factors including family history, prepregnancy body mass index, and need for insulin or oral hypoglycemics during pregnancy.[10]

Pregnant women with pre-existing diabetes are tested 6 weeks postpartum with 75 g OGTT.

Pregnant women with type 2 diabetes should also have their ophthalmic examination within 1 year postpartum.

Key Points

- Diabetes in pregnancy causes both fetal and maternal complications.
- Universal screening is recommended for pregnant women with diabetes.
- There are several diagnostic criteria used for screening and diagnosis of diabetes in pregnancy.
- Medical nutritional therapy is the first line of treatment of gestational diabetes.
- Metformin and Glyburide are the two oral hypoglycemics used in the management of gestational diabetes.
- Insulin is needed if euglycemia is not achieved with diet or oral hypoglycemics.
- Close monitoring of blood glucose is essential.

- Antenatal fetal monitoring is of paramount importance.
- Vaginal delivery is allowed after proper pelvic assessment, unless contraindicated.

REFERENCES

1. Bhide A, Arulkumaran S, Damania KR, et al. 4th ed. Arias' Practical guide to High Risk Pregnancy and Delivery: A South Asian Perspective 2015;254–66.
2. White P. Pregnancy complicating diabetes. Am J Med 1949;7:609–16.
3. Kamana KC, Shakya S, Zhang H. Gestational diabetes mellitus and macrosomia:a literature review. AnnNutr Metab 2015;66(Suppl 2):14–20.
4. Bonaventura CT, Ernest A, Hannah ED. Gestational diabetes mellitus: challenges in diagnosis and management. J Diabetes Metab Disord 2015;14:42.
5. Kampmann U, Madsen LR, Skajaa GO, et al. Gestational diabetes: A clinical update. World J Diabetes 2015;6:1065–72.
6. Kuo CH, Chen SC, Fang CT, et al. Screening gestational diabetes mellitus: The role of maternal age. PLos ONE 12:e0173049.
7. Seshiah V, Das AK, Balaji V, et al. Diabetes in Pregnancy Study Group. Gestational diabetes mellitus-guidelines 2006;54: 622–8.
8. The International Federation of Gynaecology and Obstetrics (FIGO) Intiative on Gestational diabetes mellitus. A Pragmatic guide for diagnosis, management and care 2015;131:S173–S211.
9. Purandare CN. Universal screening for Gestational diabetes mellitus. J ObstetGynaecol 2012;62: 141–43.
10. Blumar I, Hadar E, Hadden DR, et.al. Diabetes and Pregnancy: An Endocrine society clinical practice guideline. JClinEndocrinol Metab 2013;98:4227–49.
11. Macklon NS, Hop WC, Wladimiroff JW. Fetal cardiac function and septal thickness in diabetic pregnancy. Br J Obstet Gynaecol 1998;105:661–6.
12. Landon MB, Gabbe SG. Antepartum fetal surveillance in gestational diabetes mellitus. Clin Obstet Gynaecol 1985;34:50–4.
13. American College of Obstetricians and Gynaecologists, ACOG committee opinion no. 560: medically indicated late preterm and early preterm deliveries. Obstet Gynaecol 2013;121: 908–910.
14. Diagnosis and Management of GDM: Govt of India. 2018.
15. Balaji V, Balaji M, Anjalakshi C, et al. Diagnosis of gestational diabetes in Asian-Indian women. Indian J Endocr Metab 2011;15:187–90.
16. Robinson A, Nwolise C, Shawe J. Contraception for women with diabetes: Challenges and solutions. Open access journal of contraception 2016;7:11–18.
17. Management of diabetes in pregnancy: Standards of Medical Care in Diabetes 2018;41sl1:s137–43.

Section

II

Reproductive Endocrinology

- Amenorrhea: Approach to Diagnosis
- Polycystic Ovarian Syndrome and Hirsutism
- Hyperprolactinemia
- Hormone Replacement Therapy in Postmenopausal Women
- Selective Progesterone Receptor Modulators

Amenorrhea: Approach to Diagnosis

Deepti Goswami

Reproductive lifespan of a woman is characterized by regular menstruation. Amenorrhea refers to absence of menstruation. **Primary amenorrhea** implies that the woman has never achieved menstruation. It is diagnosed if a girl does not attain menarche (a) till 14 years of age and has absent secondary sexual characters or (b) till 16 years of age in presence of secondary sexual characters. **Secondary amenorrhea** is when a woman ceases to have menstruation after having achieved it earlier. It is diagnosed if a woman with previous menstrual cycles develops amenorrhea for a period of 6 months or for a period equivalent to the length of previous three menstrual cycles.[1] Though clinically a woman may be diagnosed with "primary" or "secondary" amenorrhea, it is essentially a symptom. The correct diagnosis would be the underlying cause of amenorrhea.

Causes of amenorrhea: The common causes of primary amenorrhea are Turner syndrome, physiological delay in onset of puberty, mullerian agenesis, maldevelopment of genital outflow tract, non-production of GnRH by hypothalamus, and anorexia nervosa. Secondary amenorrhea may occur due to polycystic ovarian syndrome (PCOS), hyperprolactinemia, primary ovarian insufficiency (POI), thyroid dysfunction, anorexia nervosa, Asherman syndrome and rarely Sheehan syndrome.

PATHOPHYSIOLOGY OF AMENORRHEA

A functionally competent hypothalamic-pituitary-ovarian (HPO) axis, uterus with hormonally responsive endometrium and a patent reproductive tract are the prerequisites for achieving menstruation.[2]

Hypothalamus

Hypothalamus secretes GnRH, which stimulates the secretion of gonadotropins—follicle stimulating hormone (FSH) and luteinizing hormone (LH) from the pituitary. The neurons that secrete GnRH are not formed in brain but migrate from the olfactory placode to the hypothalamus during embryonic development. Failure of these neurons to migrate to their final location will lead to absence of GnRH secretion. GnRH is secreted in pulsatile manner and loss

Table 8.1: Common causes of amenorrhea	
Level affected	*Causes*
Hypothalamus	Non-production of GnRH (Kallman syndrome), physiological delay in onset of puberty, anorexia nervosa, severe malnutrition, excessive exercise, brain tumors, psychological stress. PCOS (dysregulation of GnRH and gonadotropin secretion)
Pituitary	Adenoma, hypophysitis, Sheehan syndrome, empty sella
Ovary	Ovarian dysgenesis—Turner syndrome, primary ovarian insufficiency (idiopathic, autoimmune damage, chemotherapy or pelvic radiation)
Uterus and outflow tract	Mullerian agenesis, imperforate hymen, cervical agenesis, Asherman syndrome

of this pulsatility inhibits FSH and LH secretion. Neural influences like stress, structural causes like intracranial tumors, hormonal factors like hyperprolactinemia and other factors like anorexia nervosa, excessive physical activity, excessive weight loss, etc. affect GnRH secretion. FSH and LH levels are low in these cases (*hypogonadotropic hypogonadism*).

Pituitary Gland

This master endocrine gland is located in the sella turcica of the brain. The anterior pituitary secretes several hormones including FSH and LH. Improper GnRH stimulus, improper feedback from the ovary and structural causes like intracranial tumors, pituitary necrosis (Sheehan syndrome), hypophysitis, etc. affect the secretion of FSH and LH (*hypogonadotropic hypogonadism*).

Ovary

FSH and LH reach the ovaries through afferent vessels in infundibulopelvic ligaments. FSH is the predominant hormone in follicular phase. It promotes the secretion of estrogen from the ovary. LH is the predominant hormone in the secretory phase and promotes secretion of progesterone. Failure of proper development of ovaries (ovarian dysgenesis) as in Turner syndrome results in primary amenorrhea. Loss of ovarian function can occur later in life due to genetic, autoimmune or iatrogenic factors like radiation, chemotherapy and surgery. Absence of ovarian function causing amenorrhea is referred to as *Primary ovarian insufficiency* (POI), also known as premature ovarian failure (POF). The FSH and LH levels are raised in these cases (*hypergonadotropic hypogonadism*).

Uterus

Estrogen and progesterone act on the uterine endometrium and cause menstruation. Non-development of uterus as in mullerian agenesis presents as primary amenorrhea. Endometrial destruction and adhesion formation (*Asherman syndrome*) due to infections like tuberculosis or excessive curettage manifest as amenorrhea. The FSH and LH levels are normal in these cases (*normogonadotropic*).

Genital Outflow Tract

Congenital developmental defects like non-perforate hymen, transverse vaginal septum and cervical agenesis also manifest as amenorrhea. Menstrual blood accumulates in the genital tract proximal to the level of obstruction (*cryptomenorrhea*). Patients typically report cyclical abdominal pain.

Other Endocrine Factors

Common hormonal conditions that affect hypothalamus and pituitary and cause amenorrhea are hyperprolactinemia, hypothyroidism and PCOS. Hyperandrogenic conditions like congenital adrenal hyperplasia and Cushing's syndrome also cause amenorrhea.

APPROACH TO DIAGNOSIS

Patients presenting with amenorrhea should be asked about history of headache, cyclical abdominal pain, drug intake for other illnesses, radio or chemotherapy, history of excessive blood loss during childbirth as in postpartum hemorrhage or uterine rupture, curettage during postpartum period, history of tuberculosis. Eating disorders, emotional stresses and excessive physical activities as in athletes may also lead to amenorrhea. Any hormonal treatment given in the past should be noted. Family history regarding menstrual cycles in mother and sister should be noted.

A thorough clinical examination should be performed to assess for secondary sexual development using Tanner staging for cases of primary amenorrhea.[3] Check for other clinical features that may give a clue to the diagnosis like patient's height, stigmata of Turner syndrome, body mass index (BMI), galactorrhea, thyroid enlargement, hirsutism and clinical feature suggestive of cryptomenorrhea.

Investigations include hormonal testing, imaging and karyotype analysis.

Following cases were managed in our Gynae-Endocrinology clinic at Maulana Azad Medical College. The focus of discussion will be on establishing the cause of amenorrhea.

SECONDARY AMENORRHEA

Case 1

Mrs S, age 26 years, presented with complaint of secondary amenorrhea for 6 months. This was preceded by prolonged cycles of 2 months duration for 2 years. She was married for 4 years, had never conceived and not used any contraception. She had family history of diabetes mellitus (mother).

Her BMI was $28 kg/m^2$. There was no hirsutism or galactorrhea. Pelvic examination revealed healthy cervix and normal sized uterus and normal adnexae.

Q1. How will you establish the cause of secondary amenorrhea?

The first step in a case like this would be to exclude pregnancy.

Q2. Her urine pregnancy test is negative. How will you proceed further?

This woman is obese, has history of prolonged cycles and has not been able to conceive. Anovulation due to PCOS could be the underlying cause of her amenorrhea. However other disorders may also present in this manner. Progesterone challenge test is the first step in workup. She is advised to take tablet medroxy-progesterone acetate 10 mg once a day for 5 days. Serum thyroid stimulating hormone (TSH) and prolactin are also checked.

Q3. She has withdrawal bleeding after stopping the progesterone tablets. Her TSH and prolactin levels are normal.

Occurrence of withdrawal bleed implies presence of endogenous estrogens and amenorrhea is likely due to anovulation as in PCOS.

Q4. How would you confirm the diagnosis of PCOS?

PCOS is diagnosed on the basis of Rotterdam criteria where presence of two of the three criteria establishes the diagnosis.[4] These criteria are (a) oligo/anovulation, (b) hyper-androgenism and (c) polycystic morphology of the ovaries on transvaginal ultrasonography-ovarian volume more than 10 mL and peripherally distributed follicles numbering 12 or more and measuring 2–9 mm in diameter (Fig. 8.1).

Q5. What are the important points in management of PCOS?

The important aspects of management are:[5]

a. Investigations to rule out glucose intolerance.

b. Lifestyle management including physical activity and dietary modification to achieve weight loss. Even a small loss of 5% of body weight can help in achieving ovulation and spontaneous menstruation.

c. If the patient desires to conceive, treatment involves ovulation induction. Clomiphene is the first line of therapy.

d. If she does not want to conceive she is prescribed cyclical progesterones for at least 12 days a month to ensure regular withdrawal bleed and prevent endometrial hyperplasia. Alternatively low dose estrogen pills can be given.

e. She should be counseled about the long-term effects of PCOS, which include diabetes, endometrial hyperplasia or cancer, and cardiovascular diseases.[6]

Detailed case discussion on PCOS is covered in another chapter of the book.

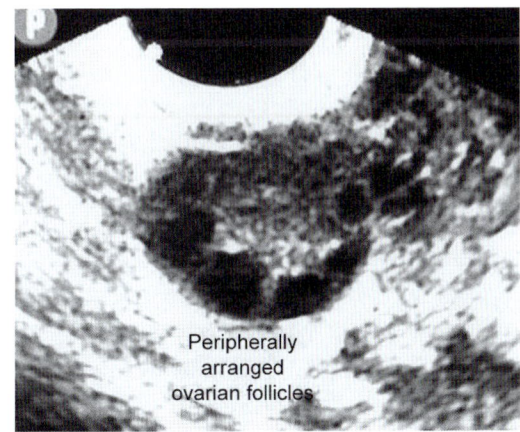

Peripherally arranged ovarian follicles

Fig. 8.1: Transvaginal sonography in a case of PCOS

Case 2

Mrs P aged 32 years, para 1 presented to the Gynae-Endocrinology clinic with complaint of secondary amenorrhea for 2 years. She had previous one vaginal delivery six years back that was uneventful. She had not taken any treatment so far and reported no other symptoms except for occasional headache.

She had normal BMI, no hirsutism or thyroid enlargement. On breast examination milky secretions were expressed. Pelvic examination revealed a healthy cervix and normal sized uterus. Bilateral adnexae were normal.

Q1. How will you establish the cause of amenorrhea?

In all cases of secondary amenorrhea one should rule out pregnancy. Once pregnancy is excluded, the presence of galactorrhea raises the possibility of hyperprolactinemia. Her serum prolactin and TSH levels should be tested. If her prolactin levels are raised one should rule out (a) use of drugs that increase serum prolactin levels and (b) pituitary adenoma. Detailed case discussion on hyper-prolactinemia is covered in another chapter of the book.

Case 3

Mrs R, aged 35 years, para 2 presented with secondary amenorrhea for three years preceded by irregular prolonged cycles for 8 years. She had two uneventful vaginal deliveries before that. She had no other medical illness. Her BMI was 23 kg/m^2, there was no thyroid enlargement, hirsutism or galactorrhea. There were no abnormal findings on pelvic examination.

Q1. How will you establish the cause of amenorrhea?

Pregnancy should always be ruled out in a woman presenting with secondary amenorrhea. The approach to diagnosis is like that in Case 1. She should be given the progesterone challenge test and her serum TSH and prolactin levels are also checked.

Q2. The patient returns after two weeks and reports no withdrawal bleeding with progesterones. Serum TSH and prolactin are normal. What should be done next?

Absence of withdrawal bleed following progesterone challenge implies either (a) lack of endogenous estrogen or (b) a non-responsive endometrium. To distinguish she should be given both estrogen and progesterone. One option is conjugated equine estrogen 0.625 mg or 1.25 mg daily for 25 days and medroxy-progesterone acetate 10 mg per day in the last 7 days.

Q3. Patient gets a withdrawal bleed. What does this indicate?

This indicates that uterus and outflow tract are normal and amenorrhea is due to lack of endogenous estrogen either due to ovarian defect or due to lack of gonadotropin secretion from the pituitary. Blood levels of FSH and LH will help in distinguishing between the two causes.

Q4. Her serum FSH is 113 mIU/mL and serum LH is 40 mIU/mL. What is the diagnosis?

This patient has amenorrhea due to primary ovarian insufficiency (earlier called as premature ovarian failure). To confirm the diagnosis levels should be rechecked after 4 weeks. Raised serum FSH >25 mIU/mL on the two occasions at least 4 weeks apart confirms the diagnosis of POI. [7]

Q5. How will you manage this case?

Women with POI are hypoestrogenic just like postmenopausal women. This adversely affects their bone health. So estrogen replacement is started.[7,8] Progesterone is added in a sequential or continuous combined manner to prevent unopposed action of estrogen on uterus. Alternatively oral contraceptive pill can be given. The treatment is continued till the age of natural menopause. A baseline dual energy X-ray absorptiometry (DEXA) helps in assessing bone health. They should have adequate calcium and vitamin D intake and follow a healthy lifestyle.

Nearly one-fourth of the cases have associated hypothyroidism.[9] Yearly review helps in detecting it. Blood tests for rheumatoid factor and anti nuclear antibodies can be advised to look for autoimmune etiology. If patient is less than 30 years of age, a karyotype is indicated.

Spontaneous pregnancy is possible but is rare and not predictable.[10] Women desiring pregnancy need to undergo assisted reproduction with donated oocytes.

Case 4

Mrs K, aged 30 years, presented with secondary amenorrhea since her vaginal delivery 5 years back. The delivery was conducted at home and the baby was stillborn. She suffered heavy blood loss and was shifted to a hospital where she received blood transfusion.

Her BMI was 20 kg/m², there was no thyroid enlargement, hirsutism or galactorrhea. The uterus was found to be small in size on pelvic examination.

Q1. How will you establish the cause of secondary amenorrhea?

In this case occurrence of amenorrhea after childbirth, which was associated with significant blood loss, should make one consider Sheehan syndrome among the differential diagnosis. The approach to diagnosis is like that in Case 1 and Case 3. She should be given the progesterone challenge test and her serum TSH and prolactin levels are also checked.

Q2. The patient does not get withdrawal bleeding after progesterone challenge. Serum TSH and prolactin are normal. What should be done next?

She should be given estrogen and progesterone in a sequential manner to induce a withdrawal bleed, as described in Case 3.

Q3. Patient gets a withdrawal bleed. What should be done next?

Serum levels of FSH and LH should be checked.

Q4. Her FSH is 1.4 mIU/mL and LH is 0.9 m IU/mL. What does this suggest?

Low levels of gonadotropins indicate that amenorrhea is due to pituitary or hypo-thalamus dysfunction. MRI of the brain is done to investigate further.

Q5. MRI of the brain revealed a very thin rim of pituitary along the floor of sella and widening of suprasellar cistern. How will you mange her?

Patient's history, examination and investigations are suggestive of hypogonadotropic hypogonadism due to Sheehan syndrome (Figs 8.2 and 8.3). She should be given hormone replacement therapy (HRT) to correct hypoestrogenemia as described in Case 3. Serum levels of other anterior pituitary hormones are also checked. Presence of other hormonal deficiencies requires consultation with an endocrinologist. Pregnancy can be achieved by ovulation induction with FSH and LH.[11]

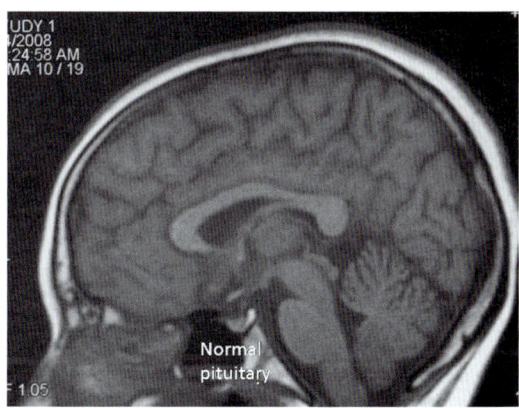

Fig. 8.2: MRI image of normal pituitary

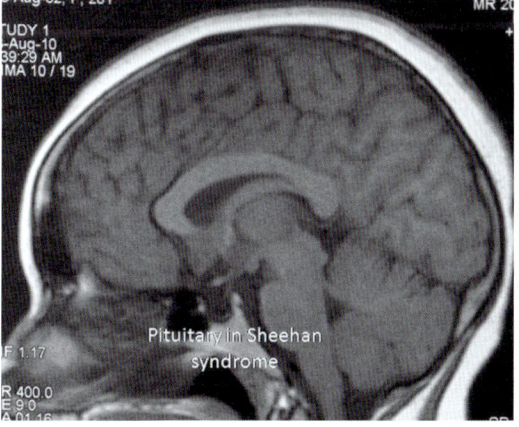

Fig. 8.3: MRI image of pituitary in Sheehan syndrome

Case 5

Mrs D, a nulliparous woman aged 28 years, presented with secondary amenorrhea of one-year duration. She had no other complaints.

Her BMI was 21 kg/m^2, there was no thyroid enlargement, hirsutism or galactorrhea. There were no abnormal findings on pelvic examination.

Q1. How will you establish the cause of secondary amenorrhea?

After ruling out pregnancy, she should be given the progesterone challenge test and her serum TSH and prolactin levels should be checked.

Q2. She has no withdrawal bleeding after progesterone challenge. Serum TSH and prolactin are normal. What should be done next?

She should be given estrogen and progesterone in a sequential manner as described in Case 3 to induce withdrawal bleed.

Q3. Patient does not have any bleeding after estrogen and progesterone treatment.

This implies that endometrium is not functional.

Q4. How will you investigate further?

Non-functional endometrial could be due to endometrial destruction and intrauterine adhesions (Asherman syndrome). Endometrial tuberculosis or excessive curettage, particularly in a postpartum woman, can destroy the endometrium and cause intrauterine adhesions. Ultrasonography of the pelvis would reveal thin, irregular or ill-defined endometrium (Fig. 8.4). Since tuberculosis is widely prevalent in our population an endometrial sampling should be done. If active tuberculosis is ruled out, hysteroscopy is done to diagnose and lyse intrauterine adhesions. After this sequential estrogen progesterone are given to encourage endometrial growth.[12]

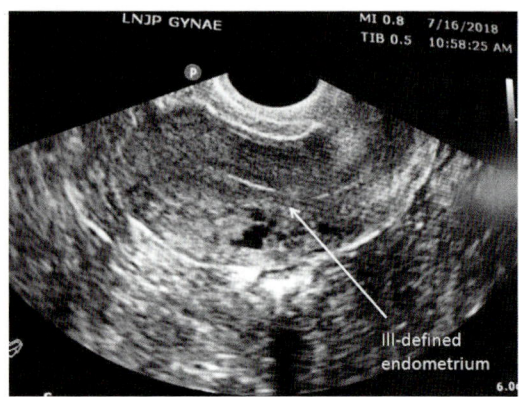

Fig. 8.4: Transvaginal sonography in a case of Asherman syndrome

PRIMARY AMENORRHEA

Case 6

Miss A, 17 years, was brought by her parents to the Gynae Endocrinology clinic for non-attainment of menses. She was a student of class 11th and had no other complaints. Her height was 156 cm and weight 56 kg. She had well developed secondary sexual characters-breasts, pubic and axillary hair. There was no thyroid enlargement, galactorrhea or hirsutism. There was no abdominal mass.

Q1. What could be the cause of primary amenorrhea in this case?

Presence of well-developed secondary sexual characters indicates that hypothalamic-pituitary-ovarian axis has been functional. One would suspect problem at the level of uterus and outflow tract in this case. Per rectal examination can be done after patient's consent to check for presence of uterus. Pelvic ultrasonography is the first modality for imaging.

Q2. Per rectal examination and pelvic ultrasonography shows absence of uterus. What is the likely diagnosis?

The findings are suggestive of mullerian agenesis also called Mayer-Rokitansky-Küster-Hauser syndrome. These patients have a non-patent genital tract and there is no vaginal opening at the introitus—"blind vagina".

Q3. How should she be managed?

Patient should be counseled about the condition and prognosis.[13] It is not possible to attain menstruation and pregnancy. However due to normal hormonal function they do not suffer from side effects of hypoestrogenemia.

X-ray of the spine and ultrasound examination of the kidneys is done to rule out congenital defects in lumbosacral spine and renal tract. Karyotype is done to rule out the differential diagnosis of androgen insensitivity syndrome.

There is a need to create neovagina to enable coitus. This can be done non-surgically with the help of dilators or surgically (vaginoplasty). Surgical treatment is usually carried out a few months before the patient plans to get married.

Such patients can have their own genetic offspring through surrogacy. A recent development in management of this condition has been the process of uterine transplantation, which is a complex procedure and is discussed in a separate chapter.

Case 7

Miss C, A 15-year, old girl presented with primary amenorrhea. She also reported abdominal pain for one year with cyclical worsening.

Her secondary sexual characters are normally developed. A 16 week size abdominal mass arising out of pelvis is palpable.

Q1. What could be the diagnosis in this case?

Presence of secondary sexual characters indicates a functional hypothalamic-pituitary-ovarian axis. Presence of cyclical abdominal pain suggests an outflow tract obstruction. Ultrasound examination would confirm the presence of hematocolpos and hematometra, which clinically appear as an abdominal mass. MRI is the gold standard investigation to identify the level of obstruction.[14,15] These patients have cryptomenorrhea where menstruation is occurring every month but menstrual blood is not discharged and accumulates proximal to the obstruction.

Q2. What is the management in these cases?

The common causes of cryptomenorrhea are imperforate hymen, transverse vaginal septum and cervical agenesis. The management is surgical. Imperforate hymen is excised. Transverse vaginal septum is also excised and raw vagina is covered with a skin graft to prevent restenosis. Postoperatively use of dilators helps in maintaining vaginal patency. Management of cervical stenosis is more challenging as restenosis is common and even hysterectomy may be required for this reason.

Case 8

Miss M, 15 years of age, a student of class 9th was brought by her parents to the Gynae-Endocrinology clinic for non-attainment of menses. Parents were concerned, as her younger sister had attained menarche. There was no complaint of cyclical abdominal pain.

Patient's height was 136 cm and weight was 36 kg. Examination showed Tanner 1 staging for breast and absence of pubic and axillary hair. Patient had short neck with suspected webbing. Systemic examination was unremarkable.

Q1. How will you establish the cause of amenorrhea?

Absence of secondary sexual characters implies a non-functional HPO axis. There could be ovarian dysgenesis as in Turner syndrome or a problem at the level of pituitary or hypothalamus. However, markedly short height raises the suspicion for Turner syndrome. Serum FSH and LH need to be checked. Their levels are (a) low in hypothalamus-pituitary defect and (b) high in ovarian dysgnesis. A karyotype would establish the diagnosis of Turner syndrome.

Q2. Her FSH is 200 mIU/mL and LH 65 mIU/mL. Karyotype is 45XO.

The findings confirm the diagnosis of Turner syndrome.

Q3. How should she be managed?

Parents and patient are counseled about the condition and its prognosis.

Her blood pressure should be checked as she may have hypertension. Investigations are done to detect other problems associated with Turner syndrome. These include fasting blood glucose, lipid profile, liver function tests, thyroid function tests, audiometry to detect hearing defect, renal ultrasound, screening for coeliac disease and echocardiography for congenital cardiac defects.[16]

Patient needs multidisciplinary care due to various associated medical issues. Management of short stature requires referral to an endocrinologist. Growth hormone therapy helps in improving height; however, the treatment is expensive.

Low dose estrogen, e.g. 2 μg/day of ethinyl estradiol or 0.3 mg of conjugated equine estrogen is started and increased incrementally. Later on progesterone is added to achieve menstruation. HRT helps in optimizing bone health and uterine size. Treatment is continued till the age of normal menopause as discussed in case 3. Adequate calcium and vitamin D intake is essential.

These patients have streak ovaries with no folliculogenesis. Pregnancy can be achieved through oocyte donation.

Case 9

Miss A, A 17-year-old girl presented with primary amenorrhea. She reported absence of breast development. There were no other complaints. She studies in class 11th and has normal eating habits. Her height was 155 cm and weight 52 kg. Breast development was at Tanner stage 2 and pubic and axillary hairs were absent.

Q1. How will you establish the cause of primary amenorrhea?

Absence of secondary sexual characters suggests hypoestrogenemia due to ovarian or pituitary/hypothalamic cause. Her serum FSH and LH should be checked.

Q2. Her FSH is 0.54 mIU/mL and LH is 0.08 mIU/mL.

Findings suggest hypogonadotropic hypogonadism due to pituitary or hypothalamic cause. MRI of brain should be done. She should

be also checked for anosmia. This patient has normal BMI. Similar clinical picture may be seen in girls with low BMI as in eating disorders.

Q3. MRI Brain is normal. How will you manage her?

She is advised low dose estrogen as discussed in case 7. The dose is increased every 3–6 months and progesterone is added later to induce menstruation. Ovaries and uterus are normal in these cases and pregnancy can be achieved by ovulation induction with FSH and LH.

Case 10

Miss S, 18 years of age, presented with primary amenorrhea. There were no other complaints. Her height was 158 cm and weight was 60 kg. She had well developed breasts but no axillary or pubic hairs. She had received some hormonal treatment from elsewhere but had no menstrual bleeding. Abdominal examination was unremarkable.

Q1. What could be the cause of primary amenorrhea in this girl?

Good breast development indicates estrogen exposure. In normal course of puberty thelarche is followed by adrenarche and menarche. Breast development may occur in response to exogenous estrogens that she may have received. Her FSH and LH levels should be checked. An ultrasound of pelvis will help assess for uterus.

Q2. Her FSH is 46 mIU/mL and LH is 38 mIU/mL. Ultrasound of pelvis shows absent uterus.

She has hypergonadotropic hypogonadism. The typical phenotype with absent uterus and no pubic or axillary hair is suggestive of androgen insensitivity syndrome (AIS). Her karyotpe should be checked.

Q3. Her karyotype is 46XY. How will you manage her?

These findings confirm the diagnosis of AIS. The condition occurs due to mutation in androgen receptor.[17] The gonads are testes and breast development occurs due to peripheral conversion of testosterone to estrogen. The most important aspect in management is not to disturb the gender identity of the girl. The gonads need to be removed, as these are prone to develop malignancy. This is followed by HRT to maintain bone health.[18] Such patients have a short blind vagina, which may achieve adequate length with coitus or dilator treatment. Some may require vaginoplasty. Pregnancy is possible only with oocyte donation and surrogacy.[19]

 Key Points

- Approach to diagnosing the cause of amenorrhea is based on an understanding of physiology of menstruation.
- Detailed history and clinical examination along with judicious use of appropriate hormonal investigations are helpful in making the diagnosis.
- Special investigations including pelvic sonography, MRI of brain and karyotype are often required.
- Management is based on the underlying cause. Reproductive needs of the patient are taken into consideration.

REFERENCES

1. Amenorrhea. In: Fritz ME, Speroff L, (eds). Clinical Gynecology, Endocrinology and Infertility. 8th ed. Philadelphia, Lippincott Williams and Wilkins 2012;435–94.
2. Regulation of menstrual cycle. In: Fritz ME, Speroff L, (eds). Clinical Gynecology, Endocrinology and Infertility. 8th ed. Philadelphia, Lippincott Williams and Wilkins 2012;199–242.
3. Marshall WA, Tanner JM. Variations in pattern of pubertal changes in girls. Arch Dis Child 1969; 44:291–303.
4. Rotterdam ESHRE/ASRM-Sponsored PCOS consensus workshop group. Revised 2003 consensus on diagnostic criteria and long-term health risks related to polycystic ovary syndrome (PCOS). Hum Reprod 2004;19:41–7.
5. Conway G, Dewailly D, Diamanti-Kandarakis E, Escobar-Morreale HF, Franks S, Gambineri A, et al; ESE PCOS Special Interest Group. The polycystic ovary syndrome: a position statement from the European Society of Endocrinology. Eur J Endocrinol 2014;171:P1–29.
6. RCOG Green-top Guideline No. 33. Polycystic Ovary Syndrome, Long-term Consequences; Nov 2014. www.rcog.org.uk/en/guidelines-research-services/guidelines/gtg33.
7. European Society for Human Reproduction and Embryology (ESHRE) Guideline Group on POI, Webber L, Davies M, Anderson R, et al. ESHRE Guideline: management of women with premature ovarian insufficiency. Hum Reprod 2016;31:926–37.
8. Goswami D, Conway GS. Premature ovarian failure. Hum Reprod Update 2005;11:391–410.
9. Goswami R, Marwaha RK, Goswami D, Gupta N, Ray D, Tomar N, Singh S. Prevalence of thyroid autoimmunity in sporadic idiopathic hypoparathyroidism in comparison to type 1 diabetes and premature ovarian failure. J Clin Endocrinol Metab 2006;91:4256–9.
10. Goswami D, Arif A, Saxena A, Batra S. Idiopathic primary ovarian insufficiency: a study of serial hormonal profiles to assess ovarian follicular activity. Hum Reprod 2011;26:2218–25.
11. Kriplani A, Goswami D, Agarwal N, Bhatla N, Ammini AC. Twin pregnancy following gonadotrophin therapy in a patient with Sheehan's syndrome. Int J Gynaecol Obstet 2000;71:59–63.
12. Salazar CA, Isaacson K, Morris S. A comprehensive review of Asherman's syndrome: causes, symptoms and treatment options. Curr Opin Obstet Gynecol 2017;29:249–256.
13. ACOG Committee Opinion No. 728 Summary: Müllerian Agenesis: Diagnosis, Management, And Treatment. Obstet Gynecol 2018;131:196–197.
14. Dietrich JE, Millar DM, Quint EH. Obstructive reproductive tract anomalies. J Pediatr Adolesc Gynecol 2014;27:396–402.
15. Acién P, Acién M. The presentation and management of complex female genital malformations. Hum Reprod Update 2016;22:48–69.
16. Gravholt CH, Andersen NH, Conway GS, Dekkers OM, Geffner ME, Klein KO, et al. International Turner Syndrome Consensus Group. Clinical practice guidelines for the care of girls and women with Turner syndrome: proceedings from the 2016 Cincinnati International Turner Syndrome Meeting. Eur J Endocrinol 2017;177:G1–G70.
17. Normal and abnormal sexual development. In: Fritz ME, Speroff L, (eds). Clinical Gynecology, Endocrinology and Infertility. 8th ed. Philadelphia, Lippincott Williams and Wilkins 2012;331–90.
18. Han TS, Goswami D, Trikudanathan S, Creighton SM, Conway GS. Comparison of bone mineral density and body proportions between women with complete androgen insensitivity syndrome and women with gonadal dysgenesis. Eur J Endocrinol 2008;159:179–85.
19. Mongan NP, Tadokoro-Cuccaro R, Bunch T, Hughes IA. Androgen insensitivity syndrome. Best Pract Res Clin Endocrinol Metab 2015;29:569–80.

Polycystic Ovarian Syndrome and Hirsutism

Madhavi M Gupta

Polycystic Ovary Syndrome (PCOS) is the commonest endocrine disorder of women in the reproductive age group globally. The prevalence is 6–10% when using the diagnostic criteria defined by the National Institute of Health (NIH). On applying the Rotterdam criteria it may be twice as high.[1] Depending on which criteria are used- NIH, Rotterdam or the AE-PCOS Society for diagnosing the condition the worldwide prevalence ranges from 4 to 21%.[2,3]

The disorder is manifested clinically as ovulatory dysfunction, hyperandrogenism, and polycystic ovarian morphology (PCOM) on ultrasound. Cutaneous manifestations of androgen excess (hirsutism) adversely affect the social interaction and quality of life of the woman and polycystic ovary syndrome is the most common cause of anovular infertility.

Case 1

A young girl of 16 years attends the OPD with complaints of irregular cycles at intervals of 2–3 months.

Q1. What history needs to be elicited?
- Age at menarche
- Details of menstrual irregularity—duration, pattern, does she require any medicine for withdrawal bleed or has spontaneous menses.
- Symptoms suggestive of hyperandrogenism—hirsutism, acne, hair loss especially frontal

- Any discharge from the breast (galactorrhea)—spontaneous or on expression
- Detailed drug history—combined oral contraceptives (COC), progestins, drugs causing menstrual irregularity or amenorrhea
- Life-style history—exercise levels, eating habits, any significant changes in the weight associated with menstrual irregularity
- Any similar history in the family—sister, mother
- History of diabetes in the family
- Symptoms indicative of disturbance of the hypothalamic-pituitary ovarian axis
- Symptoms suggestive of thyroid dysfunction—lethargy, voice change, weight gain, excessive sleepiness
- Anxiety, depression
- Any other co-morbid condition

Q2. What is to be specially looked for in the examination?
- Height, weight, body mass index (BMI)
- Clinical features of systemic illness
- Breast—galactorrhoea
- Distribution of body fat—waist-hip ratio
- Distribution and characteristics of body hair—modified Ferriman Gallwey score
- Stigmata of hyperlipidemia—xanthelesma
- Signs of thyroid disorder—skin characteristic, non-pitting edema
- External genitalia—clitoromegaly.

Q3. How is the diagnosis of polycystic ovary syndrome reached?

Diagnosis of polycystic ovary syndrome requires a careful history and clinical examination. It should be supplemented with standardized laboratory investigations including biochemical parameters and ovarian imaging. Hyperandrogenism and menstrual dysfunction are the major clinical features.

Diagnosing PCOS entails three components:

1. Establishing hyperandrogenism (clinical—hirsutism, acne and lab parameters).
2. Establishing ovulatory dysfunction—unpredictable menses at >35 days or occuring less than 8 times per year. In the presence of hyperandrogenism occurrence of regular cycles at 21–35 days does not always correspond to normal ovulatory function. It may be present in 15–40% of women with regular menses and hyperandrogenism.
3. Establishing polycystic ovarian morphology (PCOM) on ultrasound.

Diagnosis in adolescence may be tricky as there is overlap of findings with those of normal puberty. Hence, in adolescence presence of both ovulatory dysfunction inappropriate for the developmental stage and hyperandrogenism (increased free testosterone and moderate to severe hirsutism) are required for diagnosis.

Q4. What investigations are required for evaluating suspected polycystic ovary syndrome?

- Serum thyroid-stimulating hormone (TSH)
- Serum prolactin
- 2-hour oral glucose tolerance test
- Fasting lipid profile
- Serum testosterone (in those with moderate or severe hirsutism)
- Serum anti-müllerian hormone (AMH)
- Sex hormone binding globulin (SHBG)—to calculate the free androgen index (FAI)
- 17-hydroxyprogesterone (17-OHP)—morning sample in the follicular phase. Especially in women with onset of hirsutism in the pre- or perimenarcheal period or those with a history of congenital adrenal hyperplasia in the family.
- Investigations of limited value:
  - Serum LH—raised
  - Serum FSH—low to normal
  - Androsteneidione—raised in <20%
  - DHEA—S is high in 50%

Q5. How will further management be decided?

- Management is decided by the complaints of the patient.
- Lifestyle modification is the first line of management. Weight loss by means of dietary alteration and exercise is the primary therapy in PCOS. Weight loss of as little as 5% is effective in reducing androgen levels and cardiometabolic risk factors, improves menstrual function and possibly enhances the response to fertility medications.
- In cases of oligo-anovulation presenting as menstrual dysfunction-cyclical oral combined oral contraceptive pills or oral progesterones are given cyclically for 10–14 days every month. This provides protection against the unopposed high estrogen environment and results in cyclical shedding thus protecting against endometrial hyperplasia.
- **Metformin:** It is an insulin sensitizer that lowers the insulin levels and leads to 20–25% reduction in serum testosterone levels. It is recommended in women with PCOS having impaired glucose tolerance or type 2 diabetes mellitus after lifestyle modification.[4,5] Dose: 500 mg daily with meals, gradually increasing to 1000 mg twice a day with meals.
- Hirsutism—discussed further

Q6. What are the problems encountered later in life when planning pregnancy?

- Anovular infertility is most common.
- The couple should be evaluated for other common causes of infertility which may affect the choice of therapy.

- Oral clomiphene citrate is the drug of choice for inducing ovulation.
- Greater benefit has been reported in terms of live birth rate with Letrozole, an aromatase inhibitor.
- Though metformin is inferior to clomiphene in achieving live birth it may have a useful role as an adjuvant therapy in obese PCOS women.
- The second-line therapy for anovulatory infertility in PCOS is usually low-dose gonadotropin therapy.

Q7. Are women with PCOS at a higher higher risk for complications than normal women during pregnancy?

There is increased risk of gestational diabetes along with the microvascular complications of diabetes and development of pre-eclampsia.

Q8. What are the other abnormalities and risks associated with PCOS?

- Cardiometabolic abnormalities with increased risk of cardiovascular diseases.
- Risk of metabolic syndrome (MetS). Therefore, its components need to be evaluated—Type 2 DM, glucose intolerance, hypertension, hyperlipidemia, and also the possibility of clinical events like acute myocardial infarction and stroke.
- Obesity—50–80%
- Dyslipidemia—lower high-density lipoprotein (HDL), higher very-low-density lipoprotein (VLDL), higher low-density lipoprotein (LDL).
- Impaired glucose tolerance (IGT)—30–35%
- Type 2 diabetes mellitus (T2DM)—8–10%

Q9. Is any screening required for future health care purposes?

- Screening for cardiometabolic risk factors (components of MetS)
  - Measurement of blood pressure, BMI, and waist circumference to be done at each visit. Fasting lipid levels to be done every two years (earlier if the woman has gained weight). Nonalcoholic fatty liver disease should also be tested for.
  - Screening for impaired glucose tolerance and type 2 diabetes mellitus using the 2-hour oral glucose-tolerance test. Baseline oral glucose tolerance test every 1 to 2 years based on family history of T2DM and BMI. In women with IGT it should be done yearly. Glycosylated hemoglobin (HbA1c) levels are an acceptable alternative.
- Screen for anxiety, depression and obstructive sleep apnea.
- In case of persistent abnormal uterine bleeding or prolonged amenorrhea evaluate for endometrial hyperplasia.

Q10. What care should be taken prior to treating infertility?

- Women should be screened and treated for diabetes and hypertension prior to attempting conception.
- Importance of weight loss should be stressed.

HIRSUTISM

Hirsutism in women is defined as male-pattern distribution of increased terminal (coarse) hair.[6]

Race and ethnicity significantly influence the severity of hirsutism. It is seen more commonly in the Indian subcontinent and those from the Mediterranean countries than in women of east Asian or northern European descent.

The commonest cause of hirsutism is chronic anovulation and elevated androgen secretion by the ovaries. It is very uncommon to find cases of hirsutism due to adrenal cause.

Clinical assessment mandates a careful history with details regarding time of onset, progression, how frequently she has to resort to hair removal and the extent to which it negatively impacts her daily life. Cutaneous manifestations of androgen excess (hirsutism) adversely affect the social interaction and quality of life of the woman. Depending on the severity it can have a significant psychological impact leading to impaired quality of life and depressive symptoms in many women.

Case 2

A young girl of 16 years attends the OPD with complaints of extra hair growth over the face and body.

Q1. What history needs to be elicited?

- Age at menarche
- Detailed menstrual history—regularity, any change from normal pattern.
- Age of onset and severity of excessive/extra hair growth—pre- or peri-mencheal, rate of progression, use of any depilatory methods of hair removal and if so, the frequency.
- Other clinical features of hirsutism—acne, male pattern balding, voice change.
- Any discharge from the breast (galactorrhea).
- Detailed drug history—COC, progestins, drugs causing hair growth—anabolic steroids, danazol, minoxidil, diazoxide, phenytoin. Use of any supplements which may contain steroids.
- Weight changes
- Family history of menstrual irregularity, hirsutism, obesity, infertility, non-classical congenital adrenal hyperplasia (CAH).
- Assessing her quality of life and any depressive symptoms which depend on the severity of hirsutism.

Q2. What is to be specially looked for in the examination?

- Height, weight and BMI
- Clinical features of systemic illness
- Breast—galactorrhea (spontaneous or expressed)
- Distribution of body fat—central obesity, moon facies

Distribution and characteristics of body hair—modified Ferriman Gallwey score. The Ferriman-Gallwey chart is used universally to assess the severity and distribution of the excess body hair.[7] Each of the nine androgen-sensitive areas are graded visually on a scale of 0 to 4 obtaining a final score. A score of <8, 8–15 and >15 are taken as mild, moderate and severe hirsutism. Even if the score is low and the patient complains of hirsutism it may be a good practice to treat as it affects the self-esteem of the woman and has a negative impact on her quality of life.

- Other clinical features of androgen excess—seborrhea, frontal/temporal balding, acne. Acanthosis nigricans may be indicative of insulin resistance.
- Skin manifestations of hypercortisolism—striae, thin skin or easy bruising
- Signs of thyroid disorder —skin characteristic, non-pitting edema
- Signs of virilization—breast atrophy, increased muscle mass, deepening of the voice and clitoromegaly.
- Any abdominal or pelvic mass—suggestive of androgen secreting tumor.
- As serum androgens get progressively elevated, the clinical manifestations also worsen.

Q3. What investigations are required for evaluating hirsutism?

Laboratory assessment is usually recommended when hirsutism is moderate or severe, particularly in conditions when the hair growth is of sudden onset, rapidly progressive or accompanied by features of virilization

- Serum thyroid-stimulating hormone (TSH)
- Serum prolactin

  The above two tests should be done in women with menstrual irregularity

- Serum total testosterone—normal 20–80 ng/dL. If >150 ng/dL evaluate for androgen-secreting tumor.
- 17-OHP—<200 ng/dL (early morning, early follicular phase) rules out non-classical congenital adrenal hyperplasia. Higher values may be followed by the ACTH stimulation test. This test is done in patients with early onset hirsutism (pre- or peri-menarcheal onset, including those with premature adrenarche), women with a family history of the disorder, and those in high-risk ethnic groups.
- Serum DHEA-S - Though not done routinely, it is useful in cases of severe hyper-

androgenism and where there is possibility of an occult androgen-producing tumor.

- 2-hour oral glucose tolerance test—done in all women with PCOS.
- Insulin levels (fasting and two-hour along with OGTT)—to see for insulin resistance, in HAIR-AN syndrome or stromal hyperplasia (hyperthecosis).

Insulin resistance:

2-hour glucose/insulin ratio (mg/dL or µU/mL) <1

2-hour plasma insulin >100 µU/mL

Q4. What are the common causes of hirsutism?

There can be specific disorders like classical and non-classical congenital adrenal hyperplasia (CAH), androgen secreting tumors (ovary/adrenals), hyperandrogenic insulin-resistant acanthosis nigricans (HAIR-AN), and Cushing's syndrome.

Polycystic ovary syndrome (PCOS) and idiopathic hirsutism are the disorders of exclusion.

Of all the above causes PCOS is the most common cause of hyperandrogenemia in women.

Q5. What are the management options?

- Treatment should be directed towards the cause.
- Even if hirsutism is mild the woman's views should be taken into consideration if she is bothered.[8]
- Mechanical hair removal (shaving, waxing, depilatory creams, laser, electrolysis) along with medication directed to reduce the hair growth.
- The target should be to reduce the frequency of mechanically removing unwanted hair.
- Severity of the condition should be defined prior to commencing treatment for monitoring purposes.
- Counseling regarding her expectations as treatment leads to reduction in hair growth

and change in the quality of hair rather than complete cessation of hair growth.

- The woman needs to understand that the response to all pharmacological measures is slow and up to 6 months may be required to achieve significant improvement.
- Permanent hair removal methods should be resorted to once maximum benefit with medical therapy has been achieved.

Q6. What drugs are commonly used?

Estrogen-progestin Contraceptives

Combined Oral Contraceptive (COC) are considered to be the first-line agents. The COCs suppress the gonadotropin (LH) secretion and ovarian steroidogenesis.[9] SHBG production in the liver is increased by the estrogen component thus decreasing the bioavailable androgen. New terminal hair growth is reduced but these changes may take upto 6 months to be clinically visible. Low dose ethinyl estradiol (upto 30 µg) with a progestin having anti-androgenic action or low androgenic properties can be used.

- Directly or indirectly COCs can decrease adrenal DHEAS production.
- Contraceptive progestins inhibit 5α reductase activity in skin.
- The vaginal contraceptive ring (releasing 15 µg ethinyl estradiol and 120 µg etonogestrel daily) and the transdermal contraceptive patch (delivering 20 µg ethinyl estradiol and 150 µg norelgestromin daily) can also be used.[10]

In case of contraindication to use of estrogenprogestin contraceptives, medroxyprogesterone acetate can be used. It suppresses LH which in turn substantially decreases ovarian androgen production.

Antiandrogens

Effective and best used along with estrogen-progestin contraceptives or any other effective contraceptive. These drugs can also be used in combination with COC for women who do not respond well to COC alone.

- Cyproterone acetate
- Spironolactone
- Flutamide
- Finasteride

Insulin Sensitizing Drugs

Although metformin is found to lower the serum androgen levels it is not recommended for treatment of hirsutism.[11]

Eflornithine (13.9% cream)

- It inhibits ornithine decarboxylase (ODC), an enzyme responsible for catalyzing the rate-limiting step for follicular polyamine synthesis, which is necessary for hair growth.
- Improvement is gradual, occurring over a period of 4–8 weeks or longer.
- Best suited for patients with mild facial hirsutism.

Key Points

- PCOS is a common hormonal disorder affecting women in reproductive age group.
- The diagnosis is usually based on clinical features of hyperandrogenemia, anovulation and ultrasound finding of polycystic morphology of the ovaries.
- Investigations are done to rule out metabolic disorders like diabetes and dyslipidemia.
- Management is based on the clinical features and reproductive needs of the patient.

REFERENCES

1. McCartney CR, Marshall JC. Clinical practice. Polycystic Ovary Syndrome. N Engl J Med 2016;375:54–64.

2. Boyle JA, Cunningham J, O'Dea K, Dunbar T, Norman RJ. Prevalence of polycystic ovary syndrome in a sample of Indigenous women in Darwin, Australia. Med J Aust 2012;196:62–6.

3. Ma YM, Li R, Qiao J, Zhang XW, Wang SY, Zhang QF, et al. Characteristics of abnormal menstrual cycle and polycystic ovary syndrome in community and hospital populations. Chin Med J (Engl) 2010;123:2185–9.

4. Legro RS, Arslanian SA, Ehrmann DA, et al. Diagnosis and treatment of polycystic ovary syndrome: an Endocrine Society clinical practice guideline. J ClinEndocrinol Metab 2013; 98:4565–92.

5. Conway G, Dewailly D, Diamanti-Kandarakis E, Escobar-Morreale HF, Franks S, Gambineri A, et al. The polycystic ovary syndrome: a position statement from the European Society of Endocrinology. Eur J Endocrinol 2014; 171: 1–29.

6. Franks S. Polycystic ovary syndrome. N Engl J Med 1995;333: 853–861.

7. Ferriman D, Gallwey JD. Clinical assessment of body hair growth in women. J Clin Endocrinol Metab 1961;21:1440–1447.

8. DeUgarte CM, Woods KS, Bartolucci AA, Azziz R, Degree of facial and body terminal hair growth in unselected black and white women: toward a populational de nition of hirsutism. J Clin Endocrinol Metab 2006;91:1345.

9. Dewis P, Petsos P, Newman M, Anderson DC. The treatment of hirsutism with a combination of desogestrel and ethinyl oestradiol. Clin Endocrinol (Oxf) 1985;22:29.

10. White T, Jain JK, Stanczyk FZ. Effect of oral versus transdermal steroidal contraceptives on androgenic markers, Am J Obstet Gynecol 2005; 192:2055–9.

11. Martin KA, Anderson RR, Chang RJ, Ehrmann DA, Lobo RA, Murad MH, et al. Evaluation and treatment of hirsutism in premenopausal women: an Endocrine Society clinical practice guideline. J Clin Endocrinol Metab 2018;103:1233–57.

10 | Hyperprolactinemia

Sangeeta Bhasin, Rini Pachori

Hyperprolactinemia is not a disease in itself but a manifestation of disturbance in function of other organs most commonly of the hypo-thalamic-pituitary axis. It has a prevalence of 9% in women with amenorrhea and 25% in those with galactorrhea. In women having concomitant amenorrhea and galactorrhea, 70% are hyperprolactinemic.[1]

Prolactin is a 23000 Daltons molecular weight polypeptide hormone (198 amino acids) synthesized in the lactotroph cells of the anterior pituitary gland.

Its secretion is pulsatile and under the inhibitory control of dopamine which is secreted by the tuberoinfundibular dopaminergic neurons into the portal hypophyseal vessels. That is why when dopamine release from hypothalamus to pituitary is inhibited, prolactin levels rise. Prolactin production is also stimulated by thyrotropin releasing hormone, vasoactive intestinal peptide, and oxytocin.

Case 1

A 35-year-old woman presents to gynecology outpatient clinic with complaints of galactorrhea and no menses for one year. There is no history of any chronic illness or drug intake. On examination, there is milky discharge from both breasts. On pelvic examination, no abnormality is detected. On work up she is found to have an elevated prolactin level of 65 ng/mL. Her thyroid function tests are normal.

Q1. What is the normal serum level of prolactin?

- Normal serum prolactin levels vary between 5 and 25 ng/mL in women although diurnal and physiological variations occur.
- Levels are lowest in the mid morning about 2 hours after the patient wakes up and highest between 5 and 7 AM.
- A physiological increase is also seen after meals, excessive exercise, chest wall surgery or trauma, breast stimulation, venepuncture and 1–2 hours postictal.
- Because of these diurnal and physiological variations in serum levels, a mildly raised prolactin level should always be repeated.
- Hyperprolactinemia is defined as a fasting level above 25 ng/mL at least 2 hours after waking up.

Q2. What are the main actions of prolactin hormone?

- The main biological action of prolactin is inducing and maintaining lactation.
- It suppresses the pulsatile secretion of gonadotropin releasing hormone (GnRH), promotes formation of corpus luteum and directly inhibits steroidogenesis and spermatogenesis.[2]
- It also exerts metabolic effects, takes part in reproductive mammary development and stimulates immune responsiveness.

Q3. How do patients of hyperprolactinemia clinically present as?

The predominant physiologic consequence of hyperprolactinemia is hypogonadotropic hypogonadism (HH) due to suppression of pulsatile GnRH. Patients may present with:

- **Isolated galactorrhea** (non-puerperal lactation) without any menstrual abnormality may be seen in 30% of hyperprolactinemic women. Galactorrhea may be unilateral or bilateral, continuous or intermittent.

  Even though galactorrhea is considered a hallmark of hyperprolactinemia, serum prolactin levels may be normal in 50% of patients. Most likely, a transient episode of hyperprolactinemia triggers the galactorrhea that persists even after normalization of prolactin levels due to an increased sensitivity of the breast to the lactotrophic stimulus.

  Conversely, in 2/3rd of hyperprolactinemic women, galactorrhea may be absent due to inadequate estrogenic or progestational priming of the breast.

- **Ovulatory and menstrual dysfunction** results from inhibition of GnRH secretion which in turn reduces pituitary gonadotropin secretion leading to anovulation.

  Mild hyperprolactinemia (20–50 ng/mL) may cause a short luteal phase; moderately raised levels (50–100 ng/mL) may cause oligomenorrhea/amenorrhea whereas levels more than 100 ng/mL may cause frank hypogonadism with hypoestrogenism.[3]

- Both **galactorrhea and amenorrhea** together may be seen in 2/3rd of patients with hyperprolactinemia.

- **Infertility**

- **Hirsutism:** Hyperprolactinemic women may present with signs of chronic hyperandrogenism such as hirsutism and acne, possibly due to increased dehydroepiandrosterone sulfate secretion from the adrenals, as well as reduced sex hormone binding globulin leading to high free testosterone levels.

- **Sexual dysfunction, decreased libido**

- **Osteoporosis**: Prolonged hypoestrogenism secondary to hyperprolactinemia results in progressive osteopenia. Postmenopausal women with hyperprolactinemia may therefore present with back pain and loss of height. Osteopenia improves with normalization of prolactin levels though spinal bone mineral density (BMD) may not be restored completely. Women with hyperprolactinemia and normal menses have normal BMD.

- **Neurological manifestations** such as chronic headache and visual field defects like bitemporal hemianopsia may be associated with adenomas.

Q4. What are the various causes of hyperprolactinemia?

Hyperprolactinemia can be **physiological, pathological, pharmacological or idiopathic.**

A. *Physiological hyper-secretion*

- Pregnancy, lactation, chest wall stimulation, sleep, stress
- Physiological hyperprolactinemia is usually mild or moderate. During normal pregnancy, serum prolactin rises progressively to around 200–500 ng/mL.

B. *Pathological*

- Pituitary—prolactinomas, lymphocytic hypophysitis or parasellar masses, mixed cell adenomas, granulomatous hypophysitis
- Hypothalamic pituitary stalk damage
  - Tumors—craniopharyngioma, meningioma, suprasellar tumors, dysgerminoma, metastatic tumors.
  - Empty sella, granulomas, Rathke's cyst
  - Irradiation
  - Trauma—suprasellar surgery, pituitary stalk resection
- Systemic disorders

– *Chronic renal failure:* About 30% of these patients may show raised prolactin levels.
– *Hypothyroidism:* 40% patients of primary hypothyroidism show an associated hyperprolactinemia.
– Cirrhosis: Mild elevation of serum prolactin is seen in 20% cirrhotic patients.
– Polycystic ovarian syndrome: Hyperprolactinemia may be seen in 15% of the patients.
– Epileptic seizures

C. Pharmacological

Drug induced hypersecretion is seen with many antipsychotics—described later.

D. Idiopathic

In cases where all causes of hyperprolactinemia have been excluded, the hyperprolactinemia is referred to as "idiopathic".

Q5. Her repeat serum prolactin is 109 ng/mL. How will you evaluate her?

• A detailed past medical, drug and family history should be taken and a thorough physical examination should be done. In this patient there is no history of any relevant drug intake.
• After excluding pregnancy, her thyroid, kidney and liver function are assessed.
• If these tests are normal, the next step would be imaging of the hypothalamic-pituitary area.

The imaging modality of choice is MRI of the brain with gadolinium enhancement with selective pituitary cuts.

Q6. A pituitary MRI with contrast in this patient was reported as 'subtle area of delayed enhancement in the anterior pituitary, consistent with a 5 mm microadenoma' (Fig. 10.1). What does the report mean?

• Prolactin secreting pituitary adenomas or prolactinomas account for 25–30% of functioning pituitary tumors and are the most frequent cause of chronic hyperprolactinemia.
• 90% of prolactinomas are less than 1 cm in size and are called microadenomas. Tumors more than 1 cm in size are called macroadenomas and are more common in postmenopausal women (Fig. 10.2).
• Serum prolactin levels usually parallel tumor size; bigger the tumor, more the prolactin level. A level of 250 ng/mL or greater is diagnostic of a macroprolactinoma.
• A macroadenoma may sometimes show only mild elevations in prolactin levels. This could be because—(1) it is a nonfunctioning pituitary adenoma or craniopharyngioma rather than a prolactin secreting prolactinoma. (2) it is largely cystic[3], (3) very high circulating levels of prolactin as in giant prolactinomas >2 cm cause saturation of

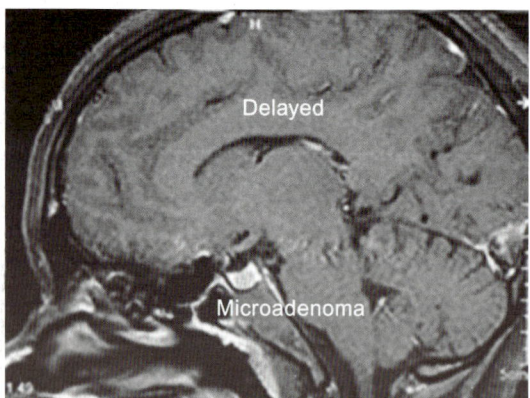

Fig. 10.1: Microadenoma (*Courtesy:* Dr D Goswami, Gyne Endocrinology Clinic, MAMC and LNH)

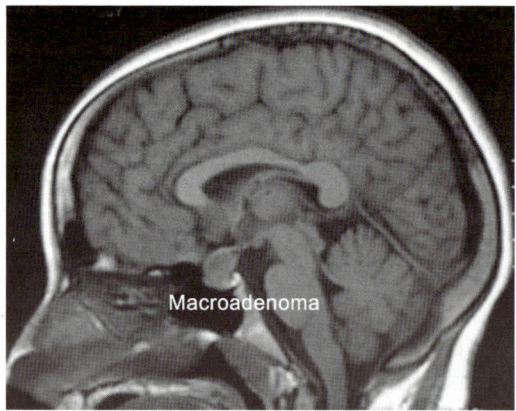

Fig. 10.2: Macroadenoma (*Courtesy:* Dr D Goswami, Gyne Endocrinology Clinic, MAMC and LNH)

antiprolactin antibodies in an immuno-radiometric assay tube causing falsely low results. This is the "hook effect". Further measurement in 1 in 100 dilution will give the true result.

Q7. How will you manage her?

- The patient should be reassured about the benign course of a microadenoma as they rarely progress to macroadenomas. However, compliance with drugs and follow up should be stressed upon.
- She should be advised to report any symptom of chronic headache, any visual disturbance (especially tunnel vision consistent with bitemporal hemianopsia) and extraocular muscle palsy immediately. Formal visual field testing at this point of time is not necessary.
- Since this patient has amenorrhea along with troublesome galactorrhea, the treatment of choice will be to prescribe **dopamine agonists** (DA) because they effectively reduce both prolactin levels as well as the size of the tumor and help ameliorate the symptoms.

Q8. Which are the commonly used DA drugs?

These are enumerated in Table 10.1.

- The most commonly used DA are cabergoline and bromocriptine and both are highly effective.

Table 10.1: Common dopamine agonist drugs

Drug	Nature	Dose
Bromocriptine	Ergot	2.5–10 mg/day
Cabergoline	Ergot	0.25 mg twice weekly 1.5 mg twice a week
Lisuride	Ergot	0.1–0.2 mg/day
Quinagolide	Ergot	25–300 micrograms/day

- Bromocriptine is a non-selective DA that binds to D1 receptors in the gut and D2 receptors in the pituitary. It is started at a dose of 1.25 mg/day at bedtime. The dose is increased by 1.25 mg/week till prolactin levels become normal or a dose of 2.5 mg twice a day is reached.
- Cabergoline, a selective dopamine receptor type 2 agonist, is given as a 0.25 mg tablet twice a week. The dose is increased gradually (guided by serial monthly prolactin levels) to avoid troublesome side effects like gastrointestinal upset and orthostatic hypotension to a maximum of 1.5 mg twice a week.
- Because of a longer half-life and fewer side effects cabergoline is better tolerated and a more favored drug. It normalizes prolactin levels in 95% and reduces tumor size in 90% of patients.

Q9. How will you follow up and for how long does the treatment continue?

- Prolactin levels start decreasing within 2–3 weeks after treatment is begun. Tumor size also reduces by 6 weeks. Menstruation, ovulation and fertility return with normalization of prolactin levels. Although galactorrhea reduces in amount, complete cessation takes more time.[4]
- Follow up is with 1–3 monthly serum prolactin and yearly MRI.
- After one year of treatment the dose of the DA can be reduced. If serum prolactin levels remain normal for 2 years and MRI does not show any evidence of tumor, the drug can be stopped.
- Follow up then includes- serum prolactin levels every 3 months for the first year and then yearly. MRI of the brain is done if prolactin increases above normal.
- However, hyperprolactinemia returns in 26–65% cases of microprolactinoma usually in the year after withdrawal.

Q10. What are the side effects of DAs?

Side effects associated with these drugs are

- Nausea, vomiting, headache, constipation, dizziness, faintness, depression, postural hypotension, digital vasospasm, and nasal stuffiness.

- Neuropsychiatric symptoms like auditory hallucinations, delusion, and mood changes. These quickly resolve with discontinuation of the drug.
- High doses of cabergoline >3 mg/week are associated with the potential risk of developing cardiac valvular regurgitation but this concern has largely been disproved for the standard doses used in prolactinomas.[5]
- Both DAs can be used vaginally to avoid troublesome side effects with oral use. Bromocriptine is also available as a long acting intamuscular injection.

Q11. If this patient did not have galactorrhea would your treatment have differed?

- Women having microadenoma with amenorrhea but no galactorrhea and not desirous of fertility can be managed expectantly.
- DA can be avoided and she can be given cyclic combined estrogen progestin therapy for amenorrhea.

Q12. If the MRI was reported as macroadenoma, how would you manage her?

- Macroprolactinomas are functional prolactin secreting pituitary tumors more than 1 cm in size. They may produce signs and symptoms of a mass effect like headaches, visual loss or visual field defects, cranial nerve neuropathies and seizures.
- Compression of the hypothalamopituitary axis by the macroprolactinoma may cause hypopituitarism. Also, about 10% of macroprolactinomas may have somatotroph cells and secrete growth hormone (GH) and rarely ACTH and TSH additionally. Conversely, some gonadotroph adenomas may co secrete prolactin. Therefore, additional evaluation with serum FSH/LH, free T4, Insulin like Growth Factor-1 (IGF-1) and morning cortisol level needs to be done.[3]
- **Medical management** with DA is the treatment of choice.[6] Rapid reduction in size and improvement in vision within 6 months is seen with cabergoline though recurrence

may occur in 36–80% of patients.[6] Factors favoring prolonged remission are—(1) when the patient has taken treatment for at least 2–3 years, (2) low prolactin levels have been achieved with low doses of DA, (3) more than 50% tumor reduction has been achieved and (4) there is no cavernous sinus invasion.[7]

- **Neurosurgical management:** Transsphenoidal surgery is less effective than medical treatment and is reserved for patients not responding to or not tolerating DA, patients with large macroadenomas >3 cm wanting to attempt pregnancy, patients having complications like pituitary apoplexy or cerebrospinal fluid leak. Complications of surgery include incomplete resection, persistent hyperprolactinemia and recurrence. A prolactin level 20 ng/mL or less on the day following surgery is a good predictor of long term cure.
- **Radiation therapy:** Is reserved for patients with significant residual tumor after surgery and aggressive prolactinomas. It may take years for prolactin levels and tumor size to decrease.
- **Temozolomide**: An oral alkylating agent may be used as a last resort for aggressive prolactinomas or prolactin secreting carcinomas.

Q13. What is an incidentaloma?

A pituitary incidentaloma is a pituitary tumor detected incidentally when a MRI brain is done for some other reason. Its overall prevalence is 10%.

Case 2

A 24-year-old-woman presents to the infertility clinic with chief complaint of inability to conceive for two years. Her menstrual cycles are prolonged, 2/45–60 days. There is no past or family history of tuberculosis.

On examination, no abnormality is detected.

On routine infertility work-up, serum prolactin level is found to be 82 ng/mL. Serum TSH is 69.5 µIU/mL.

Q1. What is the relation between serum prolactin and serum TSH? What will you do next?

Around 40% patients with primary hypothyroidism have mild elevation of serum prolactin levels as over-production of thyrotropin releasing hormone has a weak stimulating effect on the lactotroph cells of the pituitary causing a mild to moderate increase in prolactin levels.[8]

Treatment is by thyroid hormone replacement alone and serial follow up with serum TSH and serum prolactin levels, both of which will gradually decline.

Q2. The patient was started on tab thyroxine. After 6 months her serum TSH was in the normal range but her hyperprolactinemia persisted. An MRI brain was done which showed a 5 mm microadenoma. How will you proceed next?

- DA is the mainstay of treatment if fertility is desired.
- Ovulation rates of 80–90% are achieved if hyperprolactinemia is the only cause for anovulation. In the remaining women, exogenous gonadotropin stimulation can be added along with DA to achieve ovulation.

Q3. The patient conceives within 6 months of initiating cabergoline therapy and comes to you worried that the drug therapy might harm her fetus. How will you counsel her?

- The patient should be reassured that most DA are FDA Pregnancy category B drugs and cause no harm to the fetus. However, therapy should be discontinued as soon as pregnancy is confirmed except in cases of invasive macroprolactinoma.[9]
- She should be informed about the small risk– 3% of tumor enlargement and that she should report as soon as symptoms such as severe headache or visual field defects arise.
- A baseline visual field perimetry should be obtained and thereafter a clinical follow up every 2–3 months.

- If patient becomes symptomatic, visual field assessment and MRI (without gadolinium) should be done. If tumor growth is evident, Bromocriptine should be started immediately.
- Serum prolactin should be checked 2 months after delivery.
- She can continue to breastfeed.

Q4. How is the management of a macroadenoma different from a microadenoma in pregnancy?

- Small intra sellar tumor (away from optic chiasma)
  - Discontinue DA therapy.
  - Inform of high risk of tumor progression.
  - Inform about warning signs and symptoms.
  - Closer clinical monitoring with formal visual field perimetry in each trimester.
  - MRI if signs/symptoms persist/increase.
  - Initiate DA if tumor progression occurs.
- Large intra sellar tumor (abuts optic chiasma)
  - Advise against pregnancy.
  - DA therapy (bromocriptine) should be continued throughout pregnancy.
  - If enlarged tumor does not respond, start cabergoline.
  - If not responding to medical therapy, trans-nasal trans-sphenoidal surgery in the second trimester. Besides the usual surgical risks, hypopituitarism is a potential long-term effect of surgery and should be discussed with patients as part of the decision-making process. Excision is often incomplete and therefore relapse often occurs.
- External radiation therapy is only reserved for residual tumor in patients who have undergone surgery.

Case 3

A 17-year-old girl presents to the gynecology outpatient clinic with chief complaint of primary amenorrhea. She is a known case of schizophrenia on haloperidol for eight years.

On examination, breast development is normal and there is milky discharge from the nipples on pressing. On work up her serum prolactin was found to be 75 ng/mL.

Q1. What could be the cause of her hyperprolactinemia?

Her hyperprolactinemia and amenorrhea can most likely be attributed to the antipsychotic drugs that she is taking. Drug induced hyperprolactinemia is usually associated with prolactin levels <100 ng/mL.

Q2. What are the drugs that cause hyperprolactinemia?

For answer *see* Table 10.2.

Q3. How will you manage her?

These medications should be discontinued for 48–72 hours if it is safe to do so or substituted with an alternative drug and serum prolactin level repeated. Return of prolactin levels to normal clinches the diagnosis. Alternative therapy with aripiprazole, oanzapine, clozapine that rarely cause hyperprolactinemia may be started. If this is not feasible, she can be given hormone replacement for her amenorrhea or a DA could be started with caution.

Case 4

A 28-year-old lady comes to the gynecology outpatient clinic after having undergone an annual executive health checkup. She has with her a serum prolactin report of 45 ng/mL. Her menstrual cycles are regular; there is no history of any drug intake or bone pains. On examination, breasts are not active, there are no features of hypogonadism. Her repeat serum prolactin level was 50 ng/mL. Her MRI brain is normal.

Q1. What will you suspect in this case?

Prolactin circulates in blood in 3 different forms. 80% of it exists as a monomer with a molecular weight of 23 kDa. This is the most biologically active form. The remaining exists in the 'big' form and the 'big big' form which are formed when the prolactin monomers combine with immunoglobulin IgG to form PRL-IgG complexes. As they have molecular weights varying between 50 and 60–100 kDa, they have a prolonged clearance rate and are detected in blood in large amounts on prolactin assays. These "macroprolactins", however, are inactive biologically.

Macroprolactinemia should always be suspected when hyperprolactinemia is present in the absence of typical signs and symptoms. Macroprolactins can be detected in the serum if it is pre treated with polyethylene glycol before performing the assay whereby the macroprolactins get precipitated. This inexpensive test should always be done in cases of asymptomatic hyperprolactinemia.

Table 10.2: Drugs causing hyperprolactinemia		
Antipsychotics	Typical	Haloperidol, Chlorpromazine, Thioridazine, Thiothixene
	Atypical	Risperidone, Amisulpride Molindone, Zotepine
Antidepressants	Tricyclics	Amitriptyline, Desipramine Clomipramine Amoxapine
	SSRI	Sertraline, Fluoxetine, Paroxetine
	MAO-I	Pargyline, Clorgyline
Prokinetics	Metoclopramide, Domperidone	
Antihypertensives	Alpha-methyldopa, Reserpine, Verapamil	
Opiates	Morphine	
H2 antagonists	Cimetidine, Ranitidine	
Others	Fenfluramine, Physostigmine, Chemotherapies	

The highest elevation is seen with risperidone, amisulpride and paliperidone.[10]

Q2. What are the various syndromes associated with hyperprolactinemia?

1. Ahmuda-Del Castillo syndrome—refers to the association of galactorrhea and amenorrhea. It is also sometimes called amenorrhea–galactorrhea syndrome.
2. Chiari-Frommel syndrome—refers to extended postpartum galactorrhea and amenorrhea.
3. Forbes Albright syndrome—refers to galactorrhea–amenorrhea associated with a pituitary tumor.

Key Points

- Hyperprolactinemia is the commonest endocrine disorder of the hypothalamic- pituitary axis.
- Prolactin secretion exhibits diurnal and physiological variations; mildly raised prolactin levels should therefore be rechecked.
- Patients may present with oligomenorrhea, amenorrhea, infertility, galactorrhea, sexual dysfunction or headache with visual field defects.
- Prolactinomas are the most common cause of hyperprolactinemia, 90% of them being microprolactinomas.
- Asymptomatic microprolactinomas can be managed expectantly. The drug of choice for symptomatic microprolactinomas and macroprolactinomas is a dopamine agonist.
- Trans-sphenoidal surgery is reserved for macroprolactinomas not responding to medical treatment.

REFERENCES

1. Serri O, Chik CL, Ur E, Ezzat S. Diagnosis and management of hyperprolactinemia. CMAJ 2003;169:575–81.
2. Arowojolu AO, Akinloye O, Shittu OB. Serum and seminal plasme prolactin levels in male attendersof an infertility clinic in Ibadan. J Obstet Gynaecol 2004; 24:306–309.
3. Amenorrhea. In: Fritz ME, Speroff L, (eds). Clinical Gynecology, Endocrinology and Infertility. 8th ed. Philadelphia, Lippincott Williams & Wilkins 2012; 435–94.
4. Melmed S, Casanueva FF, Hoffman AR, Kleinberg DL, Montori VM, Schlechte JA, et al. Endocrine Society. Diagnosis and treatment of hyperprolactinemia: an Endocrine Society clinical practice guideline. J Clin Endocrinol Metab 2011;96: 273–88.
5. Schade R, Andersohn F, Suissa S, Haverkamp W, Garbe E. Dopamine agonists and the risk of cardiac-valve regurgitation. N Engl J Med 2007;356:29–38.
6. Casanueva FF, Molitch ME, Schlechte JA, Abs R, Bonert V, Bronstein MD, et al. Guidelines of the Pituitary Society for the diagnosis and management of prolactinomas. Clin Endocrinol (Oxf) 2006;65:265–73.
7. Maiter D. Current Challenges in the Management of Prolactinomas. Eur Endocrinol 2015; 11:39–40.
8. Goel P, Kahkasha, Narang S, Gupta BK, Goel K. Evaluation of serum prolactin level in patients of subclinical and overt hypothyroidism. J Clin Diagn Res 2015;9:BC15–7.
9. Kaiser UB. Hyperprolactinemia and infertility: new insights. J Clin Invest 2012;122:3467–8.
10. Peuskens J, Pani L, Detraux J, De Hert M. The effects of novel and newly approved antipsychotics on serum prolactin levels: a comprehensive review. CNS Drugs 2014 ;28:421–53.
11. McKenna TJ. Should macroprolactin be measured in all hyperprolactinaemic sera? Clin Endocrinol (Oxf) 2009;71:466–9.

11 | Hormone Replacement Therapy in Postmenopausal Women

Poonam Kashyap

Menopause is permanent amenorrhea resulting from cessation of follicular development and the consequent decrease in ovarian estrogen and progesterone production. It is a natural and inevitable event. It happens around 51 years of age in Caucasians though there are ethnic and regional variations. The mean age of menopause for Indian women is 46.2 years which is less than that of their western counterparts. The incidence of menopause increases rapidly after the age of 41 years. By age of 48–49 years, two-thirds of women are in menopause.

According to WHO menopause is dated from the final menstrual period regardless of whether the menopause was induced or spontaneous. The period immediately preceding and following the actual cessation of menstruation is called *perimenopause*. Menopause before the age of 40 years is considered to be premature—premature ovarian failure (POF) or primary ovarian in sufficiency (POI). It may occurr spontaneously or as a result of surgery or some other intervention (e.g. chemotherapy). Clinical implications of menopause before age of 40 years are different from menopause after 40 years of age.[1,2]

Age of menopause is an important biomarker as there is loss of fertility potential and increased risk for certain diseases. Many of these diseases can be prevented by lifestyle modification, hormone replacement therapy, and addition of supplements such as calcium, vitamin D and micronutrients. The number of women in menopause is increasing with increase in life expectancy and so is the increase in reported problems.

Case 1

A 51-year-old woman presents with troublesome hot flushes and night sweats for past 6 months. She had her last period 5 months back.

Q1. How will you manage this case?

Hormone replacement therapy (HRT) remains the most effective therapy for vasomotor symptoms. A woman having vasomotor symptoms will complain of hot flushes and night sweats. These can be present in 80% of women undergoing menopausal transition. The symptoms may be severe in 20% of women. HRT is indicated for women reporting menopausal symptoms that are debilitating and affecting the quality of life.

As per a systematic review which compaired HRT versus placebo for the relief of vasomotor symptoms, frequency of hot flushes was reduced to 75% and severity of hot flushes was reduced to 87% with HRT.[3] HRT should be given after ruling out contraindications to its use and after discussing likely risks and benefits with the patient. If there are contraindications to HRT, other non hormonal drugs like selective serotonin reuptake inhibitors (SSRIs), serotonin-norepinephrine reuptake inhibitors (SNRIs) and some anti-epileptic drugs can be given for control of symptoms.

Case 2

A 47-year-old postmenopausal woman with history of breast cancer 7 years back presents for the management of hot flushes, irritability, and reduced sleep. She reports recent onset of vaginal dryness causing dyspareunia that is not alleviated by lubricants. Her breast cancer was estrogen receptor (ER)/progesterone receptor (PR)—positive, and she received tamoxifen therapy for 5 years (now completed).

Q1. How would you manage this patient?

For such women with contraindications to HRT, selective serotonin reuptake inhibitors (SSRIs), serotonin-norepinephrine reuptake inhibitors (SNRIs), some antiepileptic drugs, and other centrally acting drugs can be given. Venlafaxine, desvenlafaxine, paroxetine, citalopram, and escitalopram are effective in reducing hot flushes in postmenopausal women and can be given to those having contraindications to HRT.[4] Paroxetine should be avoided in women receiving tamoxifen.[5] Gabapentin is a gamma - aminobutyric acid analogue. There is 18% reduction in hot flushes with 100 mg of gabapentin given three times daily and 46% reduction with 300 mg given three times daily, as compared to 18% reduction with placebo. Gabapentin is as effective but has more side-effects as compared to SSRIs/SNRIs when given in higher doses.[6] Clonidine, an α-2 adrenergic agonist is slightly more effective than placebo in reducing hot flushes but its use is associated with significant side-effects (dry mouth, dizziness, constipation, hypotension and sedation) that limit its clinical use. Transdermal hormonal preparations may be superior to oral ones as more stable hormone levels are acheived. They have less systemic side effects leading to increased compliance.

Women taking nonhormonal preparations should be evaluated periodically and the dose should be increased in a step wise manner to minimise the side effects. When planning to discontinue the therapy, these should be tapered gradually to avoid withdrawal symptoms.

Q2. How will you investigate a woman before prescribing HRT?

Proper assessment is essential before prescribing HRT.

- Assess her weight and height and calculate her body mass index (BMI). Ideal BMI is between 19 and 23 kg/m^2 for Asian women and 20–25 kg/m^2 for others.
- Take family history of osteoporosis, fragility fractures or risk factors for osteoporosis.
- History of diabetes, hypertension
- History of previous fracture
- History of any drug intake
- Family or past history of chronic heart disease.
- Any history of breast cancer in the family
- Do her Pap smear if not done so far.
- Do transvaginal sonography (TVS) if not already done or if she reports abnormal bleeding.
- ECG
- Advise mammography and breast self-examination (BSE) once in a month
- Clinical breast examination (CBE) once in a year
- Mammography annually after the age of 40 years and every 2 years after the age of 65 years.

Case 3

A 60-year-old postmenopausal lady presents with backache. She has family history of fractures.

Q1. How will you manage such a patient?

This woman needs to be screened for osteoporosis by doing bone densitometry as she is symptomatic and there is family history of fractures. The bone mineral density is graded by T score obtained on Dual-energy X-ray absorptiometry (DEXA). If the T score is ≤2.5 and fragility fractures are present, it is defined as Osteoporosis. BMD assessment is done for subjects having high risk factors for osteoporosis. This would include women with personal or family history of fractures, chronic smokers, primary ovarian insufficiency, alcohol abuse and rheumatoid arthritis. Treatment can be given to all patients with a fragility fracture or a T score of <−2.5 (osteoporosis), or a T score of <−1 and >−2.5 (osteopenia) with additional risk factors for fractures. HRT is of proven efficacy for fracture reduction in patients with osteopenia. The age at which HRT is initiated is important. In the age group 50–60 years or within 10 years after menopause, the benefits of HRT are likely to outweigh any risks.[7] Initiation of HRT in the age group 60–70 years requires balancing benefits versus risks. One can consider use of other available drugs. If HRT is required it should be given at the lowest effective dose. It should not be initiated after 70 years of age.

Standard doses of conjugated equine estrogen (CEE) and medroxyprogesterone acetate are given orally for hormone replacement. Other forms like transdermal preparations can be used, e.g. ultra-low-dose estradiol 0.14 mg patch which is given weekly. Bazedoxifene is a selective estrogen receptor modulator. When combined with CEE it effectively prevents loss of BMD and is approved for prevention of osteoporosis.[8] The additional advantage of bazedoxifene is that it does not stimulate the endometrium. Tibolone, a synthetic preparation has been found to be effective in preventing vertebral and non-vertebral fractures in in postmenopausal women with osteoporosis. It is metabolized to molecules that have affinity for the estrogen, progesterone and androgen receptors. Since Tibolone is effective in treatment of vasomotor symptoms, it should be used as an HRT substitute only in those postmenopausal women who have osteoporosis along with postmenopausal symptoms.[9]

Case 4

A 50-year-old postmenopausal lady wants to consult regarding use of HRT for preventing cardiovascular disease .

Q1. What is the role of HRT in preventing cardiovascular diseases?

HRT improves vascular function and has positive effect on glucose metabolism and lipid levels. It decreases the incidence of new - onset diabetes mellitus.[10] But all these effects depend on time of initiation of HRT. The period around the time of menopause when HRT would be most beneficial is described as 'window of opportunity' or 'timing hypothesis'. HRT may cause harm when started >10 years after menopause. Cochrane analysis, other meta-analyses, and the WHI 13-year results all show that there is a consistent reduction in coronary heart disease and all-cause mortality among women starting HRT at <60 years of age or within 10 years of menopause.[11]

Case 5

A 55-year-old lady complains of vasomotor symptoms and she has history of venous thromboembolism (VTE).

Q1. What is the importance of history of VTE?

VTE is the most important adverse effect of HRT. Oral estrogen therapy is therefore, contraindicated in women with personal history of VTE. History of thromboembolism in family, genetic thrombophilia and obesity are some of the other contraindications to HRT. The risk of thromboembolism also increases with age (>60 years). Transdermal estrogens have not been found to increase the risk of VTE and should be the first choice for obese women requiring hormone replacement.[12] The risk of VTE increases with duration of HRT. The risk of a thromboembolic event may also be affected by the type and duration of progestogen used. Medroxyprogesterone acetate may be associated with greater risk when used in oral therapy.[13] Routine screening for thrombophilia is not indicated prior to HRT use, however, selective screening may be indicated on the basis of personal and familial history.

Case 6

A 50-year-old postmenopausal lady presents with forgetfulness, inability to concentrate and depression.

Q1. What is the role of HRT in such cases?

During menopausal transition, some women may experience transient cognitive impairment but these are transitory in nature. Studies which compared conjugated equine estrogen and cyclical oral progesterone versus placebo did not show benefit or harm after treatment for a period of 2.85 years.[14] Therefore HRT should not be used to enhance cognitive function. Healthy women who are considering HRT for other indications need not worry about adverse effect of HRT on cognitive function. Estrogen therapy may provide short-term cognitive benefit to women with surgical menopause when initiated at the time of oophorectomy. Studies have found reduced Alzheimer risk for women receving HRT in younger age, but not for older postmenopausal women.[15] There is reduced Alzheimer risk if HRT is initiated within 5 years of menopause but no effect if initiated more than 5 years after menopause. If depressive symptoms occur during menopausal transition, short term estrogen therapy may increase the likelihood of remission.

Case 7

A 55-year-old postmenopausal lady on HRT presents with complaint of spotting per vaginum.

Q1. How will you manage this case?

This lady needs evaluation to rule out endometrial hyperplasia or carcinoma. Endometrial biopsy, hysteroscopy or saline infusion sonohysterography are the commonly done investigations in such cases.

There is strong association of unopposed estrogen therapy with endometrial hyperplasia and neoplasia. The risk of endometrial hyperplasia depends on the dose and duration of estrogen therapy. The risk can be reduced by adding progestogen either in continuous combined or cyclical method.[16] The use of SERMs, Ospemifene and Lasofoxifene for treatment of vulvovaginal atrophy or genito-urinary syndrome of menopause is safe for endometrium.

Case 8

A 56-year-old postmenopausal lady presents with symptoms of vulvovaginal atrophy.

Q1. How will you manage her?

The two most common symptoms of vulvovaginal atrophy are vaginal dryness and dyspareunia. These may affect sexual response and may be associated with pelvic floor dysfunction. While managing such patients, enquire about time since menopause, mood changes, vasomotor symptoms, any chronic illness and also about intrapersonal and interpersonal factors that may cause sexual dysfunction.

The treatment aims to restore urogenital physiology and alleviate symptoms. When vulvovaginal atrophy is the main symptom, local estrogen should be prescribed. Vaginal lubricants and moisturizer can also be prescribed to relieve the symptoms of vaginal dryness. Ospemifene, a SERM derived from toremifene, has also been shown to be effective in treating vulval and vaginal atrophy.[17]

Key Points

- HRT should not be recommended without a clear indication for its use, i.e. significant symptoms or physical effects of estrogen deficiency and it should be prescribed and titrated in lowest effective dose.
- The Women Health Initiative (WHI) and other studies support the safe use of HRT for 5 years if started before the age of 60 years. There are potential benefits of HRT in many conditions and risks are few which can be minimised by selecting optimal regimen.
- Women taking HRT should have at least yearly review.

REFERENCES

1. Kumar P, Malhotra N. Menopause. In Jeffcoate's Principles of Gynecology, 7th ed. New Dellhi,

India, Jaypee Brothers Medical Publishers 2008; 862–63.

2. Maninder Ahuja. Age of menopause and determinants of menopause age: A PAN India survey by IMS. J Midlife Health 2016;7:126–131.

3. MacLennan AH, Lester S, Moore V. Oral oestrogen and combined oestrogen/progestogen therapy versus placebo for hot flushes. Cochrane Database Syst Rev 2004;4:CD002978.

4. Loprinzi CL, Kugler JW, Sloan JA, et al. Venlafaxine in management of hot flashes in survivors of breast cancer: a randomised controlled trial. Lancet 2000;356:2059–63.

5. Stearns V, Beebe KL, Iyengar M, Dube E. Paroxetine controlled release in the treatment of menopausal hot flashes: a randomized controlled trial. JAMA 2003;289:2827–34.

6. Reddy SY, Warner H, Guttuso T Jr, Messing S, DiGrazio W, Thornburg L, et al. Gabapentin, estrogen, and placebo for treating hot flushes: a randomized controlled trial. Obstet Gynecol 2006; 108:41–8.

7. de Villiers TJ, Stevenson JC. The WHI: the effect of hormone replacement therapy on fracture Prevention. Climacteric 2012;15:263–6.

8. Lindsay R, Gallagher JC, Kagan R, Pickar JH, Constantine G. Efficacy of tissue-selective estrogen complex of bazedoxifene/conjugated estrogens for osteoporosis prevention in at-risk postmenopausal women. Fertil Steril 2009;92: 1045–52.

9. Hishikar R, Agrawal M, Agrawal AC. Hormone replacement therapy in prevention and treatment of postmenopausal osteoporosis. J Orthop Traumatol Rehabil 2014;7:119–22.

10. Boardman HM, Hartley L, Eisinga A, et al. Hormone therapy for preventing cardiovascular disease in post-menopausal women. Cochrane Database Syst Rev 2015;(3):CD002229.

11. Hodis HN, Collins P, Mack WJ, Schierbeck LL. The timing hypothesis for coronary heart disease prevention with hormone therapy: past, present and future in perspective. Climacteric 2012;15: 217–28.

12. Archer DF, Oger E. Estrogen and progestogen effect on venous thromboembolism in menopausal women. Climacteric 2012;15:235–40.

13. Manson JE, Chlebowski RT, Stefanick ML, Aragaki AK, Rossouw JE, Prentice RL, et al. Menopausal hormone therapy and health outcomes during the intervention and extended Post stopping phases of the Women's Health Initiative randomized trials. JAMA 2013;310: 1353–6.

14. Gleason CE, Dowling NM, Wharton W, Manson JE, Miller VM, Atwood CS, et al. Effects of hormone therapy on cognition and mood in recently postmenopausal women: findings from the randomized, controlled KEEPS-Cognitive and Affective Study. PLoS Med 2015;12:e1001833.

15. Henderson VW. Alzheimer's disease: review of hormone therapy trials and implications for treatment and Prevention after menopause. J Steroid Biochem Mol Biol 2014;142:99–106.

16. Goldstein SR, Neven P, Cummings S, et al. Postmenopausal evaluation and risk reduction with lasofoxifene (PEARL) trial: 5-year gynaecologic outcomes. Menopause 2011;18:17–22.

17. Nappi RE, Panay N, Bruyniks N, Castelo-Branco C, de Villiers TJ, Simon JA. The clinical relevance of the effect of ospemifene on symptoms of vulvar and vaginal atrophy. Climacteric 2015;18: 233–40.

Selective Progesterone Receptor Modulators

Tanuja Muthyala, Anjali Tempe

Selective progesterone receptor modulators (SPRMs) are synthetic steroids with progesterone agonist and antagonistic actions. Progesterone receptors (PR) are predominantly present in endometrial, myometrial and breast tissue and SPRMs are designed to target and treat their pathology.

Q1. What is the mechanism of action of SPRMs?

Progesterone binds to PR in cell cytoplasm. This complex then activates various genomic and non genomic signaling pathways. PR agonists bind to coactivators and stimulate transcription and PR antagonists inhibit transcription by corepressors. There are two isoforms, progesterone receptor A (PR A) and progesterone receptor B (PR B). Activation of PR A counteracts estrogen induced endometrial proliferation while PR B activation effects cellular proliferation and differentiation in the breast. SPRMs act on both PR isoforms, activate both coactivators and corepressors and produce combined agonist and antagonist effect. The functional effect depends upon the structural configuration of the specific SPRM, the proportion of PR isoforms and target tissue levels of coactivators and corepressors.

Q2. What are the different SPRM available?

Various SPRMs are shown in Table 12.1.

Among the above drugs, only Mifepristone and ulipristal acetate are approved for clinical use.

Table 12.1: SPRMs with agonistic and/or antagonistic activity	
Agonist-antagonist activity	*Pure antagonists*
Ulipristal acetate (UPA)	Mifepristone
Asoprisnil	Onapristone
Telapristone acetate	

Q3. What are the uses of SPRMs?

SPRM can be used for

a. Symptomatic treatment and preoperative preparation for fibroids: For treatment of fibroids, a drug with site-specific action is required, i.e. progestogenic action on the endometrium and anti-progestin effect on the myoma. SPRMs target the myoma cells as they have a higher proportion of PR A and PR B receptors than adjoining myometrium. Size of myoma is reduced by induction of apoptosis and anti-proliferative effect. Menstrual flow is reduced with atrophy of spiral arteries, endometrial ischemia and amenorrhea due to inhibition of ovulation.

When used preoperatively, SPRMs shrink the size of the fibroids and provide symptomatic relief, thus

- Allowing a more cosmetic pfannenstiel incision rather than a vertical one when planned for a laparotomy
- Enabling laparoscopic removal of fibroid instead of laparotomy
- Providing time to build up hemoglobin and reducing intraoperative blood loss, operating time, length of hospital stay.

- Bridge the perimenopausal period and if the patient becomes asymptomatic, the surgery can be postponed or deferred.

Cochrane Database of Systematic Review (2017) suggested that short-term SPRM use reduced morbidity by controlling menorrhagia, improved quality of life, and achieved higher rates of amenorrhea when compared to placebo. Thus, SPRMs can be an effective option for managing symptomatic fibroids.[1]

b. Endometriosis: Within the endometriotic tissue, there is increased aromatase activity and low 17β-hydroxysteroid dehydrogenase activity that increase local estradiol concentrations. SPRM inhibits estrogen receptor gene transcription, suppress ovulation, reduce endometrial bleeding and therefore can be used to treat endometriosis. Evidence from various trials show that mifepristone relieves dysmenorrhea and dyspareunia when given to patients with endometriosis.[2]

c. Adenomyosis: SPRMs reduce endometrial proliferation and suppress menstruation, which can alleviate the symptoms of adenomyosis including pain. The role of UPA in adenomyosis is currently under phase II trial.

d. Contraception: SPRMs can be used for **emergency contraception** and as a **long-term contraceptive**. They block the LH surge, inhibit ovulation, suppress endometrial development and make it out of phase for implantation. At higher doses, they cause follicular atresia by blocking follicular maturation. When taken in late luteal phase, SPRM induce endometrial bleeding and thus prevent implantation.

Mifepristone is licensed only in China as an emergency contraceptive and is effective up to 120 hours after unprotected intercourse. A WHO guided multicenter randomized controlled trial involving 4000 women compared low dose mifepristone with levonorgestrel (LNG) for emergency contraception. The results showed that 10 mg mifepristone was as effective as LNG for up to 5 days after unprotected intercourse.[3]

UPA in a dose of 30 mg can be prescribed for those who need emergency contraception provided it is taken within 120 hours of unprotected intercourse. LNG is an economically cheaper alternative but has a slightly higher risk of contraceptive failure when compared with UPA. An analysis of the three randomized trials comparing emergency contraceptive regimens suggested that UPA prevents ovulation more effectively than LNG and there is no increased risk of miscarriage, ectopic pregnancy or fetal malformations in case of contraceptive failure with UPA.[4]

SPRM can also be used as a long-term contraceptive. Low dose mifepristone (2–10 mg/day) blocks LH surge, delays follicular development and thus ovulation. When given in proliferative phase, it prevents endometrial maturation without disrupting the ovulation. When administered in the early luteal phase, i.e. 48 hours after LH surge in a high dose (200 mg), it prevents implantation without effecting ovulation or bleeding patterns. Mifepristone has also been shown to hinder tubal function, maturation of gametes and fertilization.

e. Medical termination of pregnancy and menstrual regulation: Medical abortion regimens use 200 mg oral mifepristone and misoprostol. The dose of misoprostol varies according to the gestation.

f. Mifepristone and other SPRM can be used to treat breakthrough bleeding caused by progesterone-only pills.

g. Abnormal uterine bleeding—use for this indication is under trials.

h. Treatment of hormone sensitive tumors of breast, ovary, prostate and endometrium.

i. Treatment of inoperable cases of meningioma and gliomas.

j. Cushing's syndrome

k. Alzheimer's disease and major depression with features of psychosis.

Q4. What is the role of Ulipristal Acetate in fibroids?

Uliprisal acetate (UPA) is a second generation progesterone receptor modulator with little anti-glucocortioid activity, specifically developed for emergency contraception.

Single daily dose of 5 mg UPA for three months can be prescribed before myomectomy to reduce bleeding, size of fibroids and facilitate surgery. Women with symptom relief may even postpone or defer myomectomy. This shrinkage effect on fibroids is maintained even after stopping UPA. Fertility rates may also improve. UPA inhibits ovulation without lowering estradiol levels in contrast to GnRH agonists which explains lower side-effects of UPA. UPA should be used cautiously in women with severe or uncontrolled asthma, hepatic dysfunction, and hereditary disorders of glucose and galactose intolerance. PEARL (Ulipristal Acetate/PGL4001 Efficacy Assessment in Reduction of Symptoms due to Uterine Leiomyomata) trials shown in Table 12.2, are the key studies that paved the way for use of UPA to manage symptomatic fibroids.

In our country, UPA is approved by the Ministry of Health, Social Services and Equality for preoperative use and/or for treatment of symptomatic fibroids in reproductive age women.

Q5. What are the clinical uses of other SPRMs?

Onapristone has progesterone antagonistic actions in post-menopausal women. There is no endometrial hyperplasia with its use in postmenopausal women. It is hepatotoxic and therefore was withdrawn from the trials.

Vilaprisan and telapristone acetate are currently under trials for use in fibroids.

Q6. What are the adverse effects of SPRM?

Moderate to severe hot flushes, headache, nausea, abdominal pain, acne, anemia, fatigue, insomnia can occur with SPRM use but their occurrence is less frequent as compared to treatment with Leuprolide acetate. Hypercholesterolemia and breast pain/tenderness

Table 12.2: Results from PEARL trials		
Inclusion criteria	Design	Results
PEARL-I		
Premenopausal women between 18 and 50 years with symptomatic fibroid uterus (one or more fibroids between 3 and 10 cm), menorrhagia with pictorial blood loss assessment chart score (PBAC) more than 100 during first 8 days of menses, anemic and fit for surgery if anemia is corrected.	237 women were randomized into 3 arms who received daily dose of 5 mg UPA, 10 mg UPA and placebo in each of the arms along with concomitant iron therapy for 13 weeks.	Bleeding was controlled in >90% women on UPA. Menorrhagia was settled within 7 days from treatment initiation, in 75.9% of 5 mg UPA and 82.7% of patients in the 10 mg UPA group.[5]
PEARL-II		
Similar to PEARL-I except that anemia is not must or required.	301 women were randomized into 3 arms who received daily dose of 5 mg UPA, 10 mg UPA and intramuscular Leuprorelin monthly inj. in each of the study arms along with concomitant iron therapy for 3 months.	UPA controlled menorrhagia rapidly (within 7 days) than Leuprorelin (30 days) Patients on UPA were in amenorrhea after first menstruation, while many patients on leuprorelin had further episodes of bleeding during the next 3 weeks due to flare-up effect. UPA was better tolerated.[6]

Contd...

Table 12.2: Results from PEARL trials (Contd...)		
Inclusion criteria	Design	Results
PEARL-III; Core PEARL-III with first and second extensions.		
Similar to PEARL-I	209 women with symptomatic fibroids were given UPA in a dose of 10 mg/day for 3 months followed by a 10 day course of norethisterone acetate (NETA) in one arm and placebo in other arm. In its first extension, it was given for further 3 courses. In second extension total of 8 courses were given but without continuation of NETA/placebo.	Amenorrhea after the first UPA course was seen in 80% of the women. After 4 courses: 82.3% of patients had fibroid volume reduction of $\geq$25%. 92.7% of patients achieved amenorrhea, 78.1% of patients had no bleeding/spotting and reduced fibroid volume $\geq$25%. 3.1% still had some bleeding and did not have reduced fibroid volume $\geq$25%. Multiple courses of UPA also had similar incidence of PAEC. The incidence of endometrial thickening decreased with repeated courses of UPA. PAEC is benign and reversible after stopping the drug. The routine use of NETA with UPA is not justified as it has no effect on reduction of myoma or PAEC frequency.[7,8]
PEARL-IV		
Similar to PEARL-I	451 women with menorrhagia due to fibroid uterus were treated with 4 recurrent 12 weekly courses, with a daily dose of UPA 5 mg or 10 mg.	Similar bleeding control, reduction in myoma volume and reassuring safety results with either 5 mg or 10 mg dose.[9]

occur more frequently with SPRM than with leuprolide.

Progesterone receptor modulator-associated endometrial changes (PAEC): It is a histological term coined to describe morphological alterations following treatment with SPRM like endometrial thickening, cystic glands, and adenomatous and vascular changes. It is a benign and reversible change which subsides after withdrawing UPA therapy. In most of the patients it resolves within 3 months of drug free period. Around 11% of the patients on UPA therapy had thickened endometrium to more than 16 mm. Occurrence of PAEC did not affect the benefits of UPA use for symptomatic fibroids. If other causes of abnormal uterine bleeding are ruled out, there is neither indication for a baseline biopsy prior to UPA initiation nor for a biopsy after stopping UPA treatment.[10]

SPRMs are the emerging group of drugs for medical management of symptomatic uterine fibroids and various other gynecological conditions.

Key Points

- SPRM have tissue specific agonist/antagonist actions.
- Mifepristone-mainly antagonist. Mainly used for medical abortion.
- SPRMs provide effective treatment for symptomatic fibroids. Ulipristal is approved for short-term use in several countries and is used for preoperative treatment of symptomatic fibroids.
- Ulipristal Acetate can also be used for emergency contraception.
- SPRM use causes unique endometrial changes-PAEC- which is a distinct histological entity not to be confused with hyperplasia. It is benign and reversible.

REFERENCES

1. Fu J, Song H, Zhou M, Zhu H, Wang Y, Chen H, Huang W. Progesterone receptor modulators for endometriosis. Cochrane Database Syst Rev 2017; 7:CD009881.

2. Chabbert-Buffet N, Pintiaux A, Bouchard P. The imminent dawn of SPRMs in obstetrics and gynecology. Mol Cell Endocrinol 2012;358:232–43.

3. Von Herten H, Piaggio G, Ding J, Chen J, Song S, Bártfai G, et al. WHO Research Group on Post-ovulatory Methods of Fertility Regulation. Low dose mifepristone and two regimens of levonorgestrel for emergency contraception: a WHO multicentre trial. Lancet 2002;360:1803–10.

4. Brache V, Cochon L, Deniaud M, Croxatto HB. Ulipristal acetate prevents ovulation more effectively than levonorgestrel: analysis of pooled data from three randomized trials of emergency contraception regimens. Contraception 2013; 88:611–8.

5. Donnez J, Tatarchuk TF, Bouchard P, Puscasiu L, Zakharenko NF, Ivanova T, et al. Ulipristal acetate versus placebo for fibroid treatment before surgery. N Engl J Med 2012;366:409–20.

6. Donnez J, Tomaszewski J, Vazquez F, Bouchard P, Lemieszczuk B ,Baró F, et al. Ulipristal acetate versus leuprolide acetate for uterine fibroids. N Engl J Med 2012;366:421–32.

7. Donnez J, Vazquez F, Tomaszewski J, Nouri K, Bouchard P, Fauser BC, et al. Long-term treatment of uterine fibroids with ulipristal acetate. Fertil Steril 2014;101:1565–73.

8. Fauser BCJM, Donnez J, Bouchard P, Barlow DH, Vazquez F, Arriagada P, et al. Safety after extended repeated use of ulipristal acetate for uterine fibroids. PLoS One 2017;12:e0173523.

9. Donnez J, Donnez O, Matule D, Ahrendt HJ, Hudecek R, Zatik J, et al. Long-term medical management of uterine fibroids with ulipristal acetate. Fertil Steril 2016;105:165–173.

10. Mutter GL, Bergeron C, Deligdisch L, Ferenczy A, Glant M, Merino M, et al. The spectrum of endometrial pathology induced by progesterone receptor modulators. Mod Pathol 2008;21:591–98.

Section

III

Infertility and Assisted Reproductive Technology

Female Infertility: Approach to Diagnosis and Management

Anjali Tempe, Priyanka Khandey

Infertility is a common problem that affects around 10–15% of couples in reproductive age group. The problem of infertility is on increasing trend due to urbanization, stressful life, career orientation, pollution, competitiveness and late settlement in life, etc. Management of an infertile couple is challenging and requires extensive clinical knowledge and appropriate approach to treat the cause. Assisted reproductive techniques (ART) like in vitro fertilization (IVF)/intra-cytoplasmic sperm injection (ICSI) to pre-implantation genetic screening (PGS)/pre-implantation genetic diagnosis (PGD) have revolutionized infertility management.

In this chapter, we will discuss about the evaluation of an infertile woman with the help of different case scenarios.

Q1. Define infertility.

Infertility is defined as failure to achieve a successful pregnancy after 12 months or more of appropriate, timed unprotected vaginal intercourse or therapeutic donor insemination.[1] Infertility can be further classified as primary or secondary. Primary infertility is when there is no previous pregnancy ever, whereas in secondary infertility, prior pregnancies have occurred irrespective of their outcomes, abortion or live birth.

Q2. When should you evaluate a couple seeking advice for infertility?

A woman of reproductive age, who has not conceived after 1 year of unprotected vaginal sexual intercourse, in the absence of any known cause of infertility, should be offered further clinical assessment and investigations along with her partner.[2]

Early assessment and appropriate treatment is needed if:
- The woman is aged 36 years or over.
- There is a known clinical cause of infertility.
- History of predisposing factors for infertility.

Q3. What are the common causes of infertility?

The main causes of infertility include male factor, ovulatory disorders (anovulation), decreased ovarian reserve, tubal injury or blockage, or endometriosis with evidence of tubal or peritoneal adhesions, uterine factors, systemic conditions (including infections or chronic diseases such as autoimmune conditions or chronic renal failure), cervical and immunologic factors, and unexplained factors (including endometriosis with no evidence of tubal or peritoneal adhesions).[3]

Q4. A young couple, married for 4 years came to the gyne outpatient clinic with inability to conceive. What are the important points in history and examination for the workup of infertile couples.

Couples having inability to conceive should be seen together because both partners are affected by decisions regarding investigations and treatments. Evaluation begins with a detailed history and physical examination of both the partners. Adequate psychosocial counseling should be the integral part of the management.[2]

Relevant history includes:[4]

a. *Age of both partners:* Advancing age of female partner is related to decline in fertility and increase in risk of miscarriage. There is an increased prevalence of aneuploidy in aging oocytes due to disordered meiotic spindle formation and function which leads to miscarriage. Increasing male age is also associated with decrease in fertility and pregnancy rate.

b. *Duration of infertility:* Duration of marriage and years of cohabitation should be noted.

c. *Menstrual history:* Age of menarche, cycle length and regularity, associated symptoms like dysmenorrhea, moliminal signs to detect ovulation.

d. *Obstetric history:* Any previous pregnancy, parity, abortions and associated complications.

e. *Contraceptives methods* used in past.

f. *Sexual history:* Frequency of coitus and any sexual dysfunction like dyspareunia, erectile dysfunction, retrograde ejaculation, loss of libido, etc.

g. *Medical history:*
   - History of previous infertility treatment and results.
   - Any chronic illness or history of Tuberculosis, pelvic inflammatory diseases (PID), sexually transmitted diseases (STD) or history of hospitalization, diabetes mellitus in both partners.
   - History suggestive of thyroid disorder, galactorrhea or hirsutism.
   - Any current medication
   - Allergies

h. *Past surgical history:* History of myomectomy, uterine septal resection, surgeries for endometriosis or any abdomino-pelvic surgeries.

i. Family history of early menopause, birth defects, cancers, thrombosis or any hereditary disorders.

j. Exposure to known environmental or occupational hazards.

k. Use of tobacco, alcohol, smoking, cocaine or any recreational or illicit drugs.

Physical examination should document the followings:

a. *General examination:*
   - Weight, height, body mass index (BMI), body habitus, blood pressure and pulse rate.
   - Thyroid enlargement and presence of any nodule in neck.
   - Breast examination for any secretion.
   - Signs of excessive androgens-feature of hirsutism, acne, deepening of voice.

b. *Abdominal examination* for tenderness, any palpable mass, organomegaly or scar marks of previous surgery.

c. *Pelvic examination*
   - Any abnormal vaginal or cervical secretions or discharge
   - Pap smear
   - Uterine size, shape, position, mobility
   - Adnexal masses or tenderness
   - Any nodularity or mass in cul-de-sac or tenderness.

Q5. A 30-year-old woman married for 4 years with inability to conceive came to the clinic along with her 32-year-old husband. She has regular menstrual cycles and no significant past or medical history. What are the routine tests prescribed for evaluation of infertility? Mention the specific tests that may be needed.

a. Routine preconception investigations like hemoglobin, blood group and Rh typing, Rh antibodies screening in Rh negative patients, blood sugar, urine routine microscopy and culture need to be evaluated.

b. Semen analysis provides basic information regarding semen quantity, sperm concentration, motility, morphology and viability. World health organization (WHO) in 2010 revised normal lower limit of semen parameters for fertility[5]

- Ejaculate volume : 1.5 mL
- pH : 7.2
- Sperm concentration : 15 million/mL
- Total sperm count : 39 millons per ejaculate
- Percentage motility : 40%
- Progressive motility : >32%
- Sperm morphology : 4% normal
- Sperm vitality : 58%

c. Testing for viral status like HIV, HBsAg for Hepatitis B and AntiHCV for Hepatitis C should be offered to the couple undergoing infertility treatment and planning for IVF. Screening for sexually transmitted disease like syphilis with VDRL or RPR should be done.

d. *Hormonal profile:*
- TSH for detection of thyroid disorder.
- Prolactin for hyperprolactinemia.
- FSH in case of amenorrhea/oligomenorrhea or premature ovarian failure.
- Free or total testosterone if features of hyperandrogenism present.
- AMH level for testing ovarian reserve.

e. *Screening for cervical cancer:* Pap smear is recommended for all sexually active women of reproductive age group.

f. *Screening for Chlamydia antibodies:* Detection of antibodies against Chlamydia has been associated with tubal pathology, so screening should be offered. If tested positive, couple should be treated with appropriate antibiotics.

g. Screening for immunity to rubella and varicella and immunization if no antibodies are found against the infection. Woman is advised to avoid conception for at least 3 months after of receiving vaccination.

h. Specific tests for evaluation of infertility (discussed later in this chapter along with clinical cases)
- *Tubal patency test:* HSG, HyCoSy, Laparoscopic chromotubation, fertiloscopy etc.

- *Test for documentation of ovulation:* USG monitoring of folliculogenesis, level of progesterone in luteal phase of cycle, LH kit testing.
- *Test for ovarian reserve:* AMH, Antral follicles count (AFC), FSH.
- Test to rule out uterine or cervical abnormalities.
- Hysteroscopy for evaluation of uterine abnormalities.

i. *Advanced investigations:*
- *Woman with suspected premature ovarian insufficiency:* Karyotyping, basal FSH and estradiol, AMH, antibodies for other autoimmune diseases like antiTPO antibodies, ANA, genetic testing for fragile X chromosome (FMR1 premutation).
- *Male with abnormal semen analysis:* Karyotyping, genetic testing for cystic fibrosis, Y chromosome microdeletion, hormonal assays-FSH, LH, Testosterone, TSH and prolactin, USG Doppler of scrotum, fine needle aspiration cytology (FNAC), etc.

j. Tests to detect tuberculosis infection in cases where clinical history is suspicious of TB or there is history of contact with TB. Chest X-ray (CXR), Montoux test, endometrial biopsy (EB) for acid fast bacillus (AFB) staining or BECTEC culture or TB PCR are routinely used in India.

Case 1

Mrs X, 29-year-old lady married for 9 years presented with secondary infertility. Her menstrual cycles were regular. Her husband's semen analysis was also normal. She was taking treatment for infertility for last 5 years and had received 3 cycles of ovulation induction with documented ovulation. She had taken ATT for 6 months, 3 years back for genital TB. Her tubal status was not known.

Q1. What are the risk factors for tubal involvement?

Risks factors associated with involvement of tubes are:

- Pelvic inflammatory disease (PID) is most common factor. Risk of tubal infertility increases with the number and severity of episodes of PID; the incidence is approximately 10–12% after one episode, 23–35% after two, and 54–75% after three episodes of acute PID.
- Tuberculosis: Genital tuberculosis is usually secondary to pulmonary TB or from other extrapulmonary sites like abdomen or kidney. Genital TB usually involves fallopian tubes (95–100%), uterine endometrium (50–60%), ovaries (20–30%), cervix (5–15%), uterine myometrium (2.5%) and vagina/vulva (1%).
- Endometriosis (7–14%)
- Previous surgery like appendectomy or any pelvic surgery
- Ectopic pregnancy in past whether managed surgically or medically.
- Sterilization
- Inflammation due to:
  - Prior abortions
  - Medical or surgical termination of pregnancy

Q2. What are the different tests available for the assessment of tubal patency?

Tests for tubal patency:

a. **Hysterosalphingography (HSG):** HSG is traditional and standard method of assessment of tubal patency done by using either water or lipid soluble contrast media. The positive predictive value (PPV) and negative predictive value (NPV) are 38% and 94% respectively.[4] HSG is usually done in early follicular phase (D5-D11) after giving non-steroidal anti-inflammatory drugs (NSAID) or antispasmodics, 30–60 minutes prior to the procedure. It should be done by using intensification fluoroscopy and taking 3–4 films. It is a permanent visual record of tubes and uterus. Site of tubal occlusion may be proximal, mid or distal. It can also demonstrate salpingitis isthmica nodosa, tubal architectural details, features of fimbrial phimosis or peritubular adhesions when escape of contrast is delayed or becomes loculated, respectively. Findings suggesting proximal tubal obstruction require further evaluation to exclude transient occlusion resulting from tubal spasm or myometrial contractions.

b. **Saline infusion sonosalpingography (SIS/SIONS test):** Saline is instilled via cervix inside uterine cavity and visualization of fluid in cul-de-sac by USG is suggestive of patent tubes. The test does not differentiate between unilateral versus bilateral patency.

c. **Hysterosalpingo-contrast-sonography (HyCoSy):** It is a transvaginal ultrasound guided technique, in which a contrast solution of galactose and 1% palmitic acid (Echovist-Schering-AG, Germany) or a mixture of air and saline is infused inside the uterine cavity and observed. The bright echoes generated by the Hysterosalpingo-contrast-sonography (HyCoSy) solution make tubal visualization possible. Results can be further improved by the use of color Doppler imaging or 3D technology. It is a safe outpatient procedure with relatively low cost, having sensitivity of 93.3% and specificity of 89.7%.[6]

d. **Laparoscopy and chromopertubation:** This is an invasive but more accurate method for the assessment of tubal patency. Diluted solution of methylene blue dye is injected via cervix and spillage is seen laparoscopically. This method differentiates between unilateral and bilateral blockage, identifies proximal or distal blockage, hydrosalphinx, peritubal adhesions, perifimbrial adhesions, tubo-ovarian relationship, other associated uterine anomalies, adhesions, endometriosis etc.

e. **Falloposcopy:** Falloposcopy is done transcervically by inserting a micro endoscope into the tubal lumen from the uterotubal ostium to the fimbriae. Initially, a flexible cannula is passed inside tubal lumen under hysteroscopic vision, into which the falloposcope is introduced with the help of continuous fluid irrigation through the flexible cannula (coaxial delivery system).[7]

f. **Salpingoscopy:** It can be performed during laparotomy or laparoscopy to assess the mucosa of distal tube, i.e. fimbriae, infundibulum and ampulla. It is an expensive procedure as special instrument and expertise are required.[8]

g. **Fertiloscopy:** It is a newer surgical technique used for the early diagnosis of infertility. It combines transvaginal hydropelviscopy, dye-test, optional salpingoscopy, and hysteroscopy, performed on outpatient basis under local anaesthesia. An optic device is introduced in the pouch of Douglas that allows visualization of the posterior pelvis (posterior surface of the uterus, tubes, ovaries and intestines). Small procedures like adhesiolysis, ovarian drilling, coagulation of endometriosis spots, chromosalpingoscopy and salpingoscopy can be done in the same setting.[9]

In this case, HSG was done which showed normal uterine cavity and no spillage of dye on either side with hydrosalpinx on both sides (Fig. 13.1).

Q3. What is hydrosalpinx? How does it affect pregnancy and conception?

Hydrosalpinx is a heterogeneous spectrum of distal tubal pathology characterized by

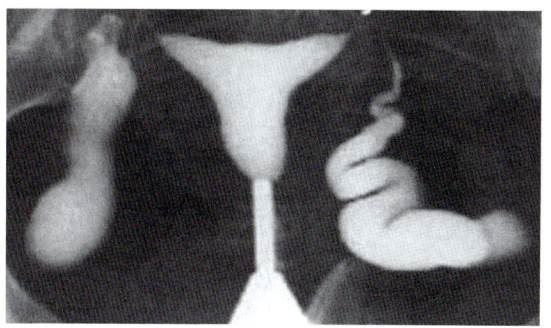

Fig. 13.1

collection of watery fluid in the uterine tube. The diagnosis of hydrosalpinx can be done by transvaginal ultrasound or HSG. Laparoscopy is an invasive but definitive method for diagnosis of hydrosalpinx and associated pathology of pelvic adhesions. No cut-off values for the size of hydrosalpinx are yet established to decide whether intervention is needed prior to IVF. Two important factors which need intervention are detection of hydrosalpinx on ultrasound examination and bilateral involvement.

Hydrosalpinx fluids is embryotoxic in nature, causes oxidative stress and impairs endometrial receptivity. Patients with hydrosalpinges have significantly lower implantation and pregnancy rates than patients suffering from other types of tubal damage.[10]

Q4. How will you manage a case of tubal infertility with hydrosalpinx?

- IVF is the treatment of choice in patients with severe tubal disease disease with hydrosalpinx and mucosal destruction.
- Laparoscopic salpingectomy followed by IVF will improve the implantation and pregnancy rates and almost double the patient's chances of success with IVF.
- In patients with extensive adhesions, where salpingectomy is difficult, proximal tubal occlusion should be done laparoscopically or hysteroscopically. If no surgical intervention is performed prior to IVF, transvaginal aspiration of the fluid can be performed in conjunction with oocyte retrieval under antibiotic cover.
- In a hydrosalpinx with preserved mucosa, salphingostomy can be done. In the presence of a unilateral hydrosalpinx and a contralateral healthy tube, a unilateral salpingectomy can be done, followed by sufficient time to await spontaneous conception, before proceeding to IVF.[10]

Another similar couple came with the HSG showing normal uterine cavity, free spillage of dye on left side and cornual block of right tube (Fig. 13.2).

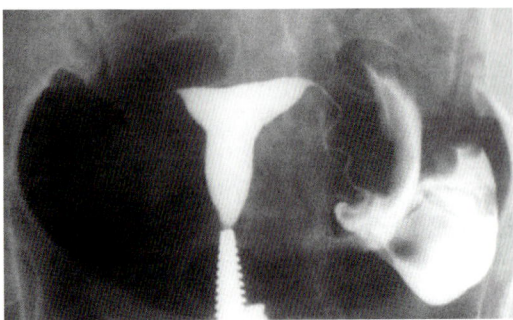

Fig. 13.2

Q5. What are the options available for the proximal tubal blockage?

- Proximal tubal occlusions constitute approximately one-third of all tubal obstructions. Histologic studies suggest that obliterative luminal fibrosis is most common, followed by salpingitis isthmica nodosa, chronic inflammation, and intratubal endometriosis.

- Proximal tubal cannulation using hystero-scopic or fluoroscopic methods can be done to relieve the obstruction. Catheterization involves passage of a soft catheter into the tubal ostia, while cannulation passes a guidewire through the ostia and injects contrast media or colored dye. Microsurgical segmental tubal resection and anastomosis is another treatment for true proximal tubal obstruction.

- In carefully selected cases, tubal cannulation alone or in conjunction with microsurgery has comparable success rates with IVF with the advantage of avoiding the risks of ovarian hyperstimulation syndrome and multiple pregnancies. Success rates with tubal surgery are also thought to depend upon the severity of the tubal damage as well as the age of the woman, duration of infertility and other associated infertility factors.

- Complications are perforation, tear of fallopian tube, failure of procedure, peritonitis.

Patients with tubal factor infertility should be treated with in vitro fertilization (IVF).

Case 2

Mrs X, 23 years old lady married for 3 years with primary infertility presented with history of irregular menstrual cycles. She has oligomenorrhea and usually takes medications for menses. She is obese with BMI of 30.2 kg/m^2 and has excessive hair growth over face and neck region. Her husband's semen analysis is within normal range. Her ultrasonography shows bilateral enlarged ovaries with multiple follicles arranged peripherally with increased stromal tissue (Fig. 13.3).

Q1. What is the most probable cause of infertility in this patient?

Young obese woman with features of hirsutism, menstrual irregularities and polycystic ovaries on USG makes the diagnosis of ovulatory dysfunction due to polycystic ovarian syndrome (PCOS).

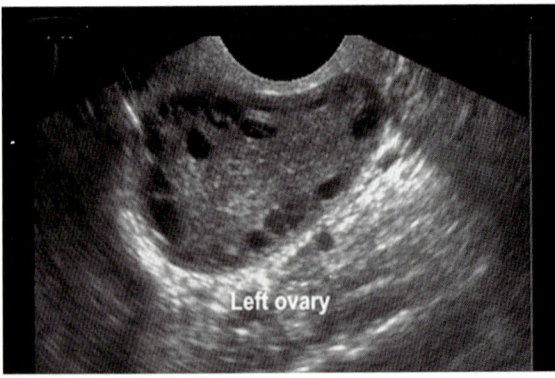
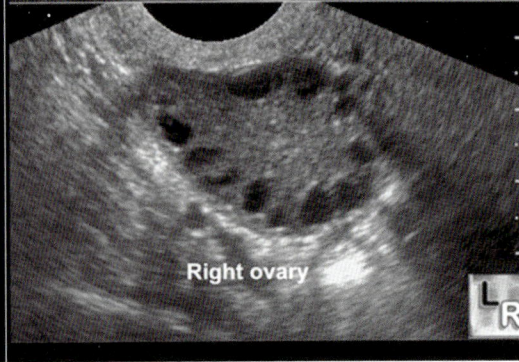

Fig. 13.3

Ovulatory dysfunction: Ovulatory dysfunction is identified in about 15% of infertile couples and accounts for 40% cases of female infertility. Common causes for ovulatory dysfunction include polycystic ovarian syndrome (PCOS), obesity, weight gain or loss, stress, thyroid disorder, hyperprolactinemia and strenuous exercise. Patient with ovulatory dysfunction presents with menstrual complaints like irregular menses, oligomenorrhea or amenorrhea.

Q2. What are the methods available to document ovulation?

Important points and tests for evaluation of ovulation:[4]

a. **Menstrual history:** Regular cycles, mid cycle spotting or pain or moliminal symptoms.

b. **Basal body temperature (BBT):** Ovulatory cycles are associated with biphasic BBT pattern whereas anovulation has monophasic pattern. Progesterone has thermogenic effect which causes rise in temperature in post ovulatory luteal phase.

c. **Cervical mucus study:** Just before ovulation cervical mucus become thin, watery, profuse, elastic and sustains stretching (Spinnbarkeit sign).

d. **Fern test:** Under influence of estrogen, cervical mucus has high level of sodium chloride. When the cervical mucus is dried on glass slide it causes crystallization and appears as Fern pattern. Disappearance of fern pattern is suggestive of ovulation.

e. **Hormonal assessments:**
   - *Serum progesterone:* Concentration of serum progesterone of more than 3 ng/mL on day 21 or one week prior to next expected menses is presumptive indicator of recent ovulation.
   - *Urinary LH:* Detection of LH by Ovulatory predictor kits provides indirect evidence of ovulation. Various commercial kits are available to identify the mid-cycle LH surge which precedes ovulation by 1–2 days.

f. **Endometrial biopsy (EB):** It is done on day 21 to 23 of cycle by curette or Karman's cannula no. 4. Secretory endometrium on histopathology report is diagnostic of ovulation.
   - EB should be subjected to acid fast bacilli (AFB) staining, culture and BACTEC to diagnose genital tuberculosis.
   - Earlier dating the endometrium using traditional histological criteria was considered the gold standard for diagnosis of luteal phase defect (LPD). However studies have demonstrated that histological dating is not a valid test and lacks accuracy and precision so EB should no longer be recommended for evaluation of luteal phase defect in infertile women.

g. **Transvaginal ultrasonography (TVS):** Monitoring of size and number of developing follicles by ultrasound is easy and direct method to document ovulation. Findings presumptive of ovulation of ovulation are sudden collapse of pre-ovulatory follicle, loss of clearly defined follicular margin, appearance of internal echoes and appearance of fluid in cul-de-sac.

Q3. What is PCOS? What are the criteria used to diagnose PCOS?

Polycystic ovarian syndrome (PCOS) is an endocrinologial disorder characterized by anovulation or oligo-ovulation, features of hyperandrogenism (hirsutism, acne, adrogenic alopecia, etc.) and ultrasonographic appearance of polycystic ovaries.

Most common criteria used to diagnose PCOS is Rotterdam criteria:[11]

At least 2 of the following must be present to diagnose PCOS

- Oligo/anovulation
- Hyperandrogenism (clinical/ biochemical) with exclusion of other causes of androgen excess
- Polycystic ovaries

Sonographic criteria for PCOS: Presence of 12 or more follicles in either ovary measuring 2 to

9 mm in diameter and/or increased ovarian volume (>10 mL).

Q4. What are the investigations advised for a patient with ovulatory dysfunction?

Documentation of biochemical hyperandrogenemia:

- Free or total testosterone in patients with hirsutism
- Sex hormone binding globulin (SHBG) level

Evaluation for metabolic abnormalities:

- 2-hour 75 gm oral glucose tolerance test: The WHO criteria for glucose intolerance can be applied to the 2-h glucose value: <140 mg/dL normal; 140–199 mg/dL impaired; ≥200 mg/dL non insulin dependent diabetes mellitus (NIDDM)
- Fasting lipid and lipoprotein level
    Ultrasound examination for determination of polycystic ovaries and follicular growth monitoring for documentation of ovulation.

Optional tests:

- Gonadotropin levels-to determine the cause of amenorrhea: Serum LH, FSH and ratio >2:1, no longer regarded as a marker.
- AMH levels are usually high in the patients with PCOS.
- Fasting insulin levels and tests for insulin resistance (IR) by euglycaemic-hyperinsulinaemic clamp or HOMA-IR- current role only in research studies.

Q5. What fertility treatment options are available for a patient having PCOS?

Lifestyle modification and weight reduction: Even 5–10% weight loss leads to restoration of ovulation. Weight reduction and exercises reduce insulin resistance and circulating free androgens by reducing insulin levels.

Insulin sensitizers: Metformin reduces hepatic production of glucose, increases peripheral sensitivity to insulin and reduces intestinal glucose absorption. A meta-analysis concluded that metformin exerts no clinical benefits on pregnancy rate or live birth rate, but it reduces the risk of OHSS, and improves implantation.[12]

Ovulation induction:

- *Clomiphene citrate:* A selective estrogen receptor modulator with week intrinsic estrogenic activity is thought to bind and block estrogen receptors in the hypothalamus, thereby decreasing the normal ovarian-hypothalamic estrogen feedback loop and increases GnRH pulsatility, leading to increased pituitary secretion of gonadotropins, which promote ovarian follicular development. A functional hypothalamic-pituitary-ovarian axis is usually required for appropriate clomiphene citrate action. The usual starting dose is 50 mg per day but dose may be increased to 100 mg to 150 mg. Therapy is typically started within the first 5 days of menses for a total of 5 days.
- *Aromatase inhibitors, letrozole and anastrazole* inhibit conversion of androgens to estrogens by inhibiting aromatase thus decreasing the level of circulating estradiol. Typical doses are 2.5 to 5 mg of letrozole or 1 mg of anastrazole daily for 5 days.
- *Gonadotropin therapy:* Anovulatory PCOS patients who fail to ovulate or conceive with oral agents should be considered for ovulation induction with exogenous gonadotropin injections.

Ovulation is triggered by injection of highly purified hCG (5000–1000 IU) once the follicle matures and attains 20–22 mm size.

Ovulation induction can be synchronized with timed intercourse or intrauterine insemination (IUI).

In-vitro fertilization (IVF) cycle with controlled ovarian hyperstimulation (COH) by exogenous gonadotropins is required for the non responsive cases.

Case 3

A 31-year-old woman came with complaint of secondary infertility for 6 years. She had one child 5 years old. She had irregular menstrual cycles for last 3–4 years, with bleeding for 1 day only. Her husband's semen analysis was normal normal and HSG showed bilateral patent tubes. She was a known case of hypothyroidism for 6 years, controlled on Tab Eltroxin 50 µg. Her investigations showed FSH level of 45 IU/L and LH of 38 IU/L. Repeat test after 6 weeks showed FSH of 40 IU/L and LH of 29 IU/L. What is the diagnosis?

Diagnosis in above case is Primary ovarian insufficiency (POI) or premature ovarian failure (POF).

- Premature ovarian insufficiency (POI) is a clinical syndrome defined by loss of ovarian activity before the age of 40. Prevalence is 1% (1 in 100) by 40 years, 1 in 1000 women by age 30 years and 1 case per 250 women by age 35 years.[13]
- The diagnosis of POI is based on presence of menstrual disturbances, i.e. oligomenorrhea/amenorrhea for at least 4 months
- Raised FSH elevated FSH level >25 IU/L on two occasions >4 weeks apart is confirmative (ESHRE 2015).[13]

Q1. Define ovarian reserve. Enumerate tests for determining ovarian reserve.

Ovarian reserve describes reproductive potential as a function of number and quality of remaining oocytes. Diminished ovarian reserve (DOR) is is suspected when a woman of reproductive age has normal menstrual cycles but reduced response to ovarian stimulation as compared to women of similar age group.

Tests for ovarian reserve:[14]

a. **Age:** Independent predictor of ovarian reserve and response to ovarian stimulation.

b. **Serum FSH and Estradiol level** on day 3:
   - High level of FSH (>10–20 IU/L) is associated associated with poor ovarian stimulation and failure to conceive.
   - Basal estradiol alone has little significance and should only be used to provide addition information along with FSH.
   - Normal FSH level with elevated estradiol concentration (>60–80 pg/mL) has increased likelihood of poor response to stimulation and less chances of pregnancy.

- According to NICE guidelines, FSH greater than 8.9 IU/L is a predictor for low response and less than 4 IU/L for a high response.

c. **Clomiphene citrate challenge test (CCT):** It is a provocative test that involves serum FSH determination before and after administration of clomiphene citrate (100 mg for 5 days - D5–D9) on day 3 and day 10. An elevated FSH concentration after CCT on day 10 suggests DOR. Serum FSH level on D10 has higher sensitivity but lower specificity than D3 serum FSH level.

d. **Antral follicle count (AFC):** AFC is the sum of antral follicles of size 2 mm to 10 mm diameters, in both the ovaries on TVS during early follicular phase. Total AFC < 4 predicts low response and >16 predicts high response to gonadotrophin stimulation in IVF cycles.

e. **Anti mullerian hormone (AMH):** AMH is produced by granulosa cells of early follicles (preantral and small antral). It is gonadotropin independent and therefore relatively constant within and between menstrual cycles. AMH of less than or equal to 5.4 pmol/L predicts low response and >25 pmol/L predicts high response to stimulation in IVF cycles.

f. Other tests which should not be used individually to predict ovarian reserve and response to outcomes of fertility treatment are:
   - Ovarian volume
   - Ovarian blood flow
   - Inhibin B
   - Estradiol level

Q2. What are the important investigations for evaluation of patients with POI?[12]

- FSH
- Karyotype
- Test for fragile X chromosome (FMR1) premutation
- Bone density by dual-energy X-ray absorptiometry (DEXA) scan
- ANA, rheumatoid factor

- Thyroid-stimulating hormone (TSH)
- Antithyroid peroxidase antibody
- Serum adrenal antibodies

Q3. How will you manage a patient with POI?

Women with POI are at an increased risk for developing the following:

- Symptoms of estrogen deficiency
- Osteopenia and osteoporosis, especially in young women
- Impaired endothelial function, increased cardiovascular morbidity and mortality
- Diminished sexual well-being
- Impaired cognition

The current approach is to treat with a hormone replacement regimen that mimics normal physiology as closely as possible until the average age of natural menopause (age 50 to 51 years). IVF with oocytes donation cycles is established option for the treatment for infertility.

Case 4

A 26-year-old lady married for 3 years came with primary infertility. She had normal menstrual cycles of 28 days interval but associated with severe dysmenorrhea. She also complained of deep dyspareunia. Her husband's semen analysis was normal. Both tubes were patent on HSG. Ultrasound of the pelvis showed a heterogeneous mass of size 4.5 × 3.6 cm in right adnexa with ground glass appearance (Fig. 13.4).

Q1. What is the diagnosis?

Endometriosis[15]

- Endometriosis is the presence of endometrium-like tissue outside the uterus, which induces a chronic, inflammatory reaction.
- Prevalence of endometriosis is unknown but estimates range from 2 to 10% within the general female population but up to 50% in infertile women.

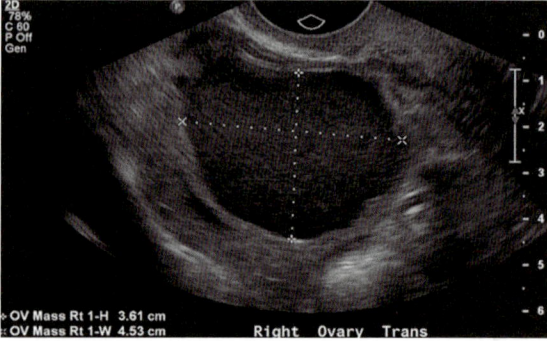

Fig. 13.4

Q2. What are the clinical features of endometriosis?

Clinical signs and symptoms: Dysmenorrhea, chronic pelvic pain, deep dyspareunia, cyclical intestinal complaints, fatigue/weariness and infertility, intestinal complaints-periodic bloating, diarrhea or constipation. Deep endometriosis of the posterior pelvis is associated with increased severity of dyschezia.

Q3. How will you diagnose a case of endometriosis?

- The diagnosis of endometriosis is first suspected based on the history; the symptoms and signs, then corroborated by physical examination and imaging techniques and finally is proven by histological examination of specimens collected during laparoscopy.
- *TVS:* Transvaginal ultrasound can identify endometriomas and deep endometriosis involving the bowel, bladder or ureter. Endometriomas can have varying features but typically appear as cystic structures with diffuse low-level internal echoes surrounded by an echogenic capsule. Some have internal septations or thickened nodular walls.
- CA-125 is usually raised in endometriosis, but should not be used to diagnose endometriosis.
- MRI is used as adjunct to TVS to diagnose deep infiltrative disease. Pelvic MRI can be done to assess the extent of deep endometriosis involving bowel, bladder or ureter.

- The combination of laparoscopy and the histological verification of endometrial glands and/or stroma is considered to be the gold standard for the diagnosis of the disease.
- Barium enema, transvaginal sonography, transrectal sonography and MRI can be used to establish the extent of disease in deep endometriosis.

Q4. Describe the staging for endometriosis.

The revised AFS classification is used to stage endometriosis.[16]

AFS classification of endometriosis.

| Patient's Name .... Date .... |
| Stage I (Minimal)—1–5 .... Laparoscopy................................. Laparotomy .... |
| Stage II (Mild)—6–15 .... Photography .... |
| Stage III (Moderate)—16–40 .... Recommended treatment |
| Stage IV (Severe)—> 40 .... |
| Total .... Prognosis............................... |

		<1 cm	1–3 cm	>3 cm
Peritoneum	Endometriosis			
	Superficial	1	2	4
	Deep	2	4	6
Ovary	R superficial	1	2	4
	Deep	4	16	20
	L superficial	1	2	4
	Deep	4	16	20
	Posterior cul-de-sac obliteration	Partial	Complete	
		4	40	
		< 1/3 enclosure	1/3–2/3 enclosure	>2/3 enclosure
Ovary	Adhesions			
	R flimsy	1	2	4
	Dense	4	8	16
	L flimsy	1	2	4
	Dense	4	8	16
TUBE	R flimsy	1	2	4
	Dense	4*	8*	16
	L flimsy	1	2	4
	Dense	4*	8*	16

*If the fimbriated end of the fallopian tube is completely enclosed, change the point assignment to 16.

Additional endometriosis	Additional pathology
....	....
....	....
To be used with normal tubes and ovaries	To be used with abnormal tubes and ovaries

Q5. How will you manage a case of endometriosis?

There are four options for the management of infertility associated with endometriosis:

a. Medical management (ovarian suppression)

b. Surgical ablation

c. Intra-uterine insemination (IUI)

d. In vitro fertilisation (IVF)

- Medical treatment of minimal and mild endometriosis does not enhance fertility and should not be offered.

- Women with minimal or mild endometriosis who undergo laparoscopy should be offered surgical ablation or resection of endometriosis and laparoscopic adhesiolysis because this improves the chance of pregnancy.

- Women with ovarian endometriomas should be offered laparoscopic cystectomy because this improves the chance of pregnancy.

- Women with moderate or severe endometriosis should be offered surgical treatment because it improves the chance of pregnancy.

- Post-operative medical treatment does not improve pregnancy rates in women with moderate to severe endometriosis and is not recommended.

Case 5

A young couple seeks advice for infertility. On basic work up there is no male factor abnormality, ovulation is documented and tubes were patent. How will you manage this case?

This is a case of unexplained infertility.

- **Unexplained infertility** is a diagnosis of exclusion when routine baseline workup shows normal semen parameters, patent tubes and evidence of ovulation. The incidence of unexplained infertility ranges from 10% to as high as 30% among infertile

populations, depending on diagnostic criteria. Most likely, unexplained infertility represents the lower extreme of normal reproductive potential of a couple or abnormalities of gamates, fertilization implantation or embryo development which can not be detected reliably by available diagnostic tests.

- Prognosis for untreated couples with unexplained infertility is affected by age of female partner, duration of infertility, ovarian reserve and is similar to that for couples with minor infertility factors, such as mild oligospermia or endometriosis.

Q1. How will you manage a case of unexplained infertility?

- As there is no identifiable cause, treatment for unexplained infertility is empirical. Whether operative laparoscopy improves pregnancy outcomes in a subject with unexplained or minimal/mild endometriosis is debatable.

Available treatment options are:

- *Ovarian stimulation:* Clomiphene citrate (CC)- One of the commonly used first-line treatments for unexplained infertility.

- *Intrauterine insemination (IUI):* Intrauterine insemination involves the placement of washed sperms into the uterine cavity around the time of ovulation. It can be performed in conjunction with natural ovulation timed with LH kit, ovulation induction using clomiphene citrate, or injectable gonadotropins.

- Controlled ovarian hyper stimulation with gonadotropins (Gn)

- CC + IUI

- Gn + IUI

- *ART-IVF:* IVF is the most effective treatment for couples with unexplained infertility, but is invasive and costly procedure and is associated with higher risks of OHSS and multifetal gestation (Table 13.1).

Table 13.1: Efficacy of treatments for unexplained infertility

Treatment	Approximate cycle fecundability
No treatment	2–4%
IUI	2–4%
Clomiphene	2–4%
Gonadotropins	5–7%
Clomiphene/IUI	5–10%
Gonadotropins/IUI	7–10%
IVF	25–45%

Newer recommendations by NICE 2013 for management of unexplained infertility:[2]

- Oral ovarian stimulation agents should not be offered (such as clomifene citrate, anastrozole or letrozole) to women with unexplained infertility.
- Women with unexplained infertility should be informed that clomifene citrate as a standalone treatment does not increase the chances of a pregnancy or a live birth.
- Women with unexplained infertility who are having regular unprotected sexual intercourse should be advised to try to conceive for a total of 2 years (this can include up to 1 year before their fertility investigations) before before going for IVF.
- IVF treatment to women with unexplained infertility should be offered to women who have not conceived after 2 years (this can include up to 1 year before their fertility investigations) of regular unprotected sexual intercourse.

Case 6

A young couple married for 3 years, came with secondary infertility. Husband's semen parameters were within normal range. Wife had one abortion at 2 months of amenorrhea 2 years back, medically managed. Her menstrual cycles were regular and routine investigations were within normal limits. Her HSG showed septate uterus with free peritoneal spill of dye on both sides (Fig. 13.5).

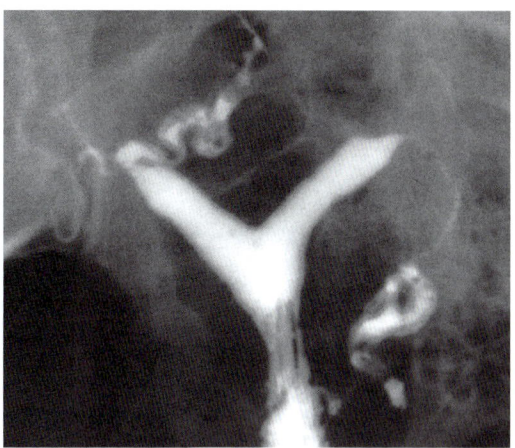

Fig. 13.5

Q1. What are the tests available for evaluation of uterine abnormalities?

a. History of recurrent abortion (septate/unicornuate uterus/myomas), abnormal uterine bleeding (polyp, submucous or intramural fibroids)

b. *Imaging:*
   - *Ultrasound:* Transabdominal or transvaginal
   - *3-D USG:* This method helps in differentiating between the septate and bicornuate uterus.
   - *MRI:* This is the most specific non-invasive method to evaluate urogenital anomalies.

c. *Hystero-salpingography (HSG):* Defines size and shape of uterine cavity and also reveals developmental anomalies like unicornuate, bicornuate or septate uterus or any filling defect lesions like polyp, submucous fibroid or adhesions (Asherman syndrome).

d. *Sonohysterography:* This procedure involves visualization of uterine the cavity by TVS after instillation of saline inside cavity.

e. Hysteroscopy is a definitive method of diagnosis and treatment of intrauterine pathology like myomas, polyps or intrauterine adhesions.

f. Laparoscopy along with hysteroscopy is the gold standard for confirmation of mullerian anomalies.

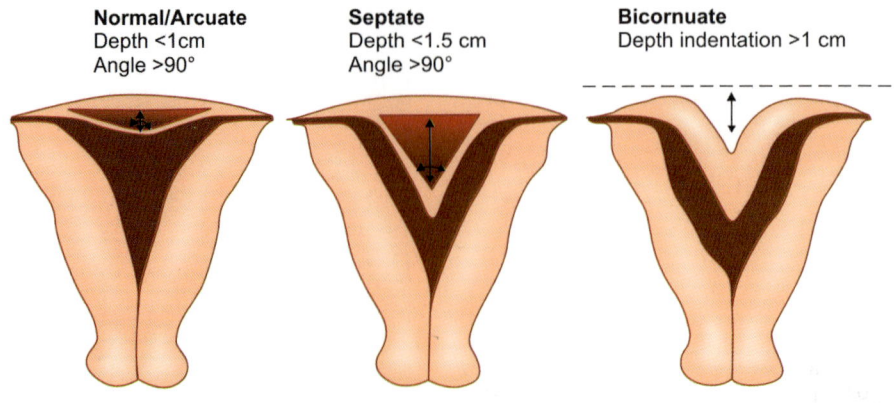

Normal/Arcuate
Depth <1cm
Angle >90°

Septate
Depth <1.5 cm
Angle >90°

Bicornuate
Depth indentation >1 cm

Fig. 13.6

Q2. How will you differentiate between septate uterus and bicornuate uterus?

A septate uterus has single uterine fundus with septum extending from top of endometrial cavity to a variable length and may extend till external os.

A bicornuate uterus has indentation at fundus, usually >1 cm. It may be associated with septum (Fig. 13.6).

Q3. What are the recommendations for the treatment of septate uterus?

Septate uterus is associated with recurrent pregnancy loss (RPL), malpresentation, preterm labour, intrauterine growth restriction, placental abruption and infertility. Hysteroscopic septum incision is associated with improved pregnancy outcome in patient with infertility and RPL.

ASRM recommends that septum incision is reasonable in women with infertility and adverse pregnancy outcomes. However, in women without infertility or any pregnancy complications, septum resection should be considered only after counseling for possible benefits and potential risks of the procedure.[17]

Case 7

A 24-year-old lady came with secondary infertility. She was married for 9 years and had 2 spontaneous abortions 6 years back followed by dilatation and evacuation. She had received 3 cycles of ovulation induction in past. Routine blood investigations and semen analysis were normal. She was advised HSG but it could not be done due to pin point os.

Q1. How will you manage such cases?

This patient has cervical stenosis which may be the cause of infertility. Prior surgical evacuation, recurrent PID and genital TB can present with cervical stenosis.

Patient may require cervical dilatation with or without hysteroscopy.

Cervical stenosis may cause difficulty in embryo transfer and intrauterine insemination, which leads to poor pregnancy outcomes. Patient with repeated difficult ET should undergo cervical dilatation on the day of ovum pick-up procedure or operative hysteroscopy prior to the IVF cycle.

Case 8

Q1. A 25-year-old lady came with inability to conceive after 2 years of unprotected vaginal intercourse. Basic work-up for infertility was normal. Describe the role of cervix in reproduction. How will you diagnose and treat the cervical pathologies causing infertility?

- Cervix acts as a reservoir of sperm. Cervix collects sperm from ejaculates and from vagina and excludes the seminal plasma and morphologically abnormal sperm. Mucin is a glycoprotein gel secreted by cervix, whose secretion is stimulated by estrogen during follicular phase. Progesterone inhibits mucin secretion and makes it opaque, viscid, and impenetrable.

- The post coital test (PCT) provides an assessment of the quantity and quality of cervical mucus, number of motile sperms per high power field, sperm-mucus interactions and the presence of antisperm antibodies. The test involves collection of cervical mucus shortly before the expected time of ovulation and within 2 to 12 hours of intercourse. Even a single motile sperm in most fields is considered as "positive" or normal test result. Abnormal or "negative" postcoital test results are usually due to improper timing. Degenerating, immotile, "shaking" or agglutinated sperms are observed in presence of antisperm antibody.

- Strategies for overcoming cervical factor infertility include treatment with exogenous estrogens (to stimulate mucus production) and intrauterine insemination (IUI).

- There is poor correlation between PCT result and pregnancy outcome. This test is subjective, has poor reproducibility, is inconvenient to the patient and rarely changes clinical management, hence, it is no longer recommended for the investigation of infertility.[4]

Key Points

1. Infertility is defined as failure to achieve a successful pregnancy after 12 months or more of appropriate, timed unprotected vaginal intercourse.

2. Couples having inability to conceive should be seen together because both partners are affected by decision regarding investigations and treatment.

3. Psychosocial counseling should be the integral part of the management.

4. Relevant points in history include age of both partners, duration of infertility, menstrual history, obstetric history, contraceptive history, sexual history, medical history, previous fertility treatment received, past surgical history, history of addiction etc.

5. Routine baseline work-up includes basic blood and urine investigations, semen analysis, tests to document tubal patency and ovulation.

6. IVF is the method of choice in patients with severe tubal disease or destroyed tubal mucosa.

7. Infertility because of ovulatory dysfunction should be treated with lifestyle modifications, ovulation inducing agents, exogenous gonadotropins and IVF.

8. IVF with oocyte donation cycles is established option to treat infertility in a patient with premature ovarian failure (POF).

9. Unexplained infertility is a diagnosis of exclusion when infertility workup shows normal semen parameters, patent tubes and evidence of ovulation.

REFERENCES

1. Definition of infertility and recurrent pregnancy loss: a committee opinion. Practice committee of American Society for Reproductive Medicine. Fertil Steril 2013;99:63.

2. National Institute for Health and Care Excellence. Fertility: assessment and treatment for people with fertility problems. London: NICE 2013. CG156.

3. Mira Aubuchon, Richard O Burney, Danny J. Schust, Mylene W.M. Yao. Infertility and Assisted Reproductive Technology. Berek & Novak's Gynecology, 15th ed. Lippincott Williams & Wilkins, Wolters Kluwer 2012;1133.

4. Practice Committee of the American Society for Reproductive Medicine. Diagnostic evaluation of the infertile female: a committee opinion. Fertil Steril 2015;103:e44-50.

5. WHO laboratory manual for the examination of human semen and processing of human semen. World Health Organization 2010.

6. Becker R, Schürmann R. Ultrasound in the investigation of tubal patency: A meta-analysis of three comparative studies of Echovist-200 including 1007 women. Zentralbl Gynakol 1997; 119:366–73.

7. Kerin J, Daykhovsky L, Segalowitz J, Surrey E, Anderson R, Stein A, et al. Falloposcopy: a microendoscopic technique for visual exploration of the human fallopian tube from the uterotubal ostium to the fimbria using a transvaginal approach. Fertil Steril 1990;54:390–400.

8. Marchino GL, Gigante V, Gennarelli G, Mazza O, Mencaglia L. Salpingoscopic and laparoscopic investigations in relation to fertility outcome. J Am Assoc Gynecol Laparosc 2001;8:218–21.

9. Watrelot A, Nisolle M,Chelli H, Hocke C, Rongieres C, Racinet C.Is laparoscopy still the gold standard in infertility assessment? A comparison of fertiloscopy versus laparoscopy in infertility. Hum Reprod 2003;18:834–9.

10. Annika S. Management of hydrosalpinx. Textbook of Assisted Reproductive Techniques. 5th ed. Taylor & Francis 2018;773–5.

11. Rotterdam ESHRE/ASRM-Sponsored PCOS Consensus Workshop Group. Revised 2003 consensus on diagnostic criteria and long-term health risks related to polycystic ovary syndrome (PCOS). Hum Reprod 2004;19:41–7.

12. Palomba S, Falbo A, La Sala GB. Effects of metformin in women with polycystic ovary syndrome treated with gonadotrophins for in vitro fertilisation and intracytoplasmic sperm injection cycles: a systematic review and meta-analysis of randomised controlled trials. BJOG 2013;120:267–76.

13. European Society for Human Reproduction and Embryology (ESHRE) Guideline Group on POI, Webber L, Davies M, Anderson R, et al. ESHRE Guideline: management of women with premature ovarian insufficiency. Hum Reprod 2016;31:926–37.

14. Testing and interpreting measures of ovarian reserve. Practice committee of American Society for Reproductive Medicine. Fertil Steril 2015; 103:e9–17.

15. Dunselman GA, Vermeulen N, Becker C, Calhaz-Jorge C, D'Hooghe T, De Bie B, et al; European Society of Human Reproduction and Embryology. ESHRE guideline: management of women with endometriosis. Hum Reprod 2014 ;29:400–12.

16. Revised American Fertility Society classification of endometriosis: 1985.Fertil Steril 1985;43:351–2.

17. Uterine septum: a guideline. Practice committee of American Society for Reproductive Medicine. Fertil Steril 2016; 106:530–40.

Male Infertility: Approach to Diagnosis and Management

Renu Tanwar, Garima Singh

Introduction

Infertility is defined as the inability of a sexually active couple to achieve pregnancy in one year.[1] About 15% of couples have difficulty in conceiving and in approximately 30% of these couples only the male partner has reproductive dysfunction.[1] In another 20%, both partners have reproductive abnormality.[1] Thus, male reproductive dysfunction contributes to about half of all cases of infertile couples.

The causes of increasing male infertility are:

1. Advanced age of marriage of both partners-with advancing age in males, there is telomeric deletion of chromosomes; this may reduce chromosomal integrity affecting spermatozoa viability.
2. Dietary habits and changing lifestyle.
3. Increasing stress in daily routine—stress induced ACTH has antigonadotrophin effect which impairs functional integrity of testes.
4. Increased use of synthetic dyes in green vegetables.
5. Use of pesticides has direct gametotoxic effect.

Q1. What are the common causes of male infertility?

Causes of male infertility (Table 14.1).

Q2. How would you evaluate the male partner?

Evaluation of male partner consists of:
- History
- Physical examination
- Specially focused investigations

Table 14.1: Causes of male infertility

- *Sexual disorders*
  Lack of libido
  Anorgasmia
  Erectile dysfunction
  Failure to have intercourse

- *Primary testicular defect in sperm production*
  Idiopathic
  Infection (e.g. mumps orchitis in nonvaccinated men)
  Trauma
  Large varicoceles
  Pelvic irradiation or surgery
  Chemotherapy
  Autoimmune Drugs
  Testicular cancer
  Orchidectomy
  Genetic mutation
  Klinefelter syndrome

- *Endocrinopathies that affect spermatogenesis*
  Obesity
  Hypothalamopituitary disease
  Hyperprolactinemia
  Thyroid dysfunction
  Cushing syndrome

- *Defects in sperm transportation*
  Congenital absence of the vasa deferens
  Acquired ejaculatory duct obstruction (e.g. recurrent infection, vasectomy)
  Ejaculatory dysfunction
  Retrograde ejaculation
  Obstruction

Relevant points in history taking:
- The age of both partners and duration of infertility.

- The gynecological cofactors of the female partner.
- *Coital history:* Frequency, erectile function, penetration and ejaculation.
- History of trauma, torsion, previous treatment or surgery for undescended testes. A history of cryptorchidism-if bilateral, it may severely affect spermatogenesis, even after correction in early life.
- *History of medical illness:* Mumps in childhood (destruction of seminiferous tubules) resulting in Sertoli cell syndrome.
- Respiratory tract infections like bronchitis, bronchiectasis and sinusitis, which could be associated with Kartagener's syndrome, Young's syndrome and cystic fibrosis.
- History of sexually transmitted diseases, history of genitourinary tuberculosis (obstruction of vas deferens and epididymis).
- *Lifestyle factors:* Long distance cycling, sauna bath, tight undergarments (cause scrotal hypothermia and trauma) stress, heavy smoking, intake of cocaine and marijuana (cause oxidative DNA damage of spermatozoa).
- *History of drug intake:* Anabolic steroids for body building, testosterone supplementation for hypogonadotrophic conditions, use of antihypertensives like alpha and beta blockers (have adverse effect on erection), antipsychotics and antidepressants (affect the hypothalamic-pituitary-gonadal axis and suppress libido), use of antibiotics (may impair sperm motility and inhibits spermatogenesis), history of any chemotherapeutic agents used (gonadotoxic).
- Professional history-agriculture (having contact with pesticides), welding, factory workers working with ceramics (may cause spermatogenetic damage).
- History of long standing diabetes can cause erectile dysfunction and retrograde ejaculation (diabetic neuropathy and vasculopathy).

Examination of infertile male includes:

a. *General examination:*
  - If male is tall with absent beard and moustache and has gynaecomastia (suggestive of hypogonadism or Klinefelters syndrome)
  - Neck swelling
  - Any palpable lymph nodes—to rule out tuberculosis
  - Any abdominal scar marks of previous surgery

b. *Local examination:*
  - *Examination of penis:* Curvature of the penis, position of the external urethral meatus to rule out hypospadias.
  - Examination of scrotal sac and testes in erect posture
  - Palpation of testes:
    – Length—should be more than 4 cm
    – Volume—should be more than 20 mL
  - Palpate for vas deferens, presence of varicocele should be checked in standing position and confirmed on USG.

c. *Digital rectal examination:* Done in suspected obstructive azoospermia or in asthenospermia of infective origin and to exclude enlarged prostate or midline prostatic cyst.

Investigations

Husband's semen analysis (HSA): The initial evaluation for male factor infertility should include at least one properly performed semen analysis. Sample should be taken after a defined abstinence period of 2–5 days. Shorter abstinence interval decreases semen volume and sperm density whereas longer abstinence interval increases the proportion of dead, immotile and morphologically abnormal sperm. Ideally semen sample should be collected by masturbation in the laboratory directly into a wide mouth sterile container made of polypropylene.

Table 14.2: Lower reference limits of seminal parameters (WHO 2010 guidelines)[2]	
Semen parameters	*Lower reference values*
Semen volume (mL)	1.5
pH value	>7.2
Sperm concentration (millions/mL)	15
Total sperm count (millions/ejaculate)	39
Sperm motility	40% motile spermatozoa (PR + NP)
Progressive sperm motility	32% rapid and slow progressive motile spermatozoa
Sperm morphology	4% normal spermatozoa
Peroxidase-positive leukocytes (millions/mL)	<1
Vitality (eosin test)	≥ 58%

Q3. When should endocrine evaluation be done for an infertile male?

A basic endocrine evaluation of infertile male includes serum measurements of testosterone, FSH, LH and prolactin levels. This is indicated in hypogonadotrophic hypogonadism, azoospermia and in infertile males with abnormal semen parameters.

Table 14.3: Normal hormone values for men[3]	
Hormone	*Normal range*
Testosterone	300–1100 ng/dL
Prolactin	7–18 ng/mL
Luteinising hormone (LH)	2–18 mIU/mL
Follicle stimulating hormone (FSH)	2–18 mIU/mL

Q4. What is the role of scrotal ultrasonography and transrectal USG in diagnosis of male infertility?

It improves the detection of scrotal pathologies in infertile men that are seen in 50.4% of cases, with varicocele being the leading diagnosis in 18.5%, epididymal pathologies 14.0%, and additional spermatoceles in 5.2% of patients.[4] The risk for testicular tumors is also increased to 1 in 200–300 men and most of these tumors may not be palpable. Testicular microlithiasis can also be seen and is a sign of spermatogenic dysfunction and is possibly associated with premalignant lesions of the testis, e.g. testicular intraepithelial neoplasia (TIN). USG is performed in high-resolution (linear) with at least a 7.5 to 12-MHz transducer, with the patient in supine position. Transrectal USG is especially useful to diagnose obstructive azoospermia.

Q5. What is the role of fine needle aspiration cytology (FNAC) in diagnosing male infertility?

It serves as minimally invasive, rapid and reliable technique and is usually done in azoospermic males or in patients with testicular mass with infertility.

Q6. When should testicular biopsy be done in male infertility?

If repeated FNAC yields no tissue then testicular biopsy needs to be done. Prior to taking biopsies, cryopreservation of spermatozoa should be offered for IVF-ICSI.[5] Testicular biopsies may be indicated if TIN is suspected in case of microlithiasis or or if there is history of a contralateral testicular tumor.

Q7. What are sperm function tests?

Sperm function tests are done to evaluate functionality of sperms when husband semen analysis reveals decreased or abnormal motility, abnormal morphology or there is repeated fertilization failure in IVF-ICSI.

Various sperm function tests are:

a. *Tests for absence of motility in viable or non viable sperms:*
  - Hypo osmotic swelling test
  - Modified hypoosmotic swelling test.

b. *Tests for acrosomal integrity:*
  - Triple stain technique
  - Monoclonal antibodies to acrosomal contents

- Radioimmunoassay
- Clinical acrosin assay

c. *Tests for nuclear DNA fragmentation:*
  - TUNEL assay
  - COMET assay
  - HALO sperm test

Q8. What is azoospermia?

Azoospermia is complete absence of sperm in two or more centrifuged semen samples four weeks apart. A sample should be considered azoospermic, if semen centrifugation at 600 G for 10 min and thorough microscopic examination of the pellet (×600) reveals no spermatozoa.

The categories of azoospermia are:
- Pre-testicular azoospermia
- Testicular failure or non-obstructive azoospermia
- Post-testicular obstruction or obstructive azoospermia.

Causes of different types of azoospermia and respective examination and investigation findings are given below.[6]

Management of azoospermia:
- Management based on FSH level and testes size
- Management based on fructose in seminal plasma.
- Management based on semen volume.

Table 14.4

	Nonobstructive		Obstructive
	Spermatogenic failure	*Hypogonadotropic hypogonadism*	*Obstructive*
Most common etiologies	Y chromosome microdeletions; Klinefelter syndrome; cryptorchidism; postinfectious (e.g. mumps orchitis); radiotherapy; chemotherapy; testicular trauma/torsion; idiopathic	Congenital (e.g. Kallman syndrome, normosmic HH), Prader-Willi), acquired (e.g. pituitary tumor, steroid abuse)	Postsurgical (e.g. vasectomy epididymal cysts removal, hernia repair, scrotal surgery, prostatectomy), CBAVD; postinfectious; ejaculatory duct obstruction; iatrogenic (e.g. urological endoscopic instrumentation); idiopathic
Physical examination	Either small-sized (volume <15 mL or long axis 4.6 cm or less) or normal epididymides and palpable vasa deferentia	Small-sized testes (volume <15 mL or testicular long axis 4.6 cm or less); small epididymides and palpable vasa deferentia	Either normal or enlarged epididymides, and palpable or nonpalpable vasa deferentia (e.g. CBAVD); normal-sized testes (volume ≥15 mL and long axis >4.6 cm)
Semen analysis	Normal (>1.5 mL) ejaculate volume and pH (>7.2); hyposermia (<1.5 mL ejaculate) may be found in males with hypogonadism	Low ejaculate volume (<1.5 mL) and normal pH	Either normal or low pH and ejaculate volume (e.g. CBAVD and EDO)
Endocrine	Either elevated (>7.6 mIU/mL) or normal FSH levels; either elevated or normal LH levels; either low (<300 ng/dL) or normal total testosterone levels	Low FSH and LH levels (<1.2 mIU/mL); low (<300 ng/dL total testosterone levels	Normal FSH (<7.6 mIU/mL) and LH levels; normal total estosterone tlevels (>300 ng/dL)
Genetic testing	Nonmosaic (47, XXY) and mosaic (46,XY/47, XXY) Klinefelter syndrome, and AZF Yq microdeletions seen in about 15% of cases	KAL-1, FGFR-1, PROK-1, PROKR-2; CHD-7 and FGF-8 gene mutations can be found in congenital HH	CFTR gene mutations usually found in males with CBAVD
Testicular biopsy	Hypospermatogenesis; maturation arrest; sertoli-cell only; tubular atrophy; mixed pattern	Not applicable	Normal spermatogenesis

CBAVD: congenital bilateral absence of the vas deferens; CFTR: cystic fibrosis transmembrane conductance regulator; CHD-7 chromodomain helicase DNA binding protein 7; EDO: ejaculatory duct obstruction; FGFR-1: fibroblast growth factor receptor 1; FGF-8: fibroblast growth factor 8; FSH: follicle-stimulating hormoen; LH: luteinizing hormone; HH: Hypogonadotropic hypogonadism; KAL-1: Kallmann syndrome 1 sequencel PROK-2: prokineticin 2; PROKR-2: Prokineticin receptor 2; YCMD: Y chromosome microdeletions; Yq: Y chromosome long arm; AZF: azoospermia factor

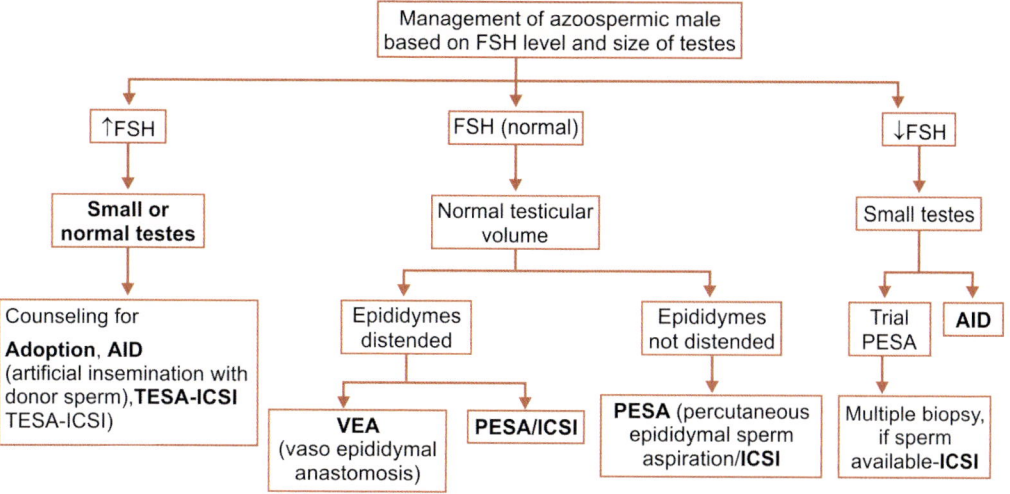

Fig. 14.1: Management based on FSH level and testes size

Table 14.5: Management based on fructose in seminal plasma	
Fructose absent	*Fructose present*
Causes	*Causes*
Congenital absence of seminal vesicles or vas deferens.	Obstruction in rete testes and epididymis.
Ejaculatory duct obstruction	Primary testicular failure
	Hypogonadotrophic hypogonadism
Management	*Management*
Seminal vesicle or vas absent-genetic counseling followed by PESA/ICSI, AID or adoption.	Depends on the size of testes and level of FSH as depicted in Fig. 14.2 above
Vas deferens palpable-TRUS, USG guided trans urethral removal of cyst plus dilation of ejaculatory duct/ICSI	

Q9. What genetic workup is required for infertile male?

Genetic workup is indicated if sperm count is severely reduced (<5 million/mL), if there is azoospermia, abnormal sperm motility and morphology and also in cases of idiopathic infertility.[8] The frequency of genetic disorders is increased in men with severe male factor infertility, varying between 4.3–20.6% for oligozoospermic and azoospermic men.

A. Chromosomal Abnormalities

a. *Chromosomal numerical anomalies*

- 47XXY—Klinefelters syndrome- most frequent sex chromosome abnormality seen in 14% of azoospermic males.

- 47XYY—rarely observed.
- 45X/46XY Mosaics—individuals present with mixed gonadal dysgenesis and phenotype may be male or female with ambiguous genitalia.

b. *Chromosomal structural anomalies-* commonest is microdeletion of Y chromosome. Another example is 46 XX male with SRY gene translocation on one arm of X chromosome at the time of fertilization.

B. Genetic Defects

These are usually deletions, mutations or polymorphic expantions.

a. Pretesticular defect—commonest X linked disorder is Kallmann syndrome.

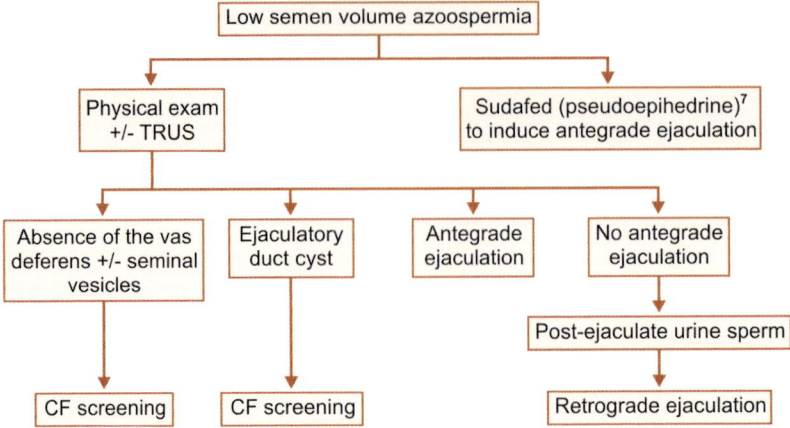

Fig. 14.2: Management for low semen volume azoospermia

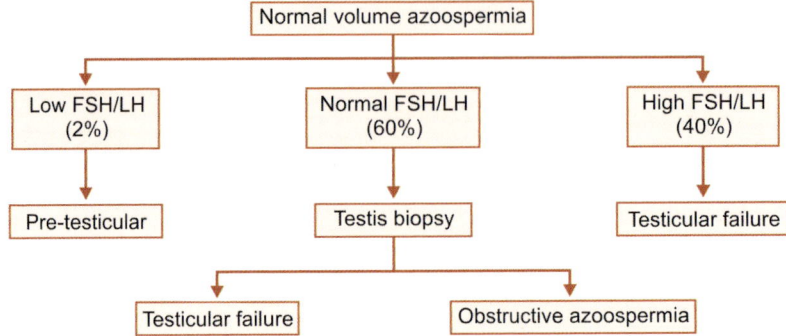

Fig. 14.3: Management for normal semen volume azoospermia

b. Testicular defect
  • Prune belly syndrome (one of the rarest variety)
  • Muscular dystrophy
c. Post testicular—commonest example is mutation or deletions in cystic fibrosis gene (CFTR gene).

How to Treat an Infertile Male

Counselling is the initial step:
  • Advice to stop smoking, alcohol abuse and use of anabolic steroids.
  • Avoid hot baths and drugs affecting spermatogenesis and to lose weight if obese.
  • Intrauterine insemination is indicated in mild to moderate male subfertility and in retrograde ejaculation.

Q10. What is the role of medical management in infertile males?

The therapeutic strategy is determined by etiology of the male infertility. Treat infections or any other medical disorder like hypo-thyroidism or hyperprolactinemia.

Drugs Commonly used in Medical Management

Clomophene Citrate[9]: When there are low testosterone levels with a normal T/E ratio, clomiphene citrate (CC) is the drug of choice. It can be started in a dose of 25 mg daily for 25 days and continued for 3 months.

Clomiphene citrate is tolerated well by most patients. More common side effects include gastrointestinal discomfort, dizziness, hair loss, gynecomastia, and minimal weight gain. There is 1.5% risk of visual disturbances such as blurred vision, photophobia and diplopia although they are reversible with cessation of the medication.[10]

Aromatase inhibitors[11]: Aromatase inhibitors (AIs) are the medication of choice for infertile males with normal testosterone levels but abnormal T/E ratios. Inhibiting the negative feedback of estrogen on the hypothalamus allows for stronger GnRH pulses that stimulate the pituitary to increase production of FSH. This increased FSH finally leads to increased spermatogenesis within the Sertoli cells. The main AIs used for infertility are Letrozole and Anastrazole (third generation nonsteroidal AIs).

Letrozole is a more potent AI than Anastrazole. There is debate over the optimal dose of Letrozole. Drastic changes in estrogen/testosterone ratio have been observed, up to 6-fold, with variable dosing ranges ranging from 2.5 mg daily to 2.5 mg three times a week. Side effects are decreased libido, headache and transient liver enzyme abnormalities.

hCG therapy[12]: Human chorionic gonadotropin (hCG) is an LH analog derived from urine or recombinant sources that stimulates intratesticular Leydig cell testosterone production and increases intratesticular and serum testosterone levels to improve spermatogenesis. It is usually recommended to a couple with idiopathic male infertility who could not achieve functional eugonadal levels on clomid and/or anastrozole or in patients who have developed clomid syndrome. Recommended doses are 1500 units of hCG IM 3 times a week as a starting dose. The dose is escalated up to 3500 units 3 times per week to achieve high normal testosterone levels (>500 ng/dL). Subsequently, semen analysis is done after 3 months to monitor the patient's response. If there is no response, donor sperm or adoption is recommended. In most cases, hypogonadotropic hypogonadism has an excellent prognosis regarding fertility options. Treatment involves substitution of substitution of gonadotropins with hCG and recombinant FSH. The hCG stimulates Leydig cells (as LH does), and FSH stimulates the germ cell compartment. This treatment normalizes gonadal function in 80% of patients, and pregnancy rates of 50–70% can be achieved.

Multivitamins[13]: Antioxidants like vitamin E and zinc have been reported to increase the clinical pregnancy rate. As per Cochrane review, oral antioxidant supplementation may improve live birth rates in subfertile males (low quality evidence), however, further trials are needed to establish their use in clinical practice.[13]

Q11. What is a varicocele?

A varicocele is an abnormal enlargement of the pampiniform venous plexus in the scrotum. It affects about 11% of men with normal semen parameters and about 25% with abnormal semen parameters.[14]

Q12. What are the surgical options for managing varicocele?

Surgical corrections available are:

A. Varicocelectomy

Varicocele repair is done in patients with abnormal semen parameters and associated clinical varicocele. Successful treatment improves semen quality in 44% of men treated.[14]

Microsurgery should be done by an experienced urologist. Epididymovasostomy is combined with microsurgical epididymal sperm aspiration (MESA) and the harvested spermatozoa **are cryopreserved for ICSI.**

Indications for epididymovasostomy are congenital and acquired obstructions at the level of the epididymis, in the presence of a normal testicular biopsy.

B. Vasovasostomy: This is performed either macroscopically or microscopically. Pregnancy rates are better with microscopic technique. The pregnancy rate is inversely proportional to the obstruction interval and becomes less than 50% after 8 years. The development of antisperm antibodies, the quality of the semen and partner's age are the important prognostic factors.

C. Microepididymal sperm aspiration (MESA): When reconstruction (vasovasostomy, epididymovasostomy) cannot be performed or is unsuccessful then MESA in combination with ICSI is indicated. Percutaneous aspiration of sperms from the caput epididymis (PESA) is another alternative. If no spermatozoa is produced or there are very low numbers of motile spermatozoa by MESA or PESA procedure then a testicular bioipsy can be performed with testicular sperm extraction (TESE) which can be used for ICSI.

D. Transurethral incision of ejaculatory ducts or midline prostatic cyst: Infections of the prostatic urethra and the accessory glands, or a cyst in the midline of the prostate causes distal obstructions of the genital tract. Transurethral incision of the cyst or ejaculatory ducts may lead to an increase in semen quality and, occasionally, spontaneous pregnancy.

 Key Points

- Incidence of male infertility has increased significantly.
- Semen analysis is the first and foremost investigation.
- Hormonal investigations are based on clinical findings.
- Chromosomal or genetic factor may be involved in majority of idiopathic male infertility.
- Proper counseling and evidence based treatment options treatment options should be given to improve fertility.

REFERENCES

1. Gnoth C, Godehardt E, Frank-Herrmann P, et al. Definition and prevalence of subfertility and infertility. Hum Reprod 2005;20:1144–1147.
2. World Health Organization. WHO laboratory manual for the examination and processing of human semen,ed 5. Geneva, Switzerland: World Health Organization 2010.
3. Sikaris K1, McLachlan RI, Kazlauskas R, et al. Reproductive hormone reference intervals for healthy fertile young men: evaluation of automated platform assays. J Clin Endocrinol Metab 2005;90:5928–36.
4. Behre HM, Kliesch S, Scha¨del F, et al. Clinical relevance of scrotal and transrectal ultrasonography in andrological patients. Int J Androl 1995;18(Suppl 2):27–31.
5. Kim ED, Gilbaugh JH, Patel VR, et al. Testis biopsies frequently demonstrate sperm in men with azoospermia and significantly elevated follicle-stimulating hormone levels. J Urol 1997; 157:144–6.
6. Clinical management of infertile men with nonobstructive azoospermia. Asian J Androl 2015; 17:459–70.
7. Shoshany O, Abhyankar N, Elyaguov J, et al. Efficacy of treatment with pseudoephedrine in men with retrograde ejaculation. Andrology 2017;5:744–748.
8. Johnson MD. Genetic risks of intracytoplasmic sperm injection in the treatment of male infertility: Recommendations for genetic counseling and screening. Fertil Steril 1998;70:397–411.
9. Ross LS, Kandel GL, Prinz LM, et al. Clomiphene treatment of the idiopathic hypofertile male: high-dose, alternate-day therapy. Fertil Steril 1980;33:618–23.
10. Bridges N, Trofimenko V, Fields S, et al. Male factor infertility and clomiphene citrate: a meta-analysis—the effect of clomiphene citrate on oligospermia. Urol Pract 2015;2:199–205.
11. Schlegel PN. Aromatase inhibitors for male infertility. Fertil Steril 2012;98:1359–62.
12. Depenbusch M, von Eckardstein S, Simoni M, et al. Maintenance of spermatogenesis in hypogonadotropic hypogonadal men with human chorionic gonadotropin alone. Eur J Endocrinol 2002;147: 617–24.
13. Showell MG, Mackenzie-Proctor R, Brown J, Yazdani A, Stankiewicz MT, Hart RJ. Antioxidants for male subfertility. Cochrane Database Syst Rev. 2014;(12):CD007411.
14. The influence of varicocele on parameters of fertility in a large group of men presenting to infertility clinics. World Health Organization. Fertil Steril 1992;57:1289–93.

Semen Preparation Techniques and Intrauterine Insemination

Pushpa Mishra, Rashmi Pillania

Introduction

The first sperm separation methods that were developed comprised of only one or two washing procedures to eliminate seminal plasma with subsequent resuspension of the male germ cells. Following it, more sophisticated methods have been developed in order to obtain sufficient amounts of motile, functionally competent spermatozoa for assisted reproductive technology (ART).

Q1. What is normal semen analysis according to WHO 2010 guidelines?

Normal semen analysis according to WHO 2010 guideline is as illustrated in Table 15.1.

Q2. What is semen preparation?

Semen contains both motile and dead spermatozoa, cells, cellular debris and microorganisms. In semen preparation, spermatozoa is separated from seminal plasma and processed to yield a high percentage of morphologically normal and motile cells, free from debris, non germ cells and dead spermatozoa[1]

Q3. What is the rationale behind separating spermatozoa from seminal plasma?

The components of seminal fluid such as prostaglandins and zinc are obstacles to conception in ART. The separation of human spermatozoa from seminal plasma yields a final preparation containing a high percentage of morphologically normal and motile cells, free from debris, non-germ cells and dead spermatozoa[1]

Q 4. Enumerate the criteria for good sperm selection technique.

Criteria for a "good" sperm selection technique are[2]:

a. Elimination of seminal plasma, and debris.

b. Elimination/reduction of dysfunctional sperm.

c. Elimination/reduction of leukocytes and bacteria.

d. Improving semen quality in terms of motility, DNA integrity, acrosome reaction, and normal sperm morphology.

e. Cost-effectiveness

f. Easy and quick to perform.

Q5. Enumerate the methods of semen sample collection

Methods of sample collection are:

a. Masturbation

b. Coitus interruptus (not preferred)

Table 15.1: Normal semen analysis according to WHO 2010 guideline	
Parameter	*Lower reference limit*
Semen volume (mL)	1.5
Sperm concentration (106/mL)	15
Total sperm number (106/ejaculate)	39
Progressive motility (PR, %)	32
Total motility (PR +NP, %)	40
Vitality (live sperms, %)	58
Sperm morphology (NF, %	4
pH	$\geq = 7.2$
Leucocyte (106/ml)	<1
MAR/Immunobead test (%)	<50

c. Assisted ejaculation, e.g. vibro ejaculation, electro ejaculation

Sterile wide mouthed container should be used for sample collection and labeled as shown in Fig. 15.1.

Q6. What factor determines the choice of method of semen preparation?

Semen quality determines the choice of semen preparation technique.

- Direct swim-up technique is used when the semen samples are considered to be largely normal with normal parameters, good count and motility.
- Density-gradient technique is used in cases of severe oligozoospermia, teratozoospermia or asthenozoospermia because of the greater total number of motile spermatozoa recovered.[1]

Q7. Enumerate the parameters for the assessment of efficiency of sperm selection technique.

The efficiency of a sperm selection technique is determined by[1]:

a. The absolute sperm number
b. The total number of motile spermatozoa
c. The recovery of morphologically normal motile spermatozoa.

Q8. What are the general principles of semen preparation?

The principles for semen preparation are[1]:

a. Semen samples like any other body fluid, should be handled as a biohazard with extreme care.
b. Semen preparation techniques should not be considered 100% effective in removing infectious agents from semen.
c. For all methods, the culture medium just like the body milieu, should be balanced for electrolytes, pH, nutrition and temperature. Therefore:
  - If the incubator contains only atmospheric air and the temperature is 37°C, the medium should be buffered with Herpes or a similar buffer, and the caps of the tubes should be tightly closed.

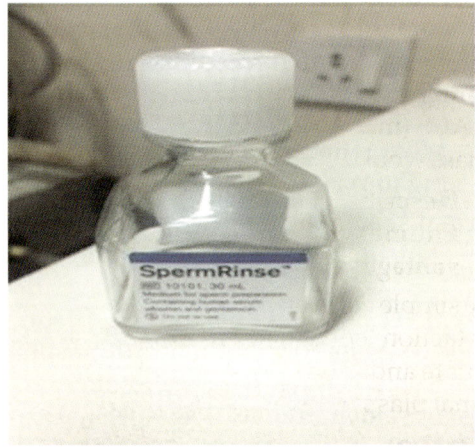

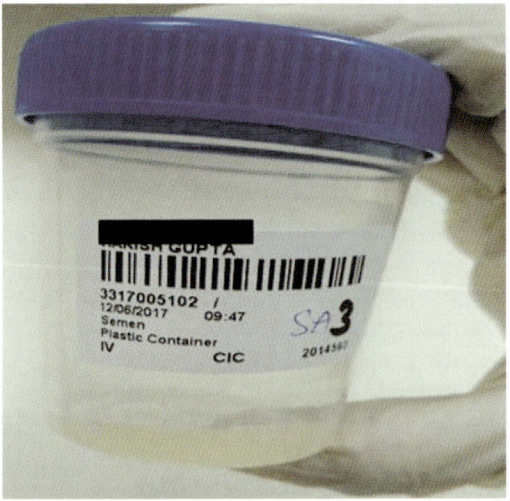

Fig. 15.1: Labeled wide mouthed container for semen collection

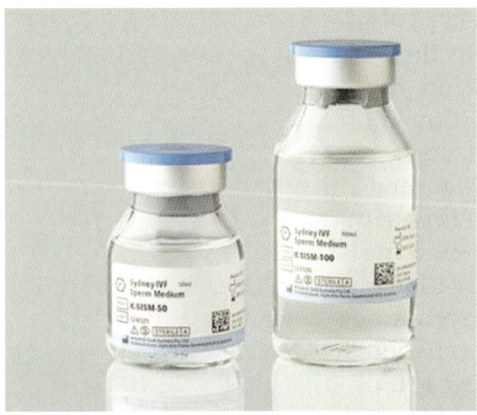

Fig. 15.2: Sperm wash medium

- If the incubator atmosphere is 5% CO_2 in air and the temperature is 37°C, then the medium is best buffered with sodium bicarbonate or a similar buffer, and the caps of the test-tubes should be loose to allow gas exchange.

d. For assisted reproduction procedures such as intracytoplasmic sperm injection (ICSI), in-vitro fertilization (IVF), artificial insemination (AI) or gamete intrafallopian transfer (GIFT) it is imperative that the human serum albumin is highly purified and free from viral, bacterial and prion contamination.

Q9. Enumerate various semen processing techniques used in IUI and IVF.

Various semen processing techniques used in IVF and IUI are:

a. Simple wash method
b. Migration based techniques
   - Swim up
   - Density gradient centrifugation
   - Migration sedimentation
c. MACS (magnetic activated cell sorting)
d. Glass wool filtration

Q10. Describe simple washing technique. Enumerate its advantages and disadvantages.

In the simple wash method, following complete liquefaction, culture medium is added to the ejaculate and centrifuged twice to remove the seminal plasma.[1]

Procedure

The steps of simple washing technique are:
a. Mix the semen sample well.
b. Dilute the entire semen sample 1 + 1 (1:2) with medium to promote removal of seminal plasma.
c. Transfer the diluted suspension into multiple centrifuge tubes, preferably not more than 3 mL per tube followed by centrifugation at 300–500 × g for 5–10 minutes.
d. Aspirate and discard the supernatants.
e. Resuspend the combined sperm pellets in 1 mL of medium by gentle pipetting and centrifuge again at 300–500 × g for 3–5 minutes.

f. Following supernatant removal by aspiration, resuspend the sperm pellet, by gentle pipetting, in a volume of medium appropriate for final disposition.

Advantages

- Easy to perform
- It provides the highest yield of spermatozoa and is adequate if semen sample is of good quality.

Disadvantages

Non-viable spermatozoa and unwanted cells that can inhibit capacitation are not removed completely.

Q11. Describe swim up technique. Enumerate its advantages and disadvantages.

Swim up technique of semen preparation is based on the ability of sperms to swin up from the seminal plasma into the culture medium. It includes:
- Direct swim up from semen
- Swim up from washed pellet

Direct Swim Up

Procedure

The steps of this method are as follows (Fig 15.3):
a. Allow specimen to liquefy completely for 15–30 minutes at 37°C in incubator before processing.
b. Measure volume using a sterile 3 mL pippete.
c. Place 1 mL of the semen sample in a sterile 15 mL conical centrifuge tube, and then layer 1.2 mL of medium over it. Alternatively, the semen sample can be placed under the culture medium using 3 mL pipette.
d. Incubate the tube for 1 hour at 37 °C.
e. Following incubation, remove the uppermost 1 mL of medium containing highly motile sperm cells.
f. Add 1.5–2.0 mL of medium to the sperm suspension and centrifuge at 300–500 × g for 5 minutes.

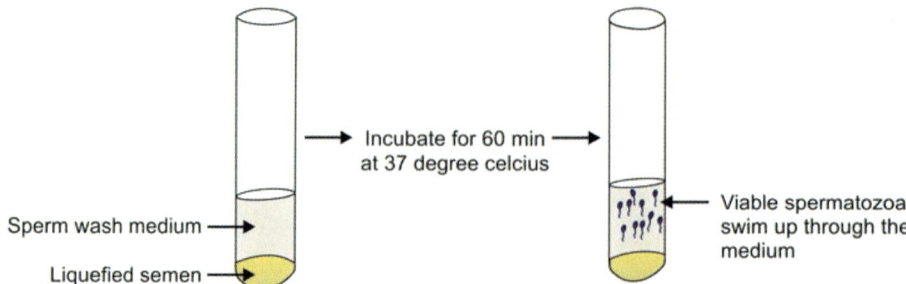

Fig. 15.3: The swim-up technique

g. Following centrifugation, discard the supernatant and resuspend the sperm pellet in 0.5 mL of medium for semen analysis and insemination.

Swim up from Washed Pellet

This technique involves the use of washed pellet prepared after double centrifugation and washing steps, resulting in a pellet of sperm on the bottom of the tube.

Procedure

a. Remove 500 microlitre aliquots of the liquefied semen sample and place in a series of round bottom sterile plastic tubes
b. Mix 1 mL of culture medium with each aliquot
c. Centrifuge for 6–10 minutes at $600 \times G$
d. Remove the supernatant from each tube
e. Resuspend 1 mL culture with the sperm pellet and centrifuge again for 6–10 minutes
f. Remove the supernatant from each tube
g. Gently overlay the sperm pellet with 1 mL culture medium

h. Place in incubator for 45–60 min
i. Gently remove 80% of the culture medium and reassess sperm concentration and motility for therapeutic use

Q12. Describe density gradient centrifugation. Enumerate its advantages and disadvantages

Density gradient centrifugation technique separates spermatozoa based on their density.
- A mature morphologically normal spermatozoa has a higher density of 1.10 g/mL compared to an immature and morphologically abnormal spermatozoa with a density between 1.06 and 1.09 g/mL.
- As a result, (a) leukocytes and cell debris at the interphases between seminal plasma and 40 percent medium and (b) morphologically abnormal sperm with poor motility in between 40 percent and upper part of the 80 percent medium are discarded. Highly motile, morphologically normal, viable spermatozoa forming a pellet at the bottom of the tube are selected for analysis and insemination.

Table 15.2: Advantages and disadvantages of swim up technique	
Advantages	*Disadvantages*
Easy to perform	Best results are obtained with ejaculates with high counts
Cost effective	Low yield
Highly motile fractions are recovered	Decrease in number of sperms with normal condensed chromatin
	Sperm can be massively damaged by ROS because of the close cell-to-cell contact during the centrifugation step particularly in patients with male genital tract infections
	Use of concentrated pellet may result in trapping of some motile spermatozoa

Steps of semen preparation by density gradient centrifugation technique (Fig. 15.4):

a. Prepare the density-gradient medium in a test-tube by layering 1 mL of 40% (v/v) density-gradient medium over 1 mL of 80% (v/v) density-gradient medium.

b. Mix the semen sample well and place 1 mL of semen above the density-gradient media and centrifuge at 300–400 × g for 15–30 minutes.

c. Remove the supernatant from the sperm pellet.

d. Resuspend the sperm pellet in 5 mL of supplemented medium and centrifuge at 200 × g for 4–10 minutes.

e. Repeat the washing procedure (steps 4 and 5 above).

f. Resuspend the final pellet in supplemented medium for semen analysis and insemination.

Q13. What is MACS? Describe its principle, technique and advantages and disadvantages

MACS, or magnetic activated cell sorting, is a new sperm selection technique that distinguishes spermatozoa with DNA fragmentation level of 30% or higher from the non fragmented ones.

Principle

In normal viable spermatozoa with intact plasma membrane, phosphatidyl serine is located on the inner leaflet of plasma membrane. Transportation of phosphatidyl serine from inner leaflet to outer leaflet, i.e externalization occurs in apoptotic cells.

Table 15.3: Advantages and disadvantages of density gradient centrifugation	
Advantages	*Disadvantages*
• Eliminates majority of leukocytes, debris, non motile spermatozoa • Higher yield of motile spermatozoa(>20%) • Effectively separates motile spermatozoa in oligozoospermic samples • Separates morphologically abnormal and fragmented sperm DNA	• Production of good interphases can take some time. • Risk of contamination from endotoxins in gradient medium. • May negatively affect sperm DNA integrity.

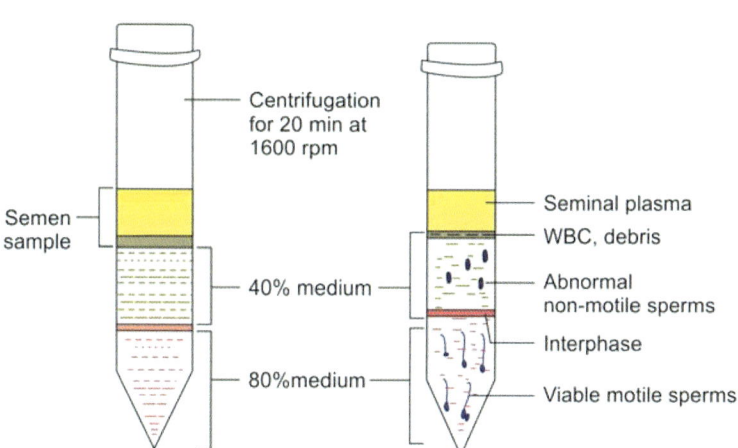

Fig. 15.4: Density gradient centrifugation

Annexin v has high affinity to phosphatidyl-serine but does not have the ability to pass intact membrane, therefore annexin v binding to spermatozoa characterizes disturbed sperm membrane integrity.

Therefore, in MACS, annexin v conjugated biodegradable microbeads (50 mm) are used to separate non apoptotic spermatozoa from those with deteriorated plasma membrane and externalization of phosphatidylserine.

Procedure

Following are the steps of sperm selection by MACS:

a. Semen sample is incubated at room temperature with annexin v conjugated microbeads for 15 min.
b. Sperm microbial suspension is loaded into a separate column containing iron spheres which is fitted in a magnet
c. Magnetic field of 5T is then applied between the poles of the magnet and up to 1.5 T within the iron spheres of column.
d. Cells which are labelled with microbeads and retained on MACS column constitute apoptotic fraction while unlabelled cells passing through the column constitute non apoptotic fraction.
e. Column is then removed from the separator and the retained cells are eluted using annexin v binding buffer.

Q14. What is glass wool filtration technique of semen preparation? Describe its principle, procedure, advantages and disadvantages.

Glass wool filtration is a technique of separation of motile from immotile sperms by means of densely packed glass wool fibres.

Principle

Self propelled movement of sperm cells along with filtration effect of glass wool fibres results in separation of motile spermatozoa from immotile spermatozoa, debris and leukocytes.

Procedure

Following are the steps of glass wool filtration technique:

a. 5–30 mg of glass wool is packed in Pasteur pipette and flushed with 2 mL sterile IVF medium
b. The glass wool column is then put on a new sterile test tube and filled with 1–3 mL of liquefied fresh semen.
c. The test tube is then placed in incubator at 37 degree Celsius where filtration occurs
d. Immediately after the semen has passed through the glass wool, the column is washed with 0.5 mL IVF medium followed by centrifugation at $300 \times g$ for 10 min
e. Following centrifugation, supernatant is discarded and pellet is suspended with IVF medium.

Table 15.4: Advantages and Disadvantages of MACS	
Advantages	*Disadvantages*
Acts at the molecular level as opposed to routine sperm preparation techniques that rely on sperm density and motility	MACS, removes only apoptotic spermatozoa To remove other substances in the ejaculate like leukocytes and debris, other techniques such as density gradient centrifugation is required along with it
Only known technique which separates apoptotic spermatozoa from non-apoptotic spermatozoa	
Rapid, convenient and non-invasive	
Optimizes the results of cryopreservation and thawing .	
Bead detachment after MACS is not necessary	

Table 15.5: Advantages and disadvantages of glass wool filtration	
Advantages	*Disadvantages*
Selects sperm cells with normal chromatin condensation	It does not result in as clean fraction
Higher percentage of spermatozoa with intact acrosome recovered	as swim up technique
Eliminates 90% leukocytes thereby reducing ROS significantly	

Q15. Describe the technique of semen preparation in HIV infected semen samples.

Viral RNA and proviral DNA are found free in seminal plasma and in non-sperm cells of HIV infected persons. HIV receptors (CD4, CCR5, CXCR4) are expressed only by non-sperm cells, therefore density-gradient centrifugation followed by swim-up technique is used to prevent infection of uninfected female partners[3]

Q16. Describe the technique of preparing semen samples obtained by PESA and TESE.

Percutaneous epididymal sperm aspiration (PESA)

- Epididymal aspirates usually have minimal contamination from red blood cells and non-germ cells.
- If large numbers of epididymal spermatozoa are obtained, the most effective technique of preparing them is by density gradient centrifugation. If less number of spermatozoa are obtained, a simple wash can be performed

Testicular sperm extraction (TESE)

- Testicular spermatozoa can be retrieved either by open biopsy (with or without microdissection) or by percutaneous needle biopsy. The testicular aspirates are usually contaminated with non-germ cells and red blood cells.
- In order to separate testicular spermatozoa, enzymatic or mechanical methods can be used.
  - In enzymatic method, the testicular tissue is incubated with collagenase (e.g. 0.8 mg of clostridium histolyticum, type 1A

per mL of medium) for 1.5–2 hours at 37°C, vortexing every 30 minutes.
  - In mechanical method, tissue is centrifuged at 100 × g for 10 minutes and pellet is examined.

Since sperm numbers are low and their motility is poor, testicular spermatozoa are prepared for ICSI.

Q17. Describe the technique of processing sperm suspensions for intracytoplasmic sperm injection (ICSI)

Steps of semen processing for ICSI are as follows:[1]

a. Add 1.5 mL of culture medium to the sample obtained and then centrifuge at 300 × g for 8–10 minutes.
b. Following centrifugation, remove the supernatant and resuspend the pellet in 0.5 mL of culture medium.
c. Remove the supernatant and resuspend the pellet in 0.5 mL of fresh culture medium.
d. Estimate the motility and number of spermatozoa in the pellet. (Some specimens with a low number of spermatozoa may need to be resuspended in a lower volume of medium).
e. Place a 5–10 microlitre droplet of culture medium in a culture dish.
f. Cover it with mineral oil (pre-equilibrated with CO2).
g. Add 5–10 microlitre of the sperm suspension into the culture medium.
h. Aspirate the motile spermatozoa found at the interface between the culture medium and oil with an ICSI pipette and transfer them to a droplet of viscous solution, e.g. polyvinylpyrrolidone 7–10% (100 g/L) medium.

Q18. What is retrograde ejaculation. Describe semen-processing technique for persons affected with retrograde ejaculation.

In retrograde ejaculation, semen passes into the bladder at ejaculation, resulting in aspermia, or no apparent ejaculate. It is diagnosed by examining the urine sample following ejaculation, for the presence of spermatozoa.

Steps of processing semen samples obtained from persons suffering from retrograde ejaculation are as following:

a. Ingestion of sodium bicarbonate prior to ejaculation .This alkalinizes the urine and increases the chances of spermatozoa passing into the urine to retain their viability.
b. At the laboratory, the person gives first urine sample without emptying the bladder completely and then produces an ejaculate by masturbation into a specimen container.
c. Following ejaculation, he gives second urine sample in a separate specimen container containing culture medium .This alkalinizes the urine further.
d. Both urine samples and the ejaculate are analysed for the presence of spermatozoa.
e. The urine sample is concentrated by centrifugation at $500 \times g$ for 8 minutes.
f. The retrograde specimen, once concentrated, and the antegrade specimen, if produced, are then processed using the density-gradient preparation method[1].

Q19. How is semen sample recovered from patients with ejaculatory dysfunction? Describe the semen processing technique of such samples?

Semen from men with disturbed ejaculation, or who cannot ejaculate, may be collected by direct vibratory stimulation of the penis or rectal electrical stimulation of the accessory organs.

Ejaculates from men with spinal cord injury will frequently have high sperm concentrations, decreased sperm motility and red and white blood cell contamination. Therefore, specimens obtained by electro-ejaculation can be processed most effectively by density-gradient centrifugation[1].

Q20. What are the new approaches for sperm selection?

New approaches for sperm selection are:
a. ICSI
b. PICSI
c. IMSI
d. Lasers to immobilize sperm

Q21. What is PICSI. Describe its principle, indication, procedure and advantages.

PICSI is physiological intracytoplasmic sperm injection.

Principle: Hyaluronan, a naturally occurring protein, is found on the membrane surrounding the egg. PICSI is based on ability of sperm to bind hyaluronan (HA) hydrogel mimicking natural binding of sperm to oocyte

Indications

- Low fertilization rate after ICSI
- Compromised embryo development in previous cycles
- History of miscarriage
- High sperm DNA fragmentation

Procedure

The drops of HA are placed in the ICSI dish. To the dish is added a drop of prepared semen. HA bound sperms are then selected for injection.

Advantages

Selects better quality, mature sperms with less DNA damage.

Q22. Write a short note on IMSI.

IMSI is a technique used in IVF treatment to examine and select sperm using a high magnification digital imaging microscope for microinjection into the egg.

The individual sperm can be examined at 6,600 times magnification in comparison to 400 times magnification in ICSI. This allows identification of spermatozoon with a normal nucleus, defined by an oval shape, smooth configuration and a normal nuclear content (with less than 4% of the nucleus occupied by vacuoles).

Indications

- High rate of sperm aneuploidy
- High levels of DNA fragmentation
- Repeated ICSI failures
- Marked alterations of seminal parameters due to severe testiculopathy

Q23. What is intrauterine insemination (IUI)?

In intrauterine insemination, the washed and processed semen sample of the male partner that contains highly motile sperms is deposited in the womb of the female partner using fine catheters at the anticipated time of ovulation.

Q24. What is the rationale behind intra-uterine insemination?

In intrauterine insemination, concentrated pellet of motile sperms is deposited into the uterine cavity close to tubal ostia around the time of ovulation thereby,

- Hostile acidic vaginal pH and cervical mucus is bypassed.
- Better quality and more number of sperms enters the uterine cavity.
- Being timed near ovulation ensures good chance of fertilization.
- Removing detrimental elements like seminal plasma, WBC and dead sperms in the seminal plasma.
- Overcoming faulty coital technique.

Q25. What are the indications of IUI?

The indications for IUI are given in Table 15.6.

Q26. What are the Indications for donor IUI?

Indications for donor IUI are:[3]
- Azoospermia with testicular failure
- Severely abnormal semen parameters
- Hereditary disease in man
- Severe untreatable Rh alloimmunisation in wife
- Same sex couples

Q27. What are the prerequisites for IUI?

Prerequisites for IUI are:
- Proper indication
- Satisfactory semen analysis
- Patent, healthy fallopian tubes
- Evidence of ovulation
- Raised FSH threshold in early follicular phase with either oral ovulation inducing agent and/or injections of exogenous gonadotropin preparations
- Identification of spontaneous LH surge
- Responsive endometrium.

Q28. What are the selection criteria for IUI?

Selection criteria for IUI are as follows:
- Female age <40 years
- Minimum of 1.5 years of infertility
- Patent fallopian tubes confirmed by laparoscopy or hysterosalpingogram
- Presumptive proof of ovulatory cycle
- Ultrasound evidence of mature follicles and ovulation
- Luteal phase progesterone (P) levels >35 nmol/L

Table 15.6: Indications for IUI	
Male factors that require IUI	*Female factors that require IUI*
• Retrograde ejaculation	• Vaginismus
• Impotence or ejaculatory dysfunction	• Cervical hostility
• Hypospadias	• Ovulatory dysfunction
• Hypospermia	• Mild Endometriosis
• Non liquefying/highly viscous semen	• Allergy to seminal plasma
• Subnormal semen parameters	• Unexplained infertility
• Seminal anti sperm antibody	
• Non-availability of partner during the fertile period due to work or other reasons	
• HIV/HBsAg/HCV positive male partner, to reduce the risk of transmission in the female partner	
• Unexplained infertility	

- Two semen analysis revealing at least 10 million recovered motile sperm/whole sample.

Q29. Describe in detail the requisites for laboratory and the equipment for IUI.

Requisites for IUI Laboratory are as following[4]:
- The room should be as close as possible to procedure room.
- The room must have its own air conditioning.
- There must not be any free access to any toxic fumes.
- Sufficient space to accommodate necessary equipments.
- There must be suitable facilities for sperm preparation.

IUI Laboratory Pieces of Equipment Include

A. Semen assessment and sperm preparation
- Makler counting chambers (Fig. 15.5)
- Microscope phase contrast microscope with resolving power 4, 10, 40, 100 with eyepiece 10x.
- Centrifuge machine with swing-out rotor, timer and RPM meter (Fig. 15.6)
- 5% CO_2 incubator with 37 degree Celsius with gas cylinder
- Laminar flow hood (horizontal/vertical) (Fig. 15.7)
- Wide mouth sterile semen collecting jar

B. Semen assessment and sperm preparation
- Sterile test tub
- Sterile conical/round bottom tubes
- Pipette
- Test tube rack
- Media
- Good light source
- CASA system

C. Gynecological equipment
- Cusco's speculum
- IUI catheter
- Uterine sound
- Cervical dilator 5/6 mm
- Allis forceps

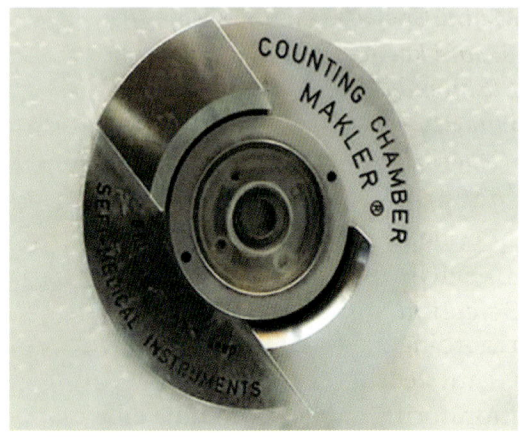

Fig. 15.5: Makler counting chamber for HSA

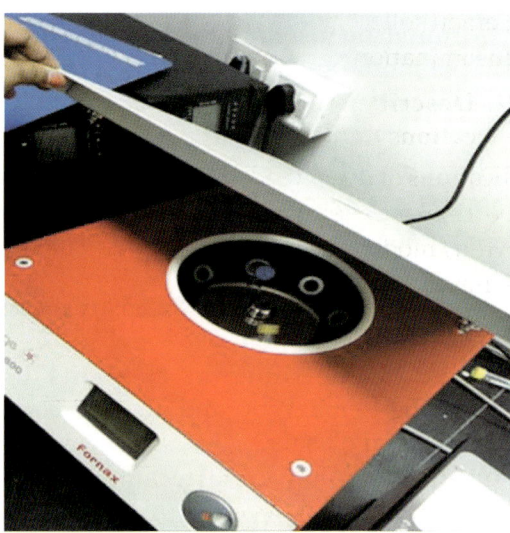

Fig. 15.6: Centrifuge machine with swing-out rotor, timer and RPM meter

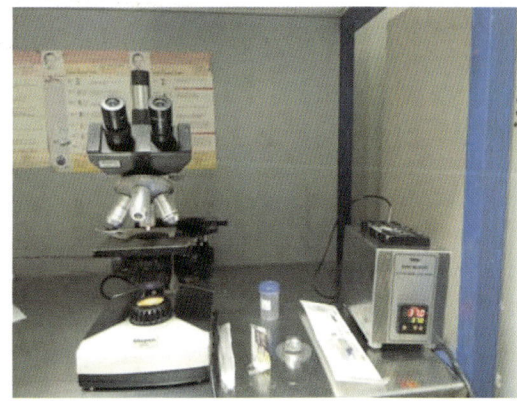

Fig. 15.7: Integrated Laminar flow IUI working station

D.*Media:* Sperm preparation media

E. *Record keeping and documentation*

F. *Maintenance of equipment*

G. *Quality control methods and laboratory asepsis should be in place*

Q30. What are the steps involved in an IUI cycle?

Steps of IUI are:

a. Selection and counseling of the couple regarding the procedure and success rate

b. Controlled ovarian Stimulation (COH)

c. Monitoring by folliculometry and endometrial thickness

d. Ovulation trigger

e. Semen collection and preparation

f. Insemination

Q31. Describe natural cycle IUI, its indications and monitoring.

Indications of natural cycle IUI are:

a. Normal female partner

b. Mild/moderate male factor

c. Unexplained infertility

Monitoring in natural cycle IUI is done either by TVS or LH surge.

- LH surge monitoring is done from D9, when positive, IUI is done after 24 hours

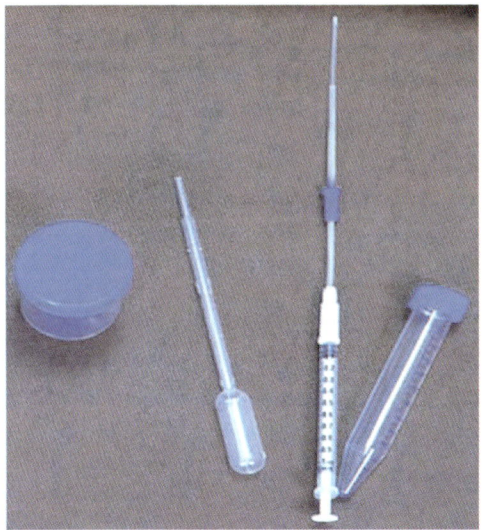

Fig. 15.8: Semen collecting jar, 3 mL pipette, IUI catheter with attached 1mL BD syringe and conical tube

- TVS is performed from D9. When dominant follicle is >/= 20 mm and the trilaminar endometrium >7–8 mm, HCG trigger is given for ovulation and IUI is done after 36 hours.[5]

Q32. What are the advantages of coupling controlled ovarian hyperstimulation with IUI?

Advantages of coupling COH with IUI are:

- Timing of HCG injection predicts ovulation better, so as to schedule IUI near ovulation
- COH offers more ova for fertilization and implantation, hence increases success

Q33. What are the criteria for optimum ovarian stimulation for IUI?

Criteria for optimum ovarian stimulation for IUI are as following[5]:

- 2–3 follicles measuring 18–19 mm.
- Serum E2 levels 150–200 pg/mL per 15 mm follicles
- Endometrium >9 mm and trilaminar
- IUI between cycle D13 and D 16

Q34. What is the cancellation criteria for IUI?

Cancellation criteria for IUI are:[6]

a. >3 follicles >15 mm or >3 follicles >12 mm

b. E2 levels >1500 pg/mL

Q35. What is the timing of ovulation trigger in stimulated IUI?

Timing of ovulation trigger is important:

- Patients undergoing stimulated IUI with gonadotropins should be administered ovulation trigger when the dominant follicle diameter reaches 18 mm.
- Patients undergoing stimulated IUI with Clomiphene should be administered trigger when the dominant follicular diameter reaches 20–24 mm.

Q36. Which drugs should be used as ovulation trigger?

Different ovulation triggers used are as following:

- Urinary HCG-5-10,000 IU
- Recombinant HCG -250 μg

- GnRH agonist -1 mg/mL
- Recombinant LH-5000 to 15000 IU.

Q37. When should insemination be done?

Single or double IUI is done:

- Single IUI should be performed 36–40 hours after administration of HCG trigger for ovulation. Alternatively, after detecting at least one follicle >17 mm, an endogenous spontaneous LH surge should be detected using urinary LH kits and IUI should be performed after 20 to 30 hours.
- Double IUI is performed at 12–18 hours and 34–42 hours of ovulation trigger assuming that first IUI provides a sufficient number of motile spermatozoa close to the first ovulated oocyte (s) and additional sperms provided by second oocyte to fertilize the oocyte ovulated subsequently.

Q38. Is double IUI advantageous over single IUI?

Most of the studies comparing single versus double IUI have concluded that single IUI is less expensive and yields similar pregnancy rates as compared to two insemination in a single cycle.[7]

Q39. Describe the technique of intrauterine insemination?

The procedure for IUI is as follows (Fig. 15.9):

- Within the target time of 90 mins from collection till insemination, patient with full bladder is placed in lithotomy position.

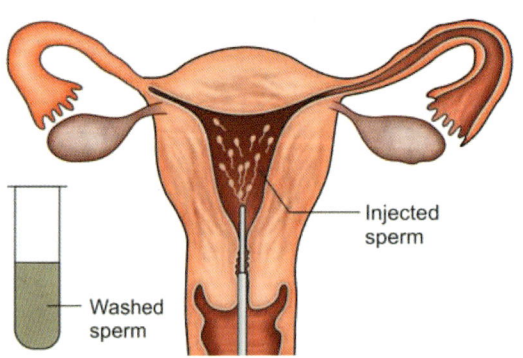

Fig. 15.9: IUI technique

- Sample is loaded in IUI catheter. There should be no free space remaining at the tip of the catheter.
- Cusco speculum is inserted in the vagina to visualize cervix and cervical mucus if present is removed.
- Insemination is then done in the uterine cavity.
- Thereafter, the patient is asked to rest for 10 mins.

Q40. Is post IUI antibiotic or progestational support required?

The couple needs to be infection free prior to IUI. If semen shows pyospermia or speculum insertion shows infection, it is better to clear it prior to IUI.IUI per se doesn't increase the risk of infection and, therefore, the antibiotic support is not required.

Luteal progestational support should be individualized and should be given only when indicated.[4]

Q41. What is the success rate of IUI?

The success rate of natural cycle IUI is 8.4%, ovulation induction and IUI is 12 to 18%. The success rate may decline with advanced maternal age.[3]

Q42. Enumerate the factors in male affecting IUI success.

Factors in male affecting IUI success are as following:[7]

a. Type of treatment.
b. Total motile sperm count (TMSC)—an average total motile sperm count in the native sperm sample of 5–10 million is the threshold value for decision about treating a couple with IUI or IVF.
c. Sperm quality—initial total sperm motility (TM) >30%, the inseminating motile sperm count (IMC) of >1 million and 4% normal morphology is critical
d. Sperm preparation technique—with abnormal semen analysis density gradient is superior to swim up technique whereas with normal semen analysis, the swim

up technique is sufficient for selecting spermatozoa

Q43. How many IUI cycles should be? What should be done following repeated IUI failure?

A patient can be offered 3–6 cycles of ovulation induction with IUI. However, the fecundity in the first three cycles of COH and IUI is significantly higher than in cycles 4–6.

If there is no conception with 3–6 ovulatory cycles in a woman in the presence of normal semen parameters, it is assumed that the cause of infertility is other than the gametes and these patients need further evaluation by laprohysteroscopy or reference to an ART center for IVF as an option[9].

Q44. What are the causes of failure of IUI?

Causes of failed IUI are:
a. Poor semen preparation
b. Poor selection of patients
c. Improper egg pick-up by fimbria due to peritubal adhesions
d. Prevalence of empty follicle syndrome or poor oocyte quality.
e. Other causes are:
   – Cause of infertility: Least pregnancy rate in male infertility and severe endometriosis
   – Age >35 years in woman and >40 years in men
   – Duration of infertility >5 years
   – Number of IUI cycles >3
   – Sperm parameters TMSC <5 million
   – Not using controlled ovarian hyperstimulation

Q45. How can IUI be made cost effective?

IUI can be made cost effective by following methods:[10]
a. Minimum investigations
b. If gonadotropins are required, low dose protocol is preferred since pregnancy rates do not differ from high dose regimen. Highly purified HMG is preferred as recombinant FSH is costlier and no difference in ongoing pregnancy rate has been found when either of the gonadotropins are used.
c. USG monitoring should be done for follicle monitoring and endometrial development. Serum estradiol levels should be performed only when
   – Woman is at risk of hyperstimulation
   – Ultrasound shows adequate follicular growth but poor endometrial growth indicating either a low estradiol levels/follicle raising questions about the health of oocyte in the follicle and possibility of empty follicle syndrome and the fault at the level of endometrium.
d. Right timing of ovulation trigger or by use of LH kit in unstimulated cycles.
e. By doing only one insemination in the cycle.
f. Proper sperm washing method which is cheaper should be used.
g. Referral to IVF unit after 3–6 IUI cycles.

Q46. What are the contraindications to IUI?

Contraindications for IUI are:
a. Blocked tubes, major tubal pathology
b. Genital tract infection in either wife or husband
c. Severe abnormality in semen parameters (low count <5 million in pre wash sample, as the nospermia, severe teratospermia)
d. Genetic reason for poor semen parameters
e. Advanced age of female partner
f. Multiple etiologies/coexisting factors for infertility
g. Multiple previous failures for IUI

Q47. What are the possible complications of IUI?

Complications are:[6]
• Ectopic pregnancy—3 to 5%
• Allergy to components of medium e.g. albumin, antibiotic—rare
• Infection—0.01 to 0.2%
• Multiple pregnancy and ovarian hyperstimulation syndrome (OHSS)—COH related
• Miscarriage rate—20 to 30%, not related to IUI but to couples which get chosen for IUI.

Key Points

- Intrauterine insemination is an important technique for assisted reproduction.
- IUI is useful for both male and female factor infertility.
- Partner's or donor semen can be used for IUI
- Semen needs to be prepared before using for IUI
- Semen is prepared for IUI by various methods in a well equipped lab.

REFERENCES

1. WHO laboratory manual of examination and processing of human semen: WHO 2010
2. Ralf Henkel. Sperm Processing for IVF, Clinical Embryology: A Practical Guide, 2013:13-21.
3. Selection, counselling and workup of patients for IUI. In: Tandulwadkar S, Mittal B, eds. Optimizing IUI results: A guide to gynecologists. 1st ed. Jaypee brothers medical publishers (P) Ltd, 2010: 15-16.
4. Setting up an IUI laboratory. In: Tandulwadkar S, Mittal B, eds. Optimizing IUI results: A guide to gynecologists. 1st ed. Jaypee brothers medical publishers (P) Ltd, 2010:133-40.
5. Bhattacharya S, Harrrild K, Mollison J, Words worth S, Tay C, Harrold A, et al. Clomiphene citrate or unstimulated intrauterine insemination compared with expectant management for unexplained infertility: pragmatic randomized controlled trial. BMJ 2008:337:a716.
6. Recombinant Gonadotropin for ovulation induction and IUI. In: Tandulwadkar S, Mittal B, eds. Optimizing IUI results: A guide to gynecologists. 1st ed. Jaypee brothers medical publishers (P) Ltd, 2010:110-113.
7. Ombelet W, Vandeput H, Van de Putte G, Cox A, Janssen M, Jacobs B et al. Intrauterine insemination after ovarian stimulation with clomiphene citrate: predictive potential of inseminating motile sperm count and sperm morphology. Human Reprod 1997;12:1458-63.
8. Cantineau AEP, Heineman MJ, Cohlen BJ. Single versus double IUI in stimulated cycle for subfertile couples. Cochrane database systematic Review 2003;(1):CD 003854
9. IUI results and coping with failure. In: Tandulwadkar S, Mittal B, eds. Optimizing IUI results: A guide to gynecologists. 1st ed. Jaypee brothers medical publishers (P) Ltd, 2010: 209–13.
10. Cost effective IUI. In: Tandulwadkar S, Mittal B, eds. Optimizing IUI results: A guide to gynecologists. 1st ed. Jaypee brothers medical publishers (P) Ltd, 2010:16–23.

IVF Protocols and Procedures

Nilanchali Singh, Komal Rastogi

The global burden of infertility remains high over the years. The National Institute for Health and Care Excellence (NICE) recommends in-vitro fertilisation (IVF) as the definitive treatment for prolonged unresolved infertility after other treatments have failed. In vitro fertilization (IVF) involves a sequence of highly coordinated steps beginning with controlled ovarian hyperstimulation with exogenous gonadotropins, followed by transvaginal ultrasound guided retrieval of oocytes, fertilization in the laboratory and transcervical transfer of embryos into the uterus. The first pregnancy resulting from IVF was reported in 1976, and was ectopic.[1] The first child resulting from IVF was born in 1978.[2]

Q1. What are the different types of ovarian stimulation regimens for IVF?

For answer see Table 16.1.

Q2. Describe the GnRH agonist and GnRH antagonist protocol and compare the two?

GnRH agonist down-regulation gonadotropin stimulation—The "Long" Protocol: Commercial preparations of GnRH agonists are deca-peptides similar to GnRH with modifications at two amino acid residues, which increases both the half-life and the receptor binding affinities.[3] Over the course of 10–14 days, agonists initially up regulate pituitary GnRH receptor activity leading to flare response which is then followed by receptor desensitization resulting in suppression of pituitary gonadotropins and with high doses and prolonged use, eventually decreases GnRH receptor numbers.[3–5]

GnRH agonists are commercially available for either depot or daily use and can be administered intramuscularly or subcutaneously (leuprolide, triptorelin, or buserelin) or intranasally (buserelin and nafarelin).

	Previous terminology	Aim	Methods
Table 16.1: The different types of ovarian stimulation regimens for IVF			
Natural cycle	Unstimulated, spontaneous cycle	Single oocyte	No medication
Modified natural cycle	Semi-natural, controlled natural cycle IVF	Single oocyte	hCG only, GnRH antagonist and FSH/HMG add-back
Mild	Soft, minimal stimulation, 'friendly' IVF	2–7 oocytes	Low dose FSH/HMG, oral compounds (clomiphene/lertozole) and GnRH anta-gonists
Conventional	Standard, routine COS	>8 oocytes	GnRH agonist or antagonist, conventional FSH/HMG dose

In the long protocol, GnRH agonist is started in the luteal phase (day 21) of the previous cycle in the dose of 1 mg or 0.5 mg daily for approximately 10 days or until onset of menses starting from day 21 of previous cycle (Fig. 16.1), decreasing to 0.5 mg or 0.2 mg daily until human chorionic gonadotropin (hCG) is administered. Gonadotropins stimulation begins from day 2 of next cycle after confirming that effective pituitary down regulation has been achieved (serum estradiol levels <30–40 pg/mL and pelvic ultrasound showing no follicles >10 mm in diameter). The starting doses of gonadotropins range between 150 and 300 IU of urinary FSH, recombinant FSH or urinary menotropins (hMG). Any of the step-up (beginning with a low dose and increasing as necessary based on response) or step-down (beginning with a higher dose and decreasing as necessary based on response) protocol can be used. Response is monitored with serial measurements of serum estradiol and transvaginal ultrasonography. The first estradiol levels are obtained after 3–5 days of stimulation. Thereafter, serum estradiol concentrations and sonography are obtained every 1–3 days and gonadotropins dosages are adjusted. Stimulation continues until at least two follicles measure 17–18 mm diameter and others typically measure 14–16 mm. Endometrial thickness is also monitored simultaneously using transvaginal ultrasound. When the cohort of ovarian follicles reaches maturity, hCG 10,000 IU im is administered to stimulate final stages of follicular development. The equivalent dose of recombinant hCG is 250 ug.

Gonadotropin-releasing hormone antagonist protocol: GnRH antagonists (cetrorelix and ganirelix) are developed by modifying the GnRH decapeptide at six positions. GnRH antagonists block the GnRH receptor in a dose dependent competitive fashion and cause immediate suppression of pituitary gonadotropins. GnRH antagonists are administered in a dose of 0.25 mg daily subcutaneously. They can also be given as 3 mg single dose, which will prevent an LH surge for 96 hours.

The treatment protocol (Fig. 16.2) may be fixed which involves starting antagonist on day (D_4–D_7) of stimulation regardless of follicular response[6] or flexible (i.e. starting antagonist when the leading follicle reaches 12–16 mm in diameter) or (when estradiol level has risen above 600 pg/mL.[7]) Fixed protocol was found to be associated with higher pregnancy rates when compared to flexible protocol in one meta-analysis involving four randomized trials, however, true superiority of one approach over the other remains to be determined.[8]

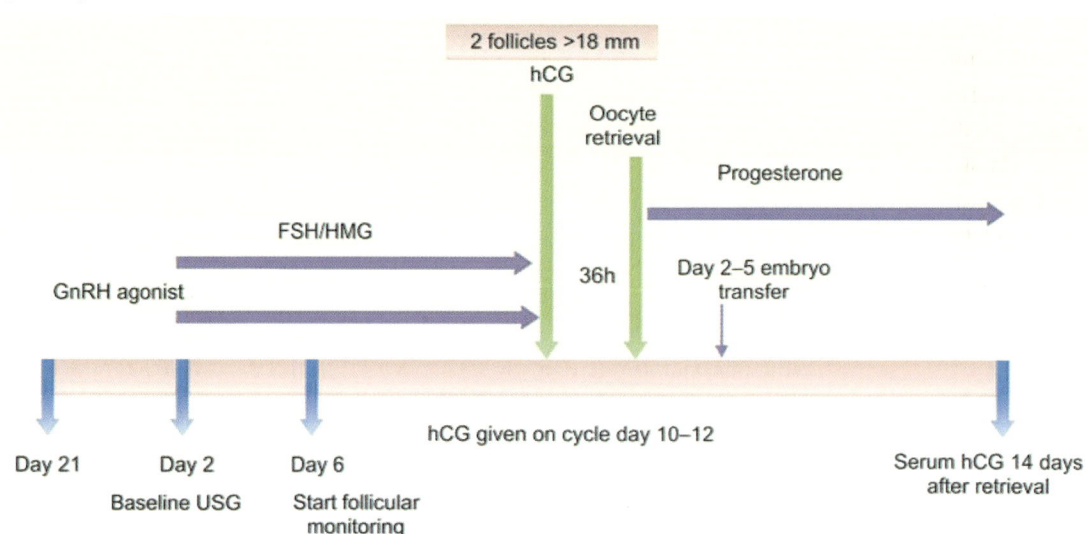

Fig. 16.1: GnRH agonist protocol—the long protocol

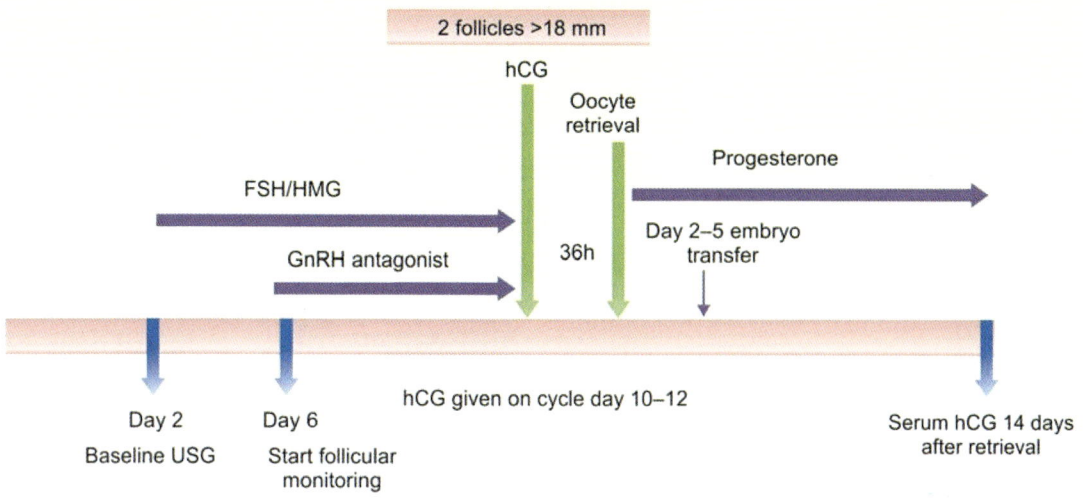

Fig. 16.2: GnRH antagonist protocol

Comparison between GnRH agonist and GnRH antagonist protocol

GnRH agonist protocol	GnRH antagonist protocol
Lengthy down regulation phase with initial flare effect	Immediate suppression
Receptor desensitization	Competitive antagonist
Increased dose of gonadotropin required, more expensive	Lesser dose of gonadotropin required, less expensive
Time consuming	Shorter regimen
Inconvenient due to more number of injections	Convenient due to lesser injections
Increased risk of OHSS	Less risk of OHSS
GnRH agonist cannot be used as trigger	GnRH agonist can be used as trigger in patients at high risk for OHSS

A Cochrane review of 27 randomized controlled trials compared the two protocols and concluded that while the number of good quality embryos produced for transfer are similar, clinical pregnancy rates are higher by 4.7% in agonist compared to antagonist cycles. The number of oocytes retrieved and live birth rates also favoured agonist usage.[9]

Q3. Describe the various GnRH agonist protocols?

GnRH agonist long protocol	GnRH agonist administration begins in mid luteal phase and continues throughout the follicular phase (described above)
Ultrashort protocol	• GnRH agonist from 1st to 3rd day of the cycle followed by gonadotropin stimulation from day 3 of the cycle • Uses initial stimulatory effect of GnRH agonist on gonadotropin secretion
Short protocol	GnRH agonist from day 1 of the cycle until the day of hCG trigger, gonadotropin stimulation begins from day 3 of the cycle
Stop protocol	GnRH agonist administration begins in the mid luteal phase and ends with the onset of menses followed by high dose stimulation with gonadotropins

The "short" or "flare" protocol uses both the brief initial flare response to a GnRH agonist and pituitary suppression following its long-term use. In a typical short protocol, leuprolide acetate is administered in a dose of 1 mg daily for three days following which the dose is reduced to half. Gonadotropin stimulation (225–450 IU daily) begins on cycle day 3. The dose of gonadotropins is adjusted depending upon ovarian response and indications for hCG administration are same as that of long protocol. This regimen may cause significant increase in serum progesterone and androgen levels due to late corpus luteum rescue thus affecting oocyte quality and pregnancy rates.

The "OC Microdose GnRH agonist flare" (Fig. 16.3) protocol is a variation of standard short protocol and involves 14–21 days of suppression with an oral contraceptive pill; followed by microdose of leuprolide acetate (40 µg BD) starting 3 days after the last pill or from day 2 after confirming pituitary down regulation. High-dose gonadotropins are started from day 3 of leuprolide therapy. This protocol does not cause rise in serum progesterone and androgen levels and may be useful in poor responders, in whom it can stimulate endogenous FSH release and may yield lower cancellation rates and higher serum estradiol levels and pregnancy rates.[10] The ultra short, short and stop protocols, all were developed in order to improve outcomes in women with poor ovarian response but there is still no one pituitary down-regulation protocol that best suits all women with such condition.

Q4. Describe the technique of oocyte retrieval?

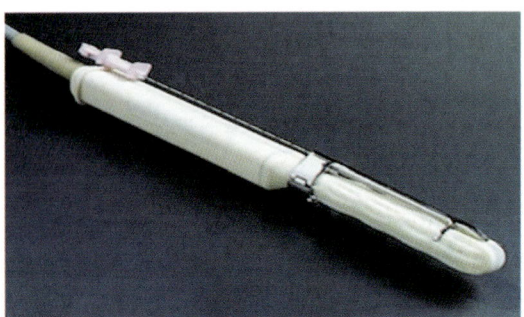

TVS probe with needle guide

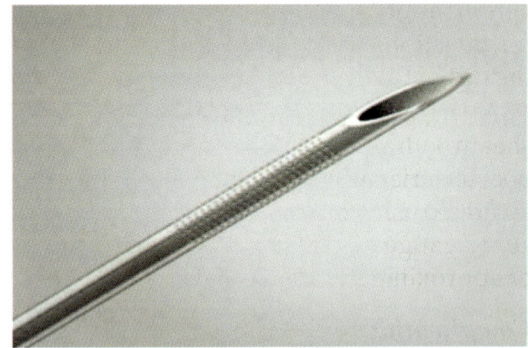

Single lumen needle for oocyte retrieval

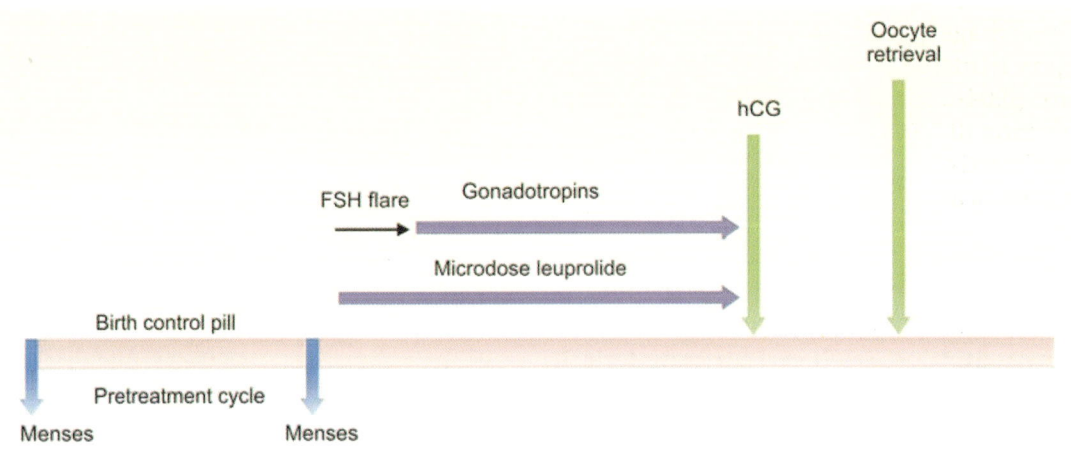

Fig. 16.3: GnRH agonist short protocol

Oocyte retrieval is generally performed approximately 34–36 hrs after hCG administration. The standard technique is transvaginal ultrasound guided aspiration of oocytes under intravenous sedation. Propofol is most commonly used but most women tolerate the procedure very well with conscious sedation using short-acting narcotics like fentanyl. Constant monitoring by pulse oximetry and automated blood pressure recordings are necessary to ensure that proper level of sedation is maintained and not exceeded.

Use of prophylactic antibiotics (cefoxitin 2 g), administered 30 minutes before the procedure is common but is controversial because of low incidence of complications associated with the procedure (0.3–0.6%).[11] Alernatively, oral antibiotics can be started after the procedure (tetracycline, doxycycline), reserving intravenous antibiotics for women at increased risk for infection, i.e. those with endometriosis or history of PID.

A vaginal probe (5–7 MHz) in a sterile plastic sheath with an attached needle guide is used for oocyte retrieval. Follicular fluid and oocytes are aspirated using a specially designed disposable 16–17 gauge needle using a vacuum pressure of approximately 100 mm of Hg.

Complications of oocyte retrieval: (a) Vaginal hemorrhage from a puncture site (8%)—usually can be controlled by direct pressure but sometimes may require a suture; (b) Acute hemorrhage from ovary or hematomas due to injury to uterine, ovarian and iliac vessels are rare (0.04-0.07%); (c) Postoperative pelvic infection (0.3–0.6%)—women with history of salpingitis and those with ovarian endometrioma are at highest risk.

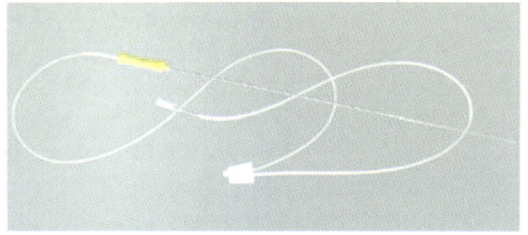

Needle with aspiration system

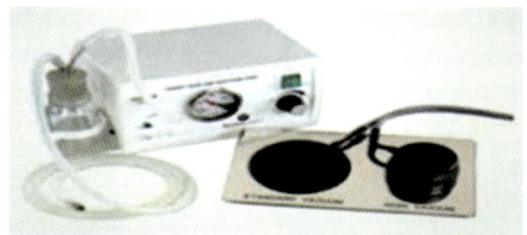

Suction apparatus with foot pump

Q5. Describe ICSI, its indications and sperm retrieval techniques for ICSI?

In the past, men with non-obstructive azoospermia were considered sterile. However, testicular biopsy specimens in such men often demonstrate sperms, suggesting low level production of sperms unable to survive epididymal transit to reach the ejaculate. ICSI has allowed such couples to achieve pregnancy outcomes comparable with those of non-male factor infertility using conventional IVF. Even grossly immature sperm (round spermatid nuclear injection; ROSNI) have now been used to achieve fertilization.

Among the many surgical methods for sperm recovery, the most widely described are microsurgical epididymal sperm aspiration (MESA), percutaneous epididymal sperm aspiration (PESA), testicular sperm extraction (TESE) and percutaneous testicular sperm fine-needle aspiration (TESA). The sperm retrieval techniques are described below:

Microsurgical epididymal sperm aspiration (MESA): It is an open surgical technique done under general or regional anesthesia. The technique involves incision of an isolated dilated tubule, gradually moving more proximally, if necessary, until sperm are obtained. Sperm are collected into a micropipette with gentle compression of the testis and epididymis by capillary action and flushed into a container with a small volume of IVF culture medium. Recovered sperm are then cryopreserved.

Percutaneous epididymal sperm aspiration (PESA): It is done using a fine needle under local anesthesia, but the technique is less reliable. Small quantities of sperm are obtained, which are sometimes inadequate to allow cryopreservation and pregnancy rates are also lower than with the open technique.

Testicular sperm extraction (TESE): This technique yields the greatest number of sperm with potential for cryopreservation and allows sperm retrieval from majority of men, even those with non-obstructive azoospermia. It is an open technique which allows identification of larger caliber tubules that are more likely to yield sperm and magnification minimizes the risk of injury to the testicular blood supply and increases the probability of retrieving a blood free biopsy specimen.[12] In men with non-obstructive azoospermia, TESE is best performed on the day of or day before oocyte retrieval as sperm retrieved in such cases may not be motile or even viable after cryopreservation and thawing and ICSI using immotile sperm may yield poorer results than when performed with motile sperm.[13] In cases where TESE is not possible near the time of oocyte retrieval, elective TESE can be done followed by sperm cryopreservation. The risk of having no viable sperm after thawing is there and donor sperm can be used if needed. If repeat sperm retrievals are needed, the minimum interval between procedures is 6 months to allow for adequate healing.

Percutaneous testicular sperm fine-needle aspiration (TESA): It is done using a fine needle under local anesthesia but is most applicable in men with normal spermatogenesis and obstructive azoospermia.[14]

Intracytoplasmic sperm injection (ICSI): ICSI has allowed couples with male factor infertility to achieve pregnancy outcomes that are comparable with those of couples with non-male factor infertility using conventional IVF treatment. In this procedure, a single selected sperm is first immobilized by compressing the sperm tail with an injection pipette and then drawn into the pipette. The oocyte is stabilized with the polar body at the 6 or 12 o'clock position and entered at 3 o'clock position. The

pipette pierces the zona and oolemma and the sperm is injected directly into the ooplasm of the mature metaphase II egg.

Indications:

- Severe oligospermia (<2 million sperm/mL)
- Asthenospermia (<5% progressive motility)
- Teratospermia (<4% normal forms by strict criteria)
- When surgically retrieved sperms are used
- When treatment includes preimplantation genetic diagnosis
- Couples with previous failed or poor fertilization with conventional IVF

Risks of ICSI:

- Oocyte degeneration can occur even after an uncomplicated procedure with rates as high as 30–50%
- ICSI is associated with a higher risk of congenital anomaly (4.2%) when compared with conventional IVF (2–3%).[15]

Q6. Describe the technique of embryo transfer?

The aim of transcervical embryo transfer is to deliver the embryos atraumatically to an optimal intrauterine location for implantation. Embryo transfer is most commonly performed 3 days after oocyte retrieval and fertilization. The ideal day 3 cleavage stage embryo has 6–8 blastomeres of equal size and no cytoplasmic fragmentation. Best results are obtained with a soft catheter, after an easy transfer and when fundal contact is avoided.[16] Soft catheters are preferred over rigid cathaters to minimize the release of prostaglandins after cervical or endometrial trauma. During embryo transfer, embryos are suspended in 20 µL media at the tip of a syringe with air on either side of the fluid. This creates an air-fluid interface easily seen with ultrasound. Embryo transfer is done under ultrasound guidance to ensure the deposit of the embryos 1.5–2 cm from uterine fundus. Following transfer, the inner and the outer sheath should be removed as a unit and checked for retained embryos.

Q7. What are the embryo transfer guidelines?

The Society for Assisted Reproductive Technology (SART) and the American Society for Reproductive Medicine (ASRM) have offered guidelines for the number of embryos to be transferred. Maternal age and embryo quality are the most important factors influencing the implantation potential of each embryo.

The Guidelines issued in 2009 for number of embryos to be transferred are summarized below:[17]

Prognosis	Age			
	<35 yrs	35–37 yrs	38–40 yrs	41–42 yrs
Cleavage-stage embryos				
Favorable*	1–2	2	3	5
All others	2	3	4	5
Blastocysts				
Favorable*	1	2	2	3
All others	2	2	3	3

*Favorable characteristics—first cycle IVF, Good quality embryo, excess embryos available for cryopreservation, previous successful IVF cycle

Q8. Discuss embryo cryopreservation and describe endometrial preparation for frozen embryo transfer (FET)?

The first pregnancy resulting from transfer of a cryopreserved embryo was reported in 1983. Embryo cryopreservation has now become an integral part of modern ART. Because transfer of cryopreserved embryos is less expensive than a second fresh cycle, overall fertility treatment costs can be optimized. Embryo cryopreservation can also be considered as a means to prevent ovarian hyperstimulation syndrome.

The cryopreservation process has two distinct stages, freezing and thawing. There are two methods for embryo cryopreservation, the "slow-freeze" technique and "vitrification". In both the techniques cellular water is gradually replaced by cryoprotectants (propanediol glycerol, dimethyl sulfoxide).

In the slow freeze method, embryos are sealed in vials, cooled to temperatures between −30°C and −110°C and then stored in liquid nitrogen. In the vitrification method, embryos are flash frozen by immersion into liquid nitrogen, creating a solid glass-like state.[18] After thawing, the process is reversed, the embryos are passed gradually through decreasing concentrations of the cryoprotectant, followed by an interval of culture before transfer. On comparing the two methods, vitrification is associated with higher post thaw survival rates (90–100%) and higher implantation and pregnancy rates.[18] Overall, success rates for frozen embryo transfer cycles are approximately one-half to two-thirds of those observed in fresh cycles as the highest quality embryos are generally selected for fresh transfer.

Endometrial preparation for frozen embryo transfer (FET): In FET cycles, estradiol is given in the early follicular phase and is continued for 13–15 days. Endometrial thickness is assessed using transvaginal ultrasound during estrogen therapy and estrogen administration continues until an optimal thickness of 8 mm is reached. Progesterone is started 48–72 hours prior to transfer when cleavage stage embryos are used and 6–7 days prior to transfer when blastocysts are used. GnRH agonists are commonly used to prevent premature LH surge that might adversely effect endometrial maturation.

Q9. Enumerate the success rates of various ART methods?

	Clinical pregnancy rate/cycle		
	Infertile	Age <35	Age ≥40
CC/TI	3–7%	8–10%	1–4%
IUI/TI	4–9%	—	—
CC/IUI	3–14%	8–19%	1–5%
INJ/IUI	13–19%	9–20%	5–9%
IVF	35%	31–46%	13%

CC, clomiphene citrate; TI, timed intercourse; IUI, intrauterine insemination; INJ, injectable gonadotropins; IVF, in vitro fertilization

Q10. What are the complications of Assisted Reproductive Technology?

a. *Multiple gestation:* The risk of multiple gestation is increased substantially in ART cycles. Multiple gestation in ART cycles occurs at higher rates than 3% rate for spontaneous conception. Success rates increase with the number of embryos transferred, to a point, beyond which only multiple pregnancy rate further increases.

b. *Cycle cancellation:* Cycle cancellation may occur in up to 6% of cycles due to inadequate stimulation response and in 1.5% of cycles because of excessive response in normal responders.

c. *Ectopic and heterotopic pregnancy:* Upto 3.4% of ART pregnancies are ectopic and require treatment with either surgery or methotrexate. The incidence of heterotopic pregnancy is 1% after IVF treatment. Smoking, multiple gestation, previous tubal surgery and prior PID are potential risk factors in addition to ART.

d. *Ovarian hyperstimulation syndrome:* Ovarian hyperstimulation syndrome (OHSS) is a rare, iatrogenic complication of ART and it occurs mostly in association with exogenous gonadotropins. The whole pathophysiology revolves around increased vascular permeability leading to abdominal distension, enlarged ovaries and ascites. Mild OHSS, which is common, occurs in about 20 to 33% in ART cycles.[4,5] Severe OHSS which is associated with extreme morbidity has been reported in 1 to 2% of ART cycles.[4,5] As OHSS is preventable condition, clinicians involved in prescribing ovarian stimulation drugs should be well versed with risk factors and strategies to minimize fatalities.

e. *Risk of cancer after fertility therapy:* Infertility by itself is a predisposing factor for ovarian cancer and breast cancer. Although treatments that promote incessant ovulation and elevated estrogen levels increase cancer risk, data regarding the impact of infertility therapy on neoplasias have been inconsistent and conflicting. A study conducted on a large british cohort of women with ovulatory disorders did not find any evidence to suggest causation for cancer of breast, ovary, colon, skin, or thyroid. However, there was a dose response relationship between development of uterine cancer and prior use of clomiphene, particularly with a lifetime exposure of 2,250 mg or more.[19]

f. *Stress:* Stress is thought to be increased among women with infertility and those undergoing infertility treatment. Stress is the most common reason for patients to terminate fertility treatment.

Key Points

- In the long protocol, GnRH agonist is started in the luteal phase of the previous cycle for approximately 10 days or until onset of menses starting from day 21 of previous cycle. Gonadotropins stimulation begins from day 2 of next cycle after confirming that effective pituitary down regulation has been achieved.
- In antagonist protocol, treatment may be fixed which involve starting antagonist on day 4–7 of stimulation regardless of follicular response or flexible, i.e. starting antagonist when the leading follicle reaches 12–16 mm in diameter or when estradiol level has risen above 600 pg/mL.
- Oocyte retrieval is generally performed approximately 34–36 hours after hCG administration. The standard technique is transvaginal ultrasound guided aspiration of oocytes under intravenous sedation.
- Among the many surgical methods for sperm recovery, the most widely described are microsurgical epididymal sperm aspiration (MESA), percutaneous epididymal sperm aspiration (PESA), testicular sperm extraction (TESE), and percutaneous testicular sperm fine-needle aspiration (TESA).
- Embryo transfer is most commonly performed 3 days after oocyte retrieval and fertilization. The ideal day 3 cleavage stage embryo has 6–8 blastomeres of equal size and no cytoplasmic fragmentation.

REFERENCES

1. Steptoe PC, Edwards RG, Reimplantation of a human embryo with subsequent tubal pregnancy. Lancet 1976;1:880–2

2. Steptoe PC, Edwards RG, Birth after the reimplantation of a human embryo. Lancet 1978; 2: 366.

3. Ortmann O, Weiss JM, Diedrich K. Gonadotrophin-releasing hormone (GnRH) and GnRH agonists: mechanisms of action. Reprod Biomed Online 2002;5:1–7.

4. Reh A, Krey L, Noyes N. Are gonadotropin releasing hormone agonists losing popularity? Current trends at a large fertility center. Fertil Steril 2010; 93:101–108.

5. Tarlatzis BC, Fauser BC, Kolibianakis EM, et al. GnRH antagonists in ovarian stimulation for IVF. Hum Reprod Update 2006;12:333–340.

6. Albano C, Smitz J, Camus M, Riethmuller-Winzen H, Van Steirteghem A, Devroey P, Comparison of different doses of gonadotropin-releasing hormone antagonist Cetrorelix during controlled ovarian hyperstimulation. Fertil Steril 1997; 67:917.

7. Ludwig M, Katalinic A, Banz C, Schroder AK, Loning M, Weiss JM, Diedrich K, Tailoring the GnRH antagonist cetrorelix acetate to individual patients' needs in ovarian stimulation for IVF: results of a prospective, randomized study. Hum Reprod 2002;17: 2842.

8. Lainas T, Zorzovilis J, Petsas G, et al. In a flexible antagonist protocol, earlier, criteria-based initiation of GnRH antagonist is associated with increased pregnancy rates in IVF. Hum Reprod 2005;20:2426–2433.

9. Al-Inany HG, Abou-Setta AM, Aboulghar M. Gonadotropin-releasing hormone antagonists for assisted conception: a Cochrane review. Reprod Biomed Online 2007;14:640–649.

10. Schoolcraft W, Schlenker T, Gee M, Stevens J, Wagley L, Improved controlled ovarian hyperstimulation in poor responder in vitro fertilization patients with a microdose follicle-stimulating hormone fl are, growth hormone protocol. Fertil Steril 1997;67: 93.

11. Dicker D, Ashkenazi J, Feldberg D, Levy T, Dekel A, Ben-Rafael Z, Severe abdominal complications after transvaginal ultrasonographically guided retrieval of oocytes for in vitro fertilization and embryo transfer. Fertil Steril 1993;59:1313.

12. Practice Committee of the American Society for Reproductive Medicine, Report on optimal evaluation of the infertile male. Fertil Steril 2006; 86:S202.

13. Dardashti K, Williams RH, Goldstein M, Microsurgical testis biopsy: a novel technique for retrieval of testicular tissue. J Urol 2000;163:1206.

14. Craft I, Tsirigotis M, Simplified recovery, preparation and cryopreservation of testicular spermatozoa. Hum Reprod 1995;10:1623.

15. Practice Committee of American Society for Reproductive Medicine; Practice Committee of Society for Assisted Reproductive Technology. Genetic considerations related to intracytoplasmic sperm injection (ICSI). Fertil Steril 2008; 90:S182–S184.

16. Mains L, Van Voorhis BJ. Optimizing the technique of embryo transfer. Fertil Steril 2010;94:785–790.

17. Stern JE, Goldman MB, Hatasaka H, MacKenzie TA, Surrey ES, Racowsky C, Optimizing the number of cleavage stage embryos to transfer on day 3 in women 38 years of age and older: a Society for Assisted Reproductive Technology database study. Fertil Steril 2009;91:767.

18. Vajta G, Nagy ZP, Cobo A, Conceicao J, Yovich J, Vitrification in assisted reproduction: myths, mistakes, disbeliefs and confusion. Reprod Biomed Online 2009;19 (suppl 3):1.

19. Goldsman MP, Pedram A, Dominguez CE, Ciuffardi I, Levin E, Asch RH. Increased capillary permeability induced by human follicular fluid: a hypothesis for an ovarian origin of the hyperstimulation syndrome. Fertil Steril 1995; 63: 268–72.

Cryopreservation of Embryos and Gametes

Anjali Tempe, Kashika Gupta Kathuria

The advent of embryo cryopreservation has been revolutionary in the field of reproductive medicine. Cryopreservation increases the cumulative pregnancy rate per in vitro fertilization (IVF) cycle, because of the ability to freeze and preserve excessive embryos obtained after ovarian stimulation and oocyte retrieval. It has also increasingly enabled clinicians to offer single embryo transfer to the patients, hence avoiding the risk of multiple pregnancy. Overall, this has translated as higher success rates of IVF in clinical practice. With the widespread availability of sperm, embryo and oocyte cryopreservation, individuals suffering from cancers and scheduled for gonadotoxic therapy can be offered fertility preservation. Cryopreservation of gametes and embryos is also done electively these days to postpone conception and child birth for non medical reasons.

Q1. What is cryopreservation?

Cryopreservation involves preserving cells and tissues by bringing them to subzero temperature in a controlled manner and storing them for use in future.

Q2. Discuss the history of cryopreservation.

The landmarks in the history of cryopreservation are listed in Table 17.1.

All these works were performed with traditional slow freezing. Vitrification was first applied in 1985 for mammalian embryos. Significant advances in the vitrification techniques and protocols for embryo and oocyte cryopreservation have made vitrification the preferred method. Presently, there is overwhelming evidence to show that vitrification produces better survival and more competent oocytes or embryos than traditional freezing.

Table 17.1: History of cryopreservation		
Year	Name of the researcher/ scientist	Landmark
1776	Spallanzani	First sperm freeze thaw(stallion semen)[1]
1930	Hammond, et al	Produced offspring from frozen thawed rabbit sperm[2]
1945	Parkes, et al	Discovered that slower rate of cooling was associated with better post thaw viability[3]
1949	Polge	Discovered glycerol as a cryoprotective agent[4]
1953	Bunge RG, et al	First human birth from frozen sperm was reported[5]
1983	Trounson A	First clinical pregnancy from frozen thawed human embryo[6]
1984	Zeilmaker GH, et al	First live births from cryopreserved embryos[7]
1986	Chen C	First human birth from cryopreserved oocytes[8]

Q3. What are the indications of cryo-preservation of gametes and embryos?

Oocyte cryopreservation[9]:

- **Fertility preservation:** In women undergoing gonadotoxic treatment for cancer (chemotherapy or radiotherapy)
- **Genetic conditions:**
  - In women with high risk of premature ovarian insufficiency (e.g.: Fragile X premutation and mosaicism for monosomy X)
  - Before prophylactic oophorectomy to decrease risk of breast or ovarian cancer (BRCA1/BRCA2 mutation carriers)
- **Lack of sperm at the time of retrieval**
  - Limited number in severe oligozoospermia
  - Failure to collect semen sample
  - Other medical emergency
- **Ethical indications**
  - In countries where there are ethical, moral or legal objections to embryo cryo-preservation
  - Ability to quarantine for donated oocytes
- **Deferred child bearing**
  - In order to defer child bearing for a later age, oocyte freezing may be done without any medical indication (social egg freezing).

Sperm cryopreservation

- **Donor semen:** Semen from screened donors is cryopreserved and stored in semen banks. It is then used anonymously for the following conditions, after written informed consent.
  - Male infertility—men with azoospermia or severe oligozoospermia, where intra-cytoplasmic sperm injection (ICSI) is not possible or not affordable.
  - To prevent transmission of a paternally inherited disorder; donor sperms can be used.
  - In cases of blood group incompatibility, semen from a compatible blood group donor can be used to prevent fetal hemolytic anaemia.
  - For single women who want to conceive, semen from a donor can be used for insemination.

  Frozen thawed anonymous donor spermatozoa are used in such cases. Based on the clinical situation, the donor sperms may be used for artificial insemination (AI), intrauterine insemination (IUI), in vitro fertilization (IVF) or intracytoplasmic sperm injection (ICSI).
- **Fertility preservation:** Cryopreservation of semen should be offered to all men who are likely to undergo any fertility impairing procedure or exposure such as:
  - Chemotherapy or radiotherapy for cancers, which is likely to impair spermatogenesis permanently.
  - Person scheduled for vasectomy (as a back up for possible future change in marital situation or desire for children).
  - Active duty in a dangerous occupation, e.g. military services.
- **Infertility treatment:** Treatment of infertile males may be facilitated by sperm cryo-preservation in the following conditions:
  - In azoospermic males: Surgical sperm retrieval can be done from epididymis or testis by testicular sperm aspiration (TESA), percutaneous epididymal sperm aspiration (PESA), testicular sperm extraction (TESE). These surgically retrieved sperms are frozen for later use in ICSI.
  - In severe oligozoospermia or variable sperm counts (intermittent presence of motile spermatozoa in the semen), spermatozoa may be frozen for use later. This is important because semen sample the day of ovum pick up may be azoospermic.
  - Transient appearance of sperms in semen as seen after gonadotropin treatment of hypogonadotropic hypogonadism or after surgery for genital tract obstruction, sperms may be present in semen for only some time (which can then be frozen for future use).

- Men with expected difficulty in giving the sample on the day of ovum pick up.
- After assisted ejaculation for patients with spinal cord injury, when sperms are frozen for use in ART procedures.

- **Minimizing infectious disease transmission**
  - In HIV discordant couples, where the male partner is seropositive but has a low viral load on antiretroviral therapy, semen samples may be frozen and later used for IUI, IVF or ICSI. This may reduce the risk of transmission of HIV to the female partner. However, this is questionable as there is limited evidence about its safety and proper consent should be taken.

Embryo cryopreservation:

- The storage of surplus embryos of good quality after fresh embryo transfer.
- Postponing embryo transfer in cases like poor endometrium or severe ovarian hyperstimulation syndrome (OHSS).
- For fertility preservation prior to chemotherapy, radiotherapy or ovariectomy.

Embryo cryopreservation increases the cumulative pregnancy rates per cycle, reduces hormone administration and the total cost of the cycle.

Q4. Describe the principles of cryopreservation?

The two main approaches to cryopreservation are slow freezing and vitrification.

Slow freezing involves gradual desiccation of the cell, based on the principle of osmotic dehydration.

- The embryos or oocytes are exposed to low concentration solutions of permeable and non permeable cryoprotectants. Permeable cryoprotectants penetrate the cell membrane, maintain chemical equilibrium and depress the freezing point of the cell, thereby decreasing risk of intracellular ice crystal formation.

- Extracellular ice crystal formation is induced by seeding the extracellular solution, which osmotically draws out water from the cells gradually.
- Embryos are loaded into 0.25 mL straw, sealed and cooled to $-6°C$ relatively rapidly by placing in a controlled rate freezer. Further cooling is carried out very slowly ($-0.3°C/minute$) to $-30°C$. Finally, the straws are immersed in liquid nitrogen for cooling and are stored at $-196°C$. Owing to the slow rate of cooling, there is gradual exchange of solution between the extracellular and intracellular fluids, thus avoiding any significant osmotic damage to the cells, hence leading to a better post thaw viability. Therefore, it is also called equilibrium freezing.[10]

In slow freezing, the toxic and osmotic damage to the cell is minimal due to the low concentrations of cryoprotectant used. However, risk of cell damage due to possibility of intracellular ice crystal formation remains a concern.

Vitrification is a method of rapid freezing, which is based on extreme elevation of solution viscosity leading to formation of a glass like, suspended state without crystallization.

- In vitrification, the cells are first exposed to a lower strength of cryoprotectant solution (usually 7.5–10%), the cryoprotective agent permeates into the cell and the process of dehydration starts.
- Subsequently, cells are exposed to higher concentration (40%) hyperosmotic solution of non permeable cryoprotectant for a very short duration (30–60 seconds) which results in complete dehydration of the cell.
- Thereafter, the sample is plunged into liquid nitrogen and stored. The process of supremely rapid cooling and use of high concentration cryoprotectant prevents ice crystal formation and causes an extreme increase in solution viscosity. As there is a relative increase in the intracellular concentration of macromolecules, this

process is described as a non-equilibrium cryopreservation method.

Q5. What are cryoprotectants?

Cryoprotectants are the agents used to minimize the damage during the freezing and thawing of slow-freeze and the vitrification processes. Cryoprotectants help in stabilizing the intracellular structures and cell membrane. There are two categories of cryoprotective agents (CPA):

- **Permeating CPA:** Those that cross the cell membrane
- **Non permeating CPA:** Those that do not cross the cell membrane

Permeating CPA: These include low molecular weight compounds like DMSO (Dimethyl sulfoxide), glycerol, ethylene glycol (EG), and propanediol (PPG or PrOH). They cross the cell membrane, causing water to leave from the cell, and also lower the freezing point of the cytoplasm. Sufficient penetration of the permeable CPA minimizes intracellular ice formation.

Non permeating CPA: They have a high molecular weight, do not cross the cell membrane and remain in the extracellular solution. Thus they cause an osmotic gradient outside the cell and water leaves the cell. Hence the cells dehydrate and shrink. They also act as an osmotic buffer and hence reduce the osmotic injury to oocytes or embryos.

These include sugars-mono-and disaccharides and other macromolecules such as sucrose, raffinose, trehalose, proteins like human serum albumin (HSA), synthetic serum substitute (SSS), polyvinylpyrrolidine (PVP).

The most commonly accepted cryoprotectant is Ethylene glycol (EG). It is least toxic and has high membrane permeability. EG and glycerol are less toxic than propanediol or DMSO. Use of high molar concentrations of CPA can result in toxicity and osmotic injury. It is preferable to use a mixture of two permeable cryoprotectants as it decreases the toxicity of one particular CPA.

Q6. What are the various tools and devices used for vitrification?

Over 25 different device systems have been developed for vitrification. These include open and closed systems. As an open or closed device is plunged into liquid nitrogen (LN2), microorganisms can attach to the device.

Open devices: These have a single container which carries the vitrified material. When immersed in liquid nitrogen for freezing, the device allows the vitrified material to have direct exposure to LN2. Thus, there is a risk of contamination of the exposed embryos or oocytes. At the time of warming, when this device is moved to the warming solution, any attached microorganisms could also be transferred to the solution. However, the risk of contamination of culture medium and/or gametes and embryos is remote and there is no documented evidence of such contamination in human cells. Open devices include plastic insemination straw (conventional), open pulled straws (OPS), cryoloop, electron microscopy (EM) grids, nylon mesh, cryotop, cryotip, gel-loading tip, minimum drop size.

Closed devices: These have an external container and an inner vitrification device. The embryos or oocytes are loaded in the inner vitrification device. At the time of freezing, only the external device is exposed to liquid nitrogen. Before warming, the external container is removed and only the 'clean' internal device is placed in the warming solution. Closed devices prevent the actual (internal) vitrification device from coming into direct contact with liquid nitrogen, hence any possible cross contamination from storage is prevented. Closed devices include Cryopette, Rapid-i, CBS-VIT high security straw.

Increasing the cooling and warming rates enables the use of a minimum concentration of cryoprotectants; hence reducing the related toxic and osmotic injuries. To accomplish an increase in the rates of cooling and warming, it is important to: (a) use the smallest volume of vitrifying solution surrounding the embryos or oocytes and (b) to establish direct contact between the sample and LN2.

The initial vitrification carriers were the plastic straws or cryovials. They required a large sample volume (0.25 mL) and provided limited cooling rates. Electron microscopy (EM grid) was one of the first devices to vitrify samples with very small volumes (<1 μL).

Cryotop is currently one of the most commonly used tool for vitrification. It consists of a transparent, plastic film which is flexible and is attached to a handle. Sample (<0.1 μL) is loaded onto the film and film is immersed in liquid nitrogen.

Cryopette is the first carrier designed to combine the benefits of a very low volume solution with the advantage of a closed system. Other satisfactory closed systems for embryo vitrification are: Rapid-i and CBS-VIT high security straw.[11,12]

Closed systems have been shown to produce adequate outcomes for embryo vitrification; however open systems provide superior results for oocyte vitrification.[13,14]

Q7. Describe the protocol for vitrification and thawing.

In vitrification, the solution is rapidly cooled so that a glass like state is formed at extremely low temperatures, without ice crystal formation. Many different protocols for vitrification exist in the field of ART.

Rapid Vit Omni and RapidWarm Omni are vitrification and warming kits respectively that are easy to use and are associated with good survival rates (Fig. 17.1). Vitrification and warming should be done at physiological temperature (37°C) in order to maintain spindle integrity and ensure viability of cells.

Rapid Vit Omni (Vitrification kit) contains three solutions for vitrification of oocytes or embryos (V1, V2, V3):

- *Vitri1 Omni:* Holding medium containing no cryoprotectants.

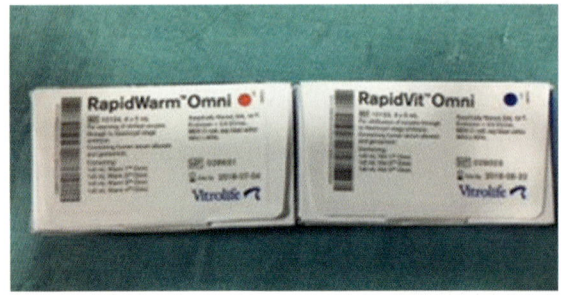

Fig. 17.1: Vitrification and warming kits

- *Vitri2 Omni:* Contains Ethylene glycol (EG) and propanediol (PrOH).
- *Vitri3 Omni:* The actual vitrification solution containing EG, PrOH and sucrose for dehydration of cell(s).

The protocol involves sequential exposure of the oocytes or embryos to the three vitrification solutions for time intervals as mentioned below (time efficient vitrification):

Table 17.2: Vitrification protocol	
Stage	*Rapid Vit Omni (duration of sequential exposure to V1, V2, V3)*
Oocytes	5′–20′, 2–5′, 45 sec
PN-stage Cleavage stage Blastocysts	5′–20′, 2′, 45 sec

After sequential exposure to the above vitrification solutions, the embryos or oocytes are loaded into a carrier tool and cooled by immersing into liquid nitrogen and stored.

Process of loading embryos into the carrier device:

- The pre labeled outer straw is placed inside the container filled with liquid nitrogen. The metal rod from the outer straw is removed (Fig. 17.2).
- The inner vitrification carrier device (rapid i) is placed inside the round dish ready for use.
- After being exposed to the third vitrification solution, the embryos are placed inside the small hole of the inner carrier device, with as

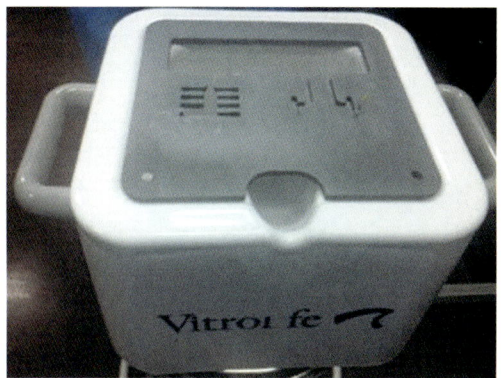

Fig. 17.2: The outer straw dipped in liquid nitrogen bath

little media as possible (Fig. 17.3)

- The inner device containing the embryos is put straight inside the outer straw.
- Thereafter, the straw is sealed with an ultrasonic sealer (Fig. 17.4).
- The straws are inserted in storage goblets (Fig. 17.5), which are then placed in liquid nitrogen flasks or tanks for storage (Fig. 17.7).

For optimal storage and handling of vitrified specimens: Clear, well-positioned, identifiable labels on vitrified samples should be there, to enable complete identification. Labels should contain: the date of cryopreservation, contents, container number, color-coding.

Warming protocol: Warming is carried out in a concentrated solution of an impermeable cryoprotectant; which is followed by exposure to decreasing concentrations of the impermeable cryoprotectant.

A commonly used warming protocol (RapidWarm Omni) uses four solutions:

- Warm 1–3 Omni contain a serial dilution of sucrose
- Warm 4 Omni contains no sucrose.

Decreasing concentrations of sucrose allows removal of intracellular cryoprotectant (EG and PrOH) and gradual rehydration of cells. The exposure to the warming solutions sequentially is for the time duration as mentioned in Table 17.3.

Table 17.3: Warming/thawing protocol	
Stage	*Rapid warm omni (4 step procedure: sequential exposure to warming media 1–4)*
Oocytes	1′, 3′, 5′, 5′–10′
PN-stage Cleavage stage Blastocysts	1′, 3′, 5′, 5′-10′

Vitrification survival is determined by the warming rate, relative to the cooling rate.

Q8. Discuss oocyte cryopreservation as used in current clinical practice.

Oocyte cryopreservation is not considered experimental anymore. Methods of oocyte vitrification have evolved over the past several

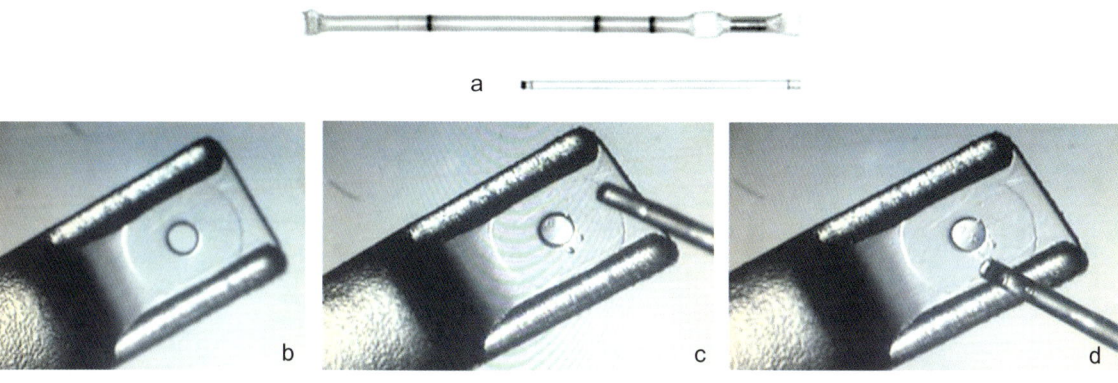

Fig. 17.3: Rapid-i kit and loading of embryos in the inner vitrification device. a: The Rapid-i kit consists of an outer straw and an inner (actual) vitrification carrier device. b: Small hole on the inner device is seen. c: Embryos being loaded into the hole in a minute volume of the vitrification solution. d: Embryos are held in place by surface tension

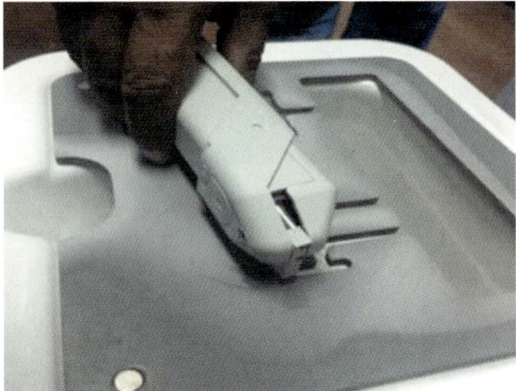

Fig. 17.4: After the inner carrier device (Rapid-i) is loaded into the outer straw, it is sealed with the ultrasonic sealer

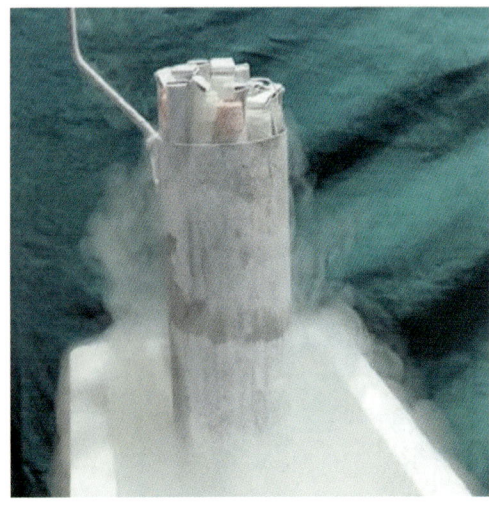

Fig. 17.6: Goblet containing frozen semen in cryovials

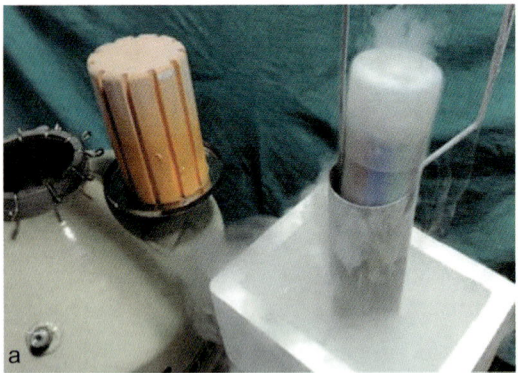

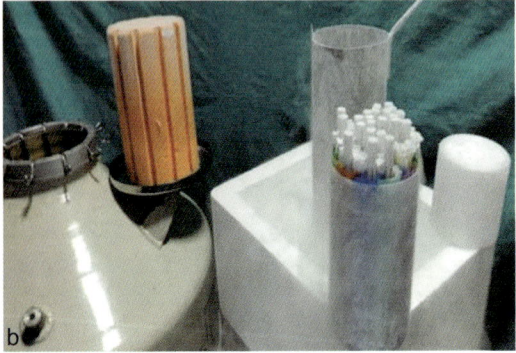

Fig. 17.5a and d: Storage goblet containing the frozen embryos in straws

years which has enabled optimum oocyte survival after freezing.[9,15,16] Evidence suggests that vitrification significantly improves oocyte survival and pregnancy rates, and is associated with faster meiotic spindle recovery, when compared with slow freezing. Similar fertilization and pregnancy rates have been demonstrated in IVF/ICSI cycles using fresh vs cryopreserved oocytes.[17,18]

There is no evidence of increased neonatal risk with the use of cryopreserved oocytes for fertility treatment compared with other assisted reproductive technologies.[19,20]

American Society for Reproductive Medicine (ASRM) recommendations:[9]

- Oocyte cryopreservation is recommended (after appropriate counseling) for patients facing infertility due to chemotherapy or other gonadotoxic therapies (Level B).
- Oocyte cryopreservation for the purpose of circumventing reproductive aging in healthy women is not yet supported by sufficient data (Level B).

Q9. Discuss the status of ovarian tissue cryopreservation in ART.

Currently ovarian tissue cryopreservation is still considered an experimental technique for fertility preservation.[21]

Indications

- Fertility preservation in women with aggressive malignancies where oocyte or embryo cryopreservation is not feasible due to paucity of time for ovarian stimulation and ovum pick up.

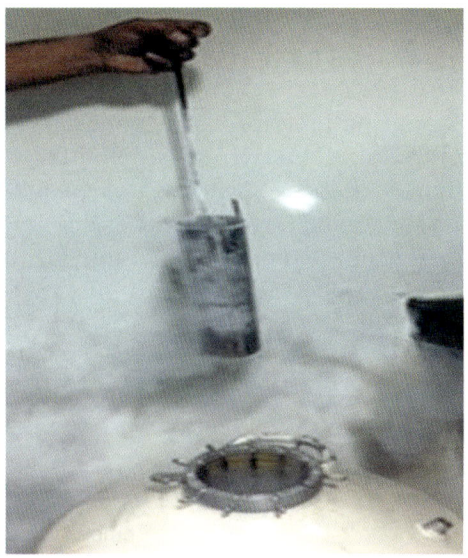

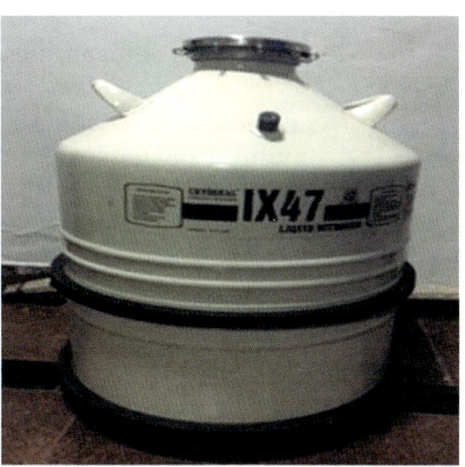

Fig. 17.7: The goblets are stored in liquid nitrogen cryocans or flasks

- Fertility preservation in pre pubertal girls or women with hormone sensitive malignancies, where ovarian stimulation and ovum pick up are not possible.
- Patients anticipating stem cell transplantation for management of hematologic malignancies.
- Prophylactic cryopreservation in women with autoimmune disease unresponsive to immunosupressants.
- Patients harboring genetic mutations that predispose them to a high risk of POI.

Techniques of ovarian tissue cryopreservation:

1. **Ovarian cortical tissue**
   - Cryopreservation of large number of oocytes can be done by obtaining a small volume of ovarian cortical tissue.
   - The tissue must be obtained prior to initiation of treatment, except in patients with leukemia where tissue has to be taken after the first remission to decrease risk of malignant cell dissemination from the re-implanted thawed tissue.
   - Most commonly, tissue is obtained by laparoscopy, though mini laparotomy may be needed in some cases.
   - The ovarian cortical tissue is transferred to the laboratory on ice and then small slivers of tissue are obtained that are 0.3–2 mm thick. These are then cryopreserved.

2. **Whole ovary cryopreservation:** May be required for patients in whom complete ovarian failure is expected after treatment. The ovary is removed by laparotomy or laparoscopically with a large vascular pedicle attached. The vascular pedicle facilitates organ transplantation after thawing.

Method of freezing: Both slow freezing and vitrification are used to cryopreserve ovarian tissue, and have shown similar oocyte survival rates. However, granulosa cell survival and stromal integrity is better with vitrification. Vitrification appears to be the favoured approach, but further studies are required.

Ovarian tissue transplantation and outcomes: Autologous ovarian cortical tissue transplantation involves attaching viable cortical ovarian tissue to pelvic (orthotopic) site or an extrapelvic (heterotopic) site, such as the forearm or anterior abdominal wall.

Orthotopic ovarian tissue transplantation involves transplantation of very thin strips (1–1.5 mm) of thawed ovarian tissue into medullary portion of remaining ovary or into the peritoneum of ovarian fossa. After orthotopic ovarian tissue transplantation, resumption of ovarian function with endogenous hormone production and normal menses has been observed. The first live birth with this technique was reported by Donnez J in 2004.[22] So far twenty four live births (spontaneous or IVF induced) have been reported with this technique worldwide.

Heterotopic transplantation of ovarian tissue has been performed over forearm, abdominal wall and chest wall with reports of restoration of ovarian function and follicular development. Pregnancy can be achieved with IVF; successful oocyte retrieval and fertilization have been demonstrated but no live births have been reported.

There is no report of whole ovary transplant in humans till date.

Q10. Briefly elaborate semen cryopreservation techniques.

After cryopreservation, semen may be used successfully indefinitely. The longest reported period of successful storage period for human sperm is 24 years.

Freezing technique: Semen is frozen using either vitrification or slow freezing. Vitrification gives superior post thaw viability and motility than slow freezing. Glycerol (10% in culture medium) is the most common cryoprotectant for semen freezing. Sucrose or other di-,trisaccharides may be added to the glycerol solution. Egg yolk or lecithin may be used as a supplement with the cryoprotectant. Glycerol Egg Yolk Cryoprotectant (GEYC) is a popular CPA used for semen freezing.

Protocol for semen freezing
- GEYC (one volume) is added to two volumes of semen and the mixture thus obtained, is incubated at 30–35 °C for 5 minutes.
- The mixture is aspirated into 0.5 mL plastic straws or placed in cryovials.
- Semen freezing is done in either programmable freezers or by manual methods. The straws or cryovials should be placed in a programmable freezer and cooling is

carried out at 1.5°C per minute from 20°C to –6°C and then at 6°C per minute to –100°C. The process takes about 40 minutes.
- Manual methods for semen freezing are less controllable than programmable freezers but been shown to give adequate results.
- The frozen straws or cryovials are placed in storage tubes (mini-goblets), which are then inserted into larger storage goblets. The goblets with the straws or cryovials are stored in liquid nitrogen flasks or tanks. (Fig. 17.6).

There is some evidence to suggest an increase in sperm DNA fragmentation and single strand breaks after semen cryopreservation, which could translate into increased risk of mutations in the offspring. However, there is no increase in chromosomal anomalies or birth defects in individuals conceived from cryopreserved sperms in long term follow up studies.

Q11. Discuss the ethical and legal dilemmas surrounding cryopreservation of gametes and embryos.

Ethical dilemmas pertaining to cryopreservation arise as some people would consider embryos as a group of cells while others would consider them to be a potential human being. Some would assert that the in vitro embryo deserves legal protection by its own. In an effort to protect life since fecundation, few countries prohibit embryo cryopreservation. Many countries allow it on the grounds of respect to women's reproductive rights.

ICMR guidelines for ART clinics in India state that:[23]
- A specific consent should be given by couples for storage and use of their embryos.
- India follows the regulations of The Human Fertilization and Embryology Act, UK (1990), which allows a 5-year storage period for embryos.
- In case the couple fails to use their embryos, consent must be taken from them for use of their stored embryos by other couples or for research. However, if the couple defaults in

payment of maintenance charges despite two reminders (sent by registered post), such a consent will not be required.

- Research on embryos should be restricted to the first fourteen days of its development only and has to be done only after permission has been sought from the owner of the embryos. No commercial transaction would be allowed for the use of embryos for research.
- Semen samples must be cryopreserved for at least six months before first use in semen banks; at this time the semen donor must be tested for HIV and hepatitis B and C again. The semen of one donor should not be supplied for more than ten successful pregnancies.
- Confidentiality must be ensured by the semen bank, with regard to the identity of the semen donor.
- A semen bank can store a semen sample for use by only the donor's wife or on any woman designated by the donor. The bank may levy an appropriate charge for such storage. In the case of non-payment of the charges when the donor is alive, the bank shall have the right to destroy the semen sample or give it to a bonafide organization where it can be used for research purposes only.

In case of death of the donor, the semen would be the property of the legal heir or the nominee of the donor. All other conditions that apply to the donor would now apply to the legal heir, except that he cannot have a woman of his choice inseminated by the frozen sperms. If there are no claimants after the donor's death, the bank can destroy the semen or give it to a bonafide organization where it should be used only for research purposes.

- Collection of gametes from a dying person (e.g. in case of malignancy) would only be allowed if the widow wishes to have a child.

Collection of gametes from a person suffering from malignancy, might translate into an increased risk of cancers in the offspring. Hence, use of cryopreserved gametes may

result in an embryo/child with inherent medical risks. Also the care of the offspring born out of the cryopreserved sperm may be compromised due to possible early death of one parent. Hence, careful counseling is essential in all cases.

 Key Points

- Cryopreservation involves preservation of cells or tissues at subzero temperature.
- Oocyte, ovarian tissue, semen and embryos can be cryopreserved for use later on to achieve pregnancy.
- The process is complex and can only be performed in a well-equipped ART center.
- The procedure is done for specific indications.
- Ethical issues must be addressed when doing this procedure.

REFERENCES

1. Spallanzani L. Observations and experiments around freezing of sperm and eggs in humans and animals. Modena; 1776.
2. Hammond J. The effect of temperature on the survival in vitro of rabbit spermatozoa obtained from the vagina. J Exp Biol 1930;7:175–195.
3. Parkes AS. Preservation of human spermatozoa at low temperatures. Br Med J 1945;2:212–213.
4. Polge C, Smith AU, Parkes AS. Revival of spermatozoa after vitrification and dehydration at low temperatures. Nature 1949;164:666.
5. Bunge RG., Sherman J.K. Fertilizing capacity of frozen human spermatozoa. Nature 1953;172: 767–768.
6. Trounson A, Mohr L. Human pregnancy following cryopreservation, thawing and transfer of an eight cell embryo. Nature 1983;305:707–9.
7. Zeilmaker GH, Alberda AT, van Gent I, Rijkmans CM, Drogendjik AC. Two pregnancies following transfer of intact frozen thawed embryos. Fertil Steril 1984;42:293–6.
8. Chen C. Pregnancy after human oocyte cryo-preservation. Lancet 1986;1: 884–6.
9. Mature oocyte cryopreservation: a guideline. Practice Committees of American Society for Reproductive Medicine; Society for Assisted Reproductive Technology. Fertil Steril 2013;99: 37–43.
10. Mazur P. Equilibrium, quasi-equlibrium and non-equilibrium freezing of mammalian embryos. Cell Biophys 1990;17:53–92.

11. Larman MG, Gardner DK. Vitrification of mouse embryos with super cooled air. Fertil Steril 2011; 95:1462–6.

12. Shu Hashimoto, Ami Amo, Satoko Hama, Kanako Ohsumi, Yoshiharu Nakaoka, Yoshiharu Morimoto. A closed system supports the developmental competence of human embryos after vitrification: Closed vitrification of human embryos. J Assist Reprod Genet 2013;30:371–6.

13. Bonetti A, Cervi M, Tomei F, Marchini M, Ortolani F, Manno M. Ultrastructural evaluation of human metaphase II oocytes after vitrification: Closed vs open devices. Fertil Steril 2011;95:928–35.

14. Papatheodorou A et al. Open vs closed oocyte vitrification system: A prospective randomized sibling oocyte study. Reprod Biomed Online. 2013; 26:595–602.

15. Oktay K, Cil AP, Bang H. Efficiency of oocyte cryopreservation: a meta-analysis. Fertil Steril 2006;86:70–80.

16. Smith GD, Serafini PC, Fioravanti J, Yadid I, Coslovsky M, Hassun P, et al. Prospective randomized comparison of human oocyte cryopreservation with slow-rate freezing or vitrification. Fertil Steril 2010; 94:2088-95.

17. Cobo A, Meseguer M, Remohi J, Pellicer A. Use of cryo-banked oocytes in an ovum donation programme: a prospective, randomized, controlled, clinical trial. Hum Reprod 2010; 25:2239–46.

18. Rienzi L, Romano S, Albricci L, Maggiulli R, Capalbo A, Baroni E, et al. Embryo development of fresh 'versus' vitrified metaphase II oocytes after ICSI: a prospective randomized sibling-oocyte study. Hum Reprod 2010; 25:66–73.

19. Noyes N, Porcu E, Borini A. Over 900 oocyte cryopreservation babies born with no apparent increase in congenital anomalies. Reprod Biomed Online 2009;18:769–76.

20. Chian RC, Huang JY, Gilbert L, Son WY, Holzer H, Cui SJ, et al. Obstetric outcomes following vitrification of in vitro and in vivo matured oocytes. Fertil Steril 2009;91:2391–8.

21. Ovarian tissue cryopreservation: A committee opinion. The practice committee of American Society for Reproductive Medicine. Fertil Steril 201;101:1237–43.

22. Donnez J, Dolmans MM, Demylle D, Jadoul P, Pirard C, Squifflet J et al. Live birth after orthotopic transplantation of ovarian tissue. Lancet 2004; 364:1405–10.

23. The Assisted Reproductive Technology (Regulation) Rules-2010. Indian Council of Medical Research, New Delhi. Ministry of Health and Family Welfare, Govt. of India.

18 | Ovarian Hyperstimulation Syndrome

Sudha Prasad, Garima Sharma, Saumya Prasad

The ovarian hyperstimulation syndrome (OHSS) is a rare iatrogenic complication of ovarian stimulation. The syndrome was first reported by Rydberg et al in 1943 and then by Davis, et al. in 1944.[1,2] It is mainly associated with exogenous gonadotropin stimulation and is rarely observed with other agents like oral ovulation induction agents and gonadotropin releasing hormone analouges. Earlier this disease was called (in French) 'syndrome d'hyperluteÂinisation massive des ovaires'. Gotzsche described the first fatal case in 1951 (EstebanAltirriba, 1961).[3]

Case 1

A 27 year old woman presented to the emergency with complaint of abdominal distension, pain abdomen, excessive nausea and vomiting for 2 days. She gave history of irregular menstrual cycles and previous 6 failed cycle of ovulation induction with intrauterine insemination. There was history of ovarian stimulation with gonadotropins. Oocyte pickup (20 oocyte retrieved 36 hr after hCG injection) was done 6 days back and embryo transfer was done 3 days back.

On examination: Pulse rate was 100/min, blood pressure was normal, chest and cardio-vascular examination was within normal limits, abdomen appeared distended.

On investigation: Blood tests were normal, on ultrasound examination-ascites present, bilateral ovaries were enlarged 10 cm in size.

Diagnosis: Early Ovarian hyperstimulation syndrome (OHSS), Severity: Moderate OHSS.

Q1. How common is OHSS?

The incidence of OHSS depends upon type of fertility treatment. Mild OHSS is seen in one third of conventional in vitro fertilisation (IVF) cycles while incidence of moderate or severe OHSS varies from 3.1 to 8%.[4] Ovulation induction drugs like clomifene, or mono-follicular ovulation induction with gonado-tropins rarely cause OHSS but a few cases have been reported. Very few cases of OHSS have also been reported in spontaneous cycle pregnancy.[5]

Q2. Who are at risk of OHSS?

Certain patient and cycle characteristics increase the risk of OHSS (ASRM Guideline 2016):[6]

- Young patients < 35 years with good ovarian reserve.
- Lean women
- Polycystic ovarian syndrome
- Women with previous history of OHSS
- Increased antral follicular count (>24)
- Increased anti müllerian hormone levels (>3.4 ng/mL)
- High or rapidly rising estradiol (E2) levels (>3500 pg/mL)
- Development of ≥25 follicles
- ≥24 oocytes retrieved

Q3. What is the etiopathogenesis of OHSS?

The primary physiological change underlying OHSS is increased capillary permeability with the resulting loss of fluid into the third space. In a high risk patient, human chorionic gonadotropin (hCG) administration for final follicular maturation and triggering of ovulation are the pivotal stimulus for OHSS. There is over expression of vascular endothelial growth factor (VEGF) in the ovary, release of vasoactive-angiogenic substances such as interleukins, tumor necrosis factor-α, endothelin-1 which cause increased vascular permeability, loss of fluid to the third space, and full-blown OHSS.[7]

Q4. How is OHSS diagnosed?

The diagnosis of OHSS is made on clinical grounds. A typical patient of OHSS presents with abdominal distension and discomfort following hCG injection which is given prior to oocyte retrieval, for final follicular maturation. Some patients give history of excessive ovarian response to stimulation in prior cycle but even if this history is absent OHSS cannot be ruled out.

OHSS can be divided into two groups-early and late OHSS. If the clinical presentation occurs within 7 days of the hCG injection it is called 'Early' OHSS which is usually associated with an excessive exogenous stimulation response. If it presents 10 or more days after hCG (trigger) injection it is 'Late' OHSS and is usually the result of endogenous hCG derived from an early pregnancy. Late OHSS is more severe and prolonged as compared to early form.[8]

Main symptoms of OHSS are:
- Abdominal bloating
- Abdominal discomfort or pain, need for analgesia
- Nausea and vomiting
- Breathlessness, inability to lie flat or talk in full sentences
- Reduced urine output
- Leg swelling
- Vulval swelling

Q5. What is differential diagnosis of OHSS?

Pelvic abscess, pelvic infection, appendicitis, ectopic pregnancy, ovarian torsion or cyst rupture and bowel perforation are important differential diagnosis of OHSS. OHSS should not, therefore, be the 'default diagnosis' for women presenting with abdominal pain during fertility treatment.

Q6. What should be asked in history of patient suspected of OHSS? (Taken from RCOG 2016 guideline)

Following points should be noted in history of patient suspected of OHSS:
- Time of onset of symptoms relative to trigger
- Medication used for trigger (hCG or GnRH agonist)
- Number of follicles on final monitoring scan
- Number of eggs collected
- Were embryos replaced and their number?
- Whether patient has polycystic ovarian syndrome?

Q7. What should the examination and investigations include in patients suspected of OHSS?

Examination
- *General:* Look for signs and symptoms of dehydration, edema (pedal, vulval and sacral); check heart rate, blood pressure, respiratory rate and body weight.
- *Abdominal:* Ascites, any palpable mass, signs of peritonism, measure abdominal girth.
- *Respiratory:* Check for pleural effusion, pneumonia, pulmonary edema.

Investigations
- Complete blood count
- Hematocrit (hemoconcentration is seen in OHSS)
- C-reactive protein (tells the severity of disease)
- Urea and electrolytes (hyponatraemia and hyperkalemia are observed in OHSS)
- Serum osmolality (OHSS is characterised by hypo-osmolality)
- Liver function tests (elevated enzymes and reduced albumin are noted)
- Coagulation profile (elevated fibrinogen and reduced antithrombin is noted in OHSS)

- hCG level (to determine if patient is pregnant or not) if appropriate
- Ultrasound scan: assess ovarian size, pelvic and abdominal free fluid. If torsion is suspected ovarian Doppler should be considered.

According to severity following tests may be indicated:

- Arterial blood gases
- D-dimers
- Electrocardiogram (ECG), echocardiogram
- Chest X-ray
- Computerised tomography pulmonary angiogram (CTPA) or ventilation/perfusion (V/Q) scan

Q8. How is severity of OHSS classified?

There have been many schemes proposed to classify severity of OHSS[9-12]. Proposed RCOG classification of severity of OHSS published in greentop guideline. 5 in February 2016:

Mild OHSS

- Abdominal bloating
- Mild abdominal pain
- Ovarian size usually <8 cm

Moderate OHSS

- Moderate abdominal pain
- Nausea ± vomiting
- Ultrasound evidence of ascites
- Ovarian size usually 8–12 cm

Severe OHSS

- Clinical ascites (± hydrothorax)
- Oliguria (<300 mL/day or <30 mL/hour)
- Haematocrit >0.45
- Hyponatraemia (sodium <135 mmol/L)
- Hypo-osmolality (osmolality < 282 mOsm/kg)
- Hyperkalaemia (potassium >5 mmol/L)
- Hypoproteinaemia (serum albumin <35 g/L)
- Ovarian size usually >12 cm

Critical OHSS

- Tense ascites/large hydrothorax
- Hematocrit >0.55
- White cell count >25 000/mL

- Oliguria/anuria
- Thromboembolism
- Acute respiratory distress syndrome

Rarely, OHSS may be associated with life-threatening complications, including renal failure, acute respiratory distress syndrome (ARDS), hemorrhage from ovarian rupture, and thrombo embolism.

Q9. How should one manage a case of OHSS?

Women with OHSS can be managed as outpatient or inpatient according to symptoms and severity (RCOG 2016 guidelines).

1. **Outpatient:** Women with mild and several cases of moderate OHSS can be managed on an OPD basis. Baseline history, examination and investigation should be done for these patients.
   a. Women should be encouraged to drink to thirst rather than to excess.[13] Fluid intake of atleast 1 litre is advised. If possible patients should be advised to maintain fluid input-output charts. Urine output of less than 1000 mL per 24 hours or a positive fluid balance of greater than 1000 mL over 24 hours should prompt medical review to assess severity.
   b. For pain relief analgesia using para-cetamol or codeine is appropriate. NSAIDS should not be used as they may compromise renal function in patients with OHSS.[14]
   c. Women should be advised to avoid strenuous activity and sexual intercourse for fear of injury or torsion of ovaries.
   d. Women can continue using progesterone for luteal support but hCG support is not to be given.
   e. Under ultrasound guidance paracentesis of ascitic fluid may be carried out on an outpatient basis by the abdominal or transvaginal route.
   f. Patient should be reviewed every 2–3 days.
   g. If the severity of OHSS worsens baseline investigations should be repeated.

Hematocrit level can be used to measure the degree of intravascular volume depletion.

Urgent clinical review is necessary if woman develops any of these signs:[15]

- If abdominal distension and pain increases
- Patient complains of shortness of breath
- There is tachycardia or hypotension
- Reduced urine output (less than 1000 mL/ 24 hours) or positive fluid balance (more than 1000 mL/24 hours)
- Weight gain and abdominal girth increases
- Increasing hematocrit (>0.45).

2. **Inpatient**
   a. Women should be considered for hospital admission if:
      - Are not able to achieve satisfactory pain control.
      - Adequate fluid intake cannot be maintained due to nausea.
      - There is worsening of severity of OHSS despite outpatient intervention.
      - They are not able to attend regular outpatient follow-up.
      - Have severe/critical OHSS.
   b. Women with critical or severe OHSS should be looked after by multidisciplinary team.
   c. Women with critical OHSS may require intensive care (ICU admission).
   d. A clinician experienced in the management of OHSS should remain in overall charge of the woman's care.
   e. *Monitoring:* Woman admitted with OHSS should be monitored closely. Blood pressure, pulse, respiratory rate should be monitored 4 hourly. Body weight, abdominal girth, and fluid intake and output should be measured on a daily basis, along with complete blood count, hematocrit, serum electrolytes, osmolality, coagulation profile and liver function tests and ultrasound to assess ovarian size and ascites.

   f. *Management of symptoms:* Relief of abdominal pain and nausea constitute important part of the supportive care of women with OHSS. Analgesia with paracetamol and opiates, if required, is appropriate, while NSAIDs should be avoided as renal function may be compromise.[14] Antiemetic drugs should be used if there is possibility of early pregnancy—prochlorperazine, metoclopramide and cyclizine.

   g. *Management of fluid balance:*
      - Women should be allowed to drink to thirst as it represents the most physiological approach to replacing volume.
      - Invasive monitoring and discussion with the anesthetist may be required in women with severe OHSS having persistent oliguria and hemoconcentration despite initial fluid therapy.
      - I/V crystalloids such as normal saline should be used for initial fluid therapy. Fluid intake of 2–3 litres in 24 hours is generally required by most women but this should be guided by a strict fluid balance chart.
      - As diuretics further deplete intravascular volume they should be avoided, but they may have a role if oliguria persists despite adequate fluid replacement and ascites drainage, after discussion with multidisciplinary team.
      - Colloids may benefit women with persistent hemoconcentration and/or urine output less than 0.5 mL/kg. Human albumin, haemaccel, 6% hydroxyethylstarch (HES), dextran and mannitol have been used for this purpose. These hyperosmotic agents act by increasing intravascular oncotic pressure which draws third-space fluid back into the intravascular space.

h. *Management of ascites and effusion:* Paracentesis is indicated if there is:
- Severe abdominal distension and abdominal pain secondary to ascites.
- Shortness of breath and respiratory compromise secondary to ascites and increased intra-abdominal pressure.
- Oliguria despite adequate volume replacement, secondary to increased abdominal pressure causing reduced renal perfusion.

Paracentesis can be performed abdominally or vaginally but it should always be carried out under ultrasound guidance.

i. *Management of risk of thrombosis:* Severe OHSS is a prothrombotic state due to hemoconcentration and vascular endothelial dysfunction. The incidence of thrombosis in women with severe OHSS is between 0.7% and 10%.[16] Women with severe or critical OHSS and those admitted with OHSS should receive LMWH prophylaxis. The duration of LMWH prophylaxis should be individualised according to risk factors and outcome of treatment.

j. *Role of GnRH antagonist and cabergolin:* one observational study has suggested that GnRH antagonist (cetrorelix, ganirelix) 0.25 mg daily administered from days 5 to day 8 post oocyte retrieval in women with established severe early OHSS may result in quicker regression of the syndrome.[17] Another observational study suggests that dopamine agonist (cabergolin) 0.5 mg daily for 8 days may have a beneficial role in the treatment of established OHSS.[18]

k. *Role of surgery:* Patients with OHSS may require surgery if there is a coincident problem such as ectopic pregnancy, adnexal torsion or ovarian rupture.

Q10. What are the risks associated with pregnancy and OHSS?

Cases complicated with severe OHSS have high incidence of multiple pregnancies, gestational diabetes, preeclampsia, placental abruption, prematurity and low birth weight. Such pregnancies should therefore be considered as high risk and manged as such.[19]

Q11. Can anything be done to prevent OHSS?

Risk of OHSS should be assessed in all patients undergoing ovarian stimulation. Methods that can be used in order to prevent OHSS in these patients are:[6] (ASRM 2016)

a. **Primary**
- *Insulin-sensitizing agents:* Metformin suppresses insulin levels and decreases ovarian androgen production which results in improved ovulation rates. By improving intraovarian hyperandrogenism, metformin reduces the number of nonperiovulatory follicles and thereby reduce estradiol secretion and preventing OHSS. Dose: 500 mg three times daily or 850 mg twice daily during IVF stimulation.
- *Reducing dose of Gonadotropins (Mild/Minimal protocol):* Using low dose of gonadotropins for stimulation in high risk patients reduces the risk of OHSS.
- *GnRH antagonists protocols:* The use of antagonist compared with long GnRH agonist protocols was associated with a large reduction in incidence of OHSS without affecting the live-birth rates.
- *Low dose of hCG:* Using low dose of hCG for trigger of oocyte maturation in high-risk patients reduces the risk of OHSS.
- *Alternative agents to hCG for trigger:* Use of GnRH agonists (0.2–0.3 mg triptorelin, 0.5–4 mg leuprolide acetate or 0.5 mg buserelin) instead of hCG for trigger results in a lower incidence of OHSS.
- Avoiding hCG for luteal phase support
- *In vitro oocyte maturation (IVM):* It involves retrieval of immature oocytes at the germinal-vesicle stage followed by IVM and ICSI.
- *Aspirin:* Aspirin decreases the level of histamine, serotonin, platelet-derived

growth factor, or lysophosphatidic acid, that can further potentiate the physiologic cascade of OHSS. Dose: 100 mg aspirin given from the first day of the menstrual cycle when IVF was performed, and continued until menstruation, a negative pregnancy test, or the ultrasonographic detection of embryonic cardiac activity.

b. **Secondary**
  - Cycle cancellation
  - *Coasting:* Coasting involves withholding further gonadotropin stimulation and delaying hCG administration until E2 levels plateau or decrease significantly. Coasting should not be more than 3 days as it is detrimental for oocyte quality.
  - *Cryopreservation/segmented cycle:* Cryopreservation involves freezing of all embryos to be thawed and transferred at a later date. Early OHSS may occur but it almost eliminates the risk of late OHSS.
  - Intravenous albumin and HES
  - *Dopamine agonists:* Dopamine-receptor agonist such as cabergoline may result in a reduction of VEGF production and a subsequent reduction in incidence of OHSS. Dose: 0.5 mg daily for 8 days starting from the day of hCG trigger.
  - *Calcium gluconate infusion:* Calcium infusion (10 mL of 10% Ca gluconate in 200 mL saline on the day of oocyte retrieval and day 1–3 after oocyte retrieval) helps in preventing severe OHSS and decreases OHSS occurrence rates.
  - *Luteal phase GnRH antagonist:* 0.25 mg daily from day 5–8 post ovum pick up with or without embryo transfer causes rapid resolution of early onset severe OHSS by decreasing the serum estradiol level.

Q12. What are OHSS free clinics?

The concept of OHSS free clinic is need the hour in ART today. This approach includes pituitary down-regulation using a GnRH antagonist, ovulation triggering with a GnRH agonist, vitrification of oocytes or embryos and transfer of embryos later in unstimulated cycle (frozen embryo transfer).[20]

Case 2

A 25-year-old woman presented to the emergency with complaints of severe pain abdomen and distension, excessive nausea and vomiting, difficulty in breathing and not able to pass urine for one day. She gave history of ovarian stimulation with gonadotropins, oocyte pick up done 15 days back and embryo transfer done 10 days back.

On examination patient was breathless, her pulse rate was 118 per minute, blood pressure was 120/70 mm Hg. General examination was normal. Abdominal examination revealed the presence of ascites. Respiratory system examination revealed moderate left pleural effusion. Other systems were normal.

Laboratory investigations: hemoglobin 12.5 gm%, total count 17520/mm^3 LFT and KFT were within normal limits, serum albumin 3.1 gm%, serum sodium 129 mEq/L, serum potassium 5.1 mEq/L, Chest X-ray revealed moderate left sided pleural effusion and ECG showed sinus tachycardia without any ST-T abnormalities. Transabdominal and transvaginal sonogram showed moderate ascites. Endometrial thickness was increased and both ovaries were enlarged to 14 cm in size with multiple cysts. Urine pregnancy test was positive and Beta hCG was 1200 mIU/mL.

Diagnosis: Late OHSS, severity: Severe OHSS. This patient requires admission in ICU and management on the lines of severe OHSS.

Key Points

- Ovarian hyperstimulation syndrome is mostly iatrogenic and self-limiting disorder which is seen in ART cycles.
- Women who are at high risk of this disorder should be identified prior to stimulation, and various preventive methods should be selected to minimize the risk of OHSS.
- When signs of OHSS occur, the patient must be adequately informed and hospitalization should be proposed at slightest deterioration.

- Fluid resuscitation and prophylactic anticoagulation are the mainstay of treatment for OHSS. When a large amount of ascites is present paracentesis or culdocentesis may be recommended.
- A few cases of severe OHSS can be life threatening and multidiciplinary team should be involved in their management.
- Each ART centre must try for OHSS free clinic with all precautions.

REFERENCES

1. Rydberg E and Pedersen-Bjergaard K. Effect of serum gonadotropin and chorionic gonadotropin on the human ovary. JAMA 1943;121:1117–1122.

2. Davis E and Hellebaum AA. Observations on the experimental use of gonadotropic extracts in the human female. J. Clin. Endocrinol 1944; 4: 400–409.

3. Esteban-Altirriba, J. Le syndrome d'hyperstimulation massive des ovaires. Rev. FrancÉaise de GyneÂcologie et d'ObsteÂtrique 1961;7: 555–564.

4. Delvigne A, Rozenberg S. Epidemiology and prevention of ovarian hyperstimulation syndrome (OHSS): a review. Hum Reprod Update 2002;8: 559–77.

5. Sridev S, Barathan S. Case report on spontaneous ovarian hyperstimulation syndrome following natural conception associated with primary hypothyroidism. J Hum Reprod Sci 2013;6:158–61.

6. Prevention and treatment of moderate and severe ovarian hyperstimulation syndrome: a guideline. Fertil Steril 2016; 106: 1634–47.

7. Elchalal U, Schenker JG. The pathophysiology of ovarian hyperstimulation syndrome-views and ideas. Hum Reprod. 1997;12:1129–37.

8. Mathur RS, Akande AV, Keay SD, Hunt LP, Jenkins JM. Distinction between early and late ovarian hyperstimulation syndrome. Fertil Steril 2000; 73:901–7.

9. Schenker JG, Weinstein D. Ovarian hyperstimulation syndrome: a current survey. Fertil Steril 1978;30:255–68.

10. Golan A, Ron-el R, Herman A, Soffer Y, Weinraub Z, Caspi E. Ovarian hyperstimulation syndrome: an update review. Obstet Gynecol Surv 1989; 44:430–40.

11. Navot D, Bergh PA, Laufer N. Ovarian hyperstimulation syndrome in novel reproductive technologies: prevention and treatment. Fertil Steril 1992;58:249–61.

12. Mathur R, Evbuomwan I, Jenkins J. Prevention and management of ovarian hyperstimulation syndrome. Curr Obstet Gynaecol 2005;15:132–8.

13. Evbuomwan I. The role of osmoregulation in the patho physi ology and management of severe ovarian hyperstimulation syndrome. Hum Fertil (Camb) 2013;16:162–7.

14. Balasch J, Carmona F, Llach J, Arroyo V, Jové I, Vanrell JA. Acute prerenal failure and liver dysfunction in a patient with severe ovarian hyperstimulation syndrome. Hum Reprod 1990;5: 348–51.

15. Practice Committee of the American Society for Reproductive Medicine. Ovarian hyperstimulation syndrome. Fertil Steril 2008;90:S188–93.

16. Royal College of Obstetricians and Gynaecologists (RCOG). The Management of Ovarian Hyperstimulation Syndrome Green-top Guideline No. 5;2016.

17. Lainas GT, Kolibianakis EM, Sfontouris IA, Zorzovilis IZ, Petsas GK, Tarlatzi TB, et al. Outpatient management of severe early OHSS by administration of GnRH antagonist in the luteal phase: an observational cohort study. Reprod Biol Endocrinol 2012;10:69.

18. Rollene NL, Amols MH, Hudson SB, Coddington CC. Treatment of ovarian hyperstimulation syndrome using a dopamine agonist and gonadotropin releasing hormone antagonist: a case series. Fertil Steril 2009;92:1169.e15–17.

19. Arieh Raziel, Morey Schachter et al. Outcome of IVF pregnancies following severe OHSS. Reproductive BioMedicine Online 2009 ;19:61–65.

20. Paul Devroey, Nikolaos P. Polyzos, Christophe Blockeel; An OHSS-Free Clinic by segmentation of IVF treatment, Human Reproduction 2011; 26: 2593–2597.

Fertility Preservation in Women Requiring Cancer Treatment

Rashmi Pillania, Anjali Tempe

Cancer usually affects elderly persons. However, many young women and men are also diagnosed with cancer every year. They need treatment with surgery, chemotherapy or radiotherapy which results in unwanted side effects such as reduced fertility.[1] The treatment-related infertility can lead to psychological distress and affects their treatment decisions. Thus, physicians should discuss with these patients and their parents the risk of infertility from the disease and/or treatment and options for fertility preservation.[2,3]

Q1. Enumerate the indications of fertility preservation therapies.

Indications of fertility preservation are:[4]
- **Gonadotoxic treatment of malignancy**
  (i) Chemotherapy/radiotherapy
  (ii) Reproductive tract surgery
- **Genetic conditions**
  (i) Turner syndrome, (ii) Fragile X per-mutation, (iii) X chromosome aberrations
- **Surgery for reproductive tract disease**
  (i) Ovarian endometriosis, (ii) Ovarian neoplasms, (iii) Cervical/uterine neoplasia
- **Autoimmune conditions**
  (i) Autoimmune oophoritis, (ii) Treatment of connective tissue disease
- **Counteract effects of ovarian aging**: Social fertility preservation

Q2. Enumerate factors affecting chemo-therapy and radiotherapy induced gonadotoxicity.

Type, duration and dose of chemotherapy determines the extent of chemotherapy induced gonadotoxicity. Gonadotoxicity, induced by chemotherapy is almost irreversible.

Factors affecting the extent of radiotherapy induced gonadotoxicity are—patient's age, dose of radiation (breaking point 300 cGy), extent and type of radiation (abdominal, pelvic external beam, brachytherapy).

Q3. Describe the mechanism of chemo-therapy related decreased fertility.

Normal premenopausal ovary has low level of recruitment of primordial follicles. Cytotoxic chemotherapy causes oocyte toxicity resulting in decreased serum estradiol and increased FSH levels. Increased FSH causes recruitment of more follicles thereby resulting in diminished ovarian reserve.

Q4. Classify anticancer therapies on the basis of their risk for causing infertility.

Various anticancer therapies have different effects on fertility:[5]
a. *High risk:* Total body irradiation, high dose cyclophosphamide, chlorambucil, melphalan, busulfan, nitrogen mustard, procarbazine
b. *Intermediate risk:* Cisplatin, carboplatin, doxorubicin
c. *Low or no risk:* Methotrexate, 5-fluorouracil, vincristine, vinblastine, bleomycin, actinomycin
d. *Unknown risk:* Taxanes, oxaliplatin, irinotecan, monoclonal antibodies, tyrosine kinase inhibitors

Case 1

A 15-year-old boy is diagnosed with high risk acute lymphocytic leukaemia (ALL) and is planned for chemotherapy.

Q1. How would you counsel his parents regarding future fertility following treatment with chemotherapeutic agents? What fertility preserving options can be offered to them?

The parents should be counseled about the option of semen cryopreservation. The parents of the boy should be informed that the sperm quality in the boy might be poor even prior to treatment due to the disease itself. ALL is usually treated with cyclophosphamide containing drug protocols. Relapse may occur while they are on therapy or shortly after completing therapy for which they require more aggressive chemotherapy and even hematopoietic stem cell transplant. At that time, they may not have recovered their sperm count to have an adequate specimen to cryopreserve. So, all teenaged boys newly diagnosed with cancer should be counseled to cryopreserve sperm before any treatment. Intracytoplasmic sperm injection (ICSI) for these patients allows the future use of small sample.[6]

The other option for gonadoprotection is through hormonal manipulations, however, it has not been successful in preserving fertility in men when highly sterilizing chemotherapy is given.

Potential future options not tested in humans till now are (a) Testicular tissue cryopreservation or reimplantation, (b) Testicular tissue removal followed by grafting in experimental mice.

Case 2

A 29-year-old woman, married for a year, is diagnosed with right solid ovarian mass measuring 6 to 7 cm. Her left ovary and uterus are normal and there is no ascites. Her CA125 is 360 U/mL and other tumor markers are normal.

Q1. How would you manage this patient?

This woman is likely to have an ovarian cancer that requires staging laparotomy. This involves peritoneal wash for cytology, right salpingo-oophorectomy, infracolic omentectomy and peritoneal biopsies. If the patient requires chemotherapy after surgery, she will be referred to reproductive medicine unit for fertility preserving options.

Q2. What are the criteria for fertility preservation in epithelial ovarian cancer (EOC)?

Criteria for fertility preservation in EOC are:
- Patient desirous of preserving fertility
- Patient and family consent and agree to close follow-up
- No evidence of dysgenetic gonads
- Stage I invasive epithelial tumour grade 1, grade 2

Q3. What fertility preserving option would be offered to a patient following surgery for early stage ovarian cancer?

The fertility preserving management includes ovarian stimulation by antagonist protocol followed by oocyte retrieval and embryo cryopreservation and subsequent gonadotrophin-releasing hormone (GnRH) analogue therapy during chemotherapy for ovarian protection.

Ovarian stimulation is conventionally initiated at the beginning of the follicular phase. 'Random-start' cycles as an alternative, are as effective as conventional cycles.[4]

Random start cycle protocol varies according to the phase of menstrual cycle in which the patient presents (Fig. 19.1).

a. *If the patient presents in luteal phase,* GnRH antagonist is administered for accelerated luteolysis and menses. Gonadotropin stimulation with or without aromatase inhibitors is started from second or third day of menstrual cycle. Follicle monitoring is done by ultrasound. When the lead follicle reaches 12–14 mm, GnRH antagonist is initiated to prevent premature LH surge. When at least two follicles reach 17–18 mm, ovulation trigger is given by human chorionic gonadotropin (hCG) or GnRH agonist. Oocyte retrieval is done 34–36 hours following trigger.

b. *If the patient presents in late follicular phase with lead follicle <12 mm,* immediate stimulation without GnRH antagonist is commenced. After endogenous LH surge, once secondary follicle cohort reaches 12–14 mm, GnRH antagonist is introduced to prevent premature secondary LH surge. Final maturation is achieved by hCG or GnRH agonist when follicles reach 17–18 mm which is followed by oocyte retrieval 34–36 hours later.

c. *If patient presents in late follicular phase with lead follicle exceeding 12 mm,* ovulation is induced with hCG or GnRH agonist and stimulation is started after 2–3 days.

In all these protocols, use of aromatase inhibitor along with gonadotropin for ovarian stimulation has an advantage of lowering peak estradiol levels and decreasing gonadotrophin requirement. However, there is no difference in oocyte or embyo yield[7] (Fig. 19.1).

Q4. What are the pharmacological agents used for preventing chemotherapy induced premature ovarian failure (POF)?

Pharmacological agents for preventing chemotherapy induced POF are GnRH agonist and Sphingosine 1 phosphate

a. GnRH agonist—GnRH agonist administration prior to chemotherapy decreases follicular recruitment, thus reducing the risk of toxicity.

b. Sphingosine 1 phosphate is an inhibitor of apoptosis.[8] However, its use in fertility preservation is still under investigation

Q5. Describe fertility sparing surgery in epithelial ovarian cancer (EOC).

Fertility sparing surgery is possible only in early stage EOC and involves unilateral salpingo-oophorectomy and complete staging, with preservation of the uterus and contralateral ovary. Biopsy of normal looking contralateral ovary is avoided. Pelvic and para-aortic lymph nodes must be palpated and any suspicious node must be removed. Adjuvant

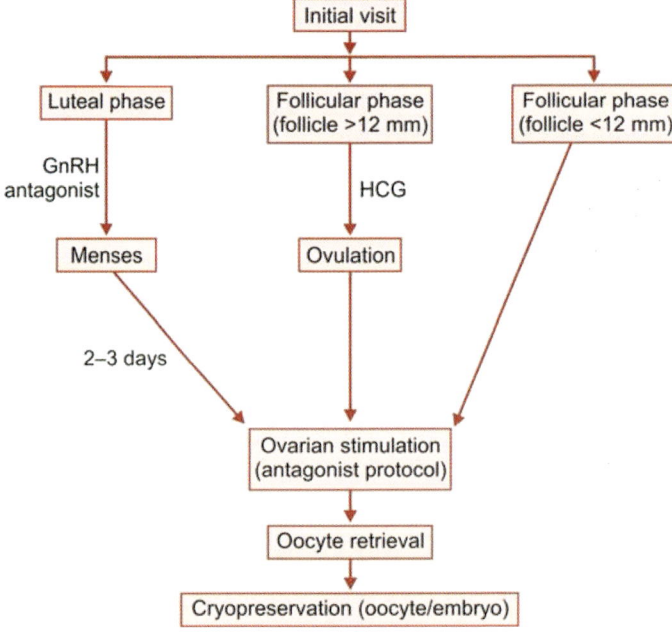

Fig. 19.1: Random start cycle

chemotherapy is indicated in high risk group (Grade 2 and grade 3, Stage 1c).

Case 3

A 13-year-old girl presents to the gynaecology outpatient clinic with a huge 25 × 18 cm mass in the abdomen with raised values of human chorionic gonadotropin (hCG), alphafeto-protein (AFP) and lactate dehydrogenase (LDH).

Q1. What is the diagnosis?

The likely diagnosis is malignant mixed germ cell tumor.

Q2. Describe the fertility sparing surgical management in malignant germ cell tumor.

The surgical management of malignant germ cell tumor in young girls include:[9]

Comprehensive surgical staging with unilateral salpingo-oophorectomy as for EOC. Benign cystic teratomas are managed with ovarian cystectomy.

Post-surgical treatment guidelines for malignant germ cell tumors are as illustrated in Table 19.1.

Q3. What is the rate of recurrence following fertility sparing management in malignant germ cell tumors? How would you follow-up such patients?

The rate of recurrence after fertility sparing management in germ cell tumors is 15–20%

over two years. The 5-year survival rate in Stage I is around 95.6% and 73.2% in advanced stage disease.

Follow-up in patients undergoing fertility sparing management is monthly for 1 year, every 2 months for next 1 year followed by every 3 months for 1 year and later 6 monthly is done by clinical assessment, tumor markers and if required by contrast enhanced computer tomography (CECT) or ultrasonography (USG).

Case 4

A 9-year-old prepubertal girl with history of sickle cell disease since 5 months of age has to undergo autologous stem cell transplant (SCT) as a treatment for severe sickle cell disease due to increased frequency of vaso-occlusive crisis. Her mother is concerned regarding her future fertility perspective.

Q1. How would you counsel her parents? What fertility preserving strategy would be offered to this prepubertal girl?

They are counseled regarding the benefits and side effects of chemotherapeutic agents and SCT particularly the risk of infertility and premature ovarian failure. Ovarian tissue cryopreservation followed by transplantation later is the only available option for fertility preservation. Ovarian stimulation with oocytes or embryo banking is not possible in prepubertal girls.

Table 19.1: Treatment guidelines of malignant germ cell tumors			
Stage	*Histology*	*Residual disease*	*Treatment*
1 to 3	Non dysgerminoma (endodermal sinus tumor, mixed germ cell, embryonal carcinonima)	Nil or ≤ = 1 cm	BEP-3 cycles
3 To 4	Any of the above	≥ = 1 cm	BEP-4 cycles
1 A grade 1	Immature teratoma	NIL	Observation
1A grade 2–3 1B–3	Immature teratoma	Nil or ≤ = 1 cm	BEP-3 cycles
3–4	Immature teratoma	≥ = 1 cm	BEP-4 cycles
1A	Dysgerminoma	NIL	Observation
Any stage	Dysgerminoma	≥ = 1 cm	BEP-4 cycles

Q2. What is ovarian tissue cryopreservation? Describe its role in fertility preservation.

Primordial follicles are less sensitive to cryodamage because of low metabolic rate, absence of zona pellucida and a high surface–volume ratio. In ovarian tissue cryopreservation, ovarian cortex containing primordial follicles is harvested laparoscopically, cut into thin strips of tissue, typically 0.3–2 mm thick and cryopreserved for transplantation later.

Limitations of ovarian tissue cryopreservation are:

- It requires surgical procedure to remove ovary or piece of ovary
- It may increase risk of infertility in low risk situation as initial ischemia encountered after transplantation destroys a significant proportion of these available follicles.
- Risk for reintroduction of malignant cells at reimplantation
- Highly experimental procedure

Ovarian tissue cryopreservation is discussed in detail in the chapter on cryopreservation.

Q3. What are the types of ovarian transplantation?

Types of ovarian transplantation are:

a. **Orthotopic transplantation**, in which the tissue is placed onto the remaining ovary or into a peritoneal pocket within the pelvic peritoneum or ovarian fossa. It has advantage of allowing natural conception and is the method with the most success. The first successful live birth using this technique was reported by Donnez in year 2004.[10]

b. **Heterotopic transplantation**, in which the tissue is placed outside the peritoneal cavity in sites like abdominal wall, forearm and chest. It is less successful due to less favorable environment for follicular development, with differences in temperature, pressure, vascular supply and paracrine effects. There are documented reports of hormonal function restoration, follicle development and oocyte retrieval from such sites however no successful live birth has been reported so far with this process.[11]

Q4. How long does it take for ovarian function to return in the transplanted tissue?

The ovarian function returns after 12–18 weeks following heterotopic transplantation and 8–18 weeks after orthotopic transplantation. The return of ovarian function depends on factors like freezing protocol, baseline ovarian reserve, vascularization of the graft, site of the graft and ischemia time after thawing prior to transplantation.

Case 5

A 26-year-old nulliparous is diagnosed with stage 1A1 poorly differentiated squamous cell carcinoma of cervix. She is concerned about her fertility preservation.

Q1. What measures can be taken for fertility preservation in this case?

Fertility preservation is best done by ovarian stimulation by antagonist protocol followed by oocyte retrieval and embryo freezing. However, this has the disadvantage of delaying cancer management.

Alternatively, radical trachelectomy with pelvic lymph node dissection can be performed along with bilateral oophorexy wherein ovaries are fixed higher up in the abdomen so that they stay outside the field of pelvic radiation. Later, following completion of treatment including radiotherapy, ovarian stimulation and trans abdominal retrieval of oocytes can be performed. However, patient should be counseled regarding the possibility of POF despite oophorexy due to radiation scatter and vascular compromise.

Case 6

A 30-year-old unmarried woman with family history of carcinoma ovary is recently diagnosed with invasive ductal breast carcinoma. She expresses her desire for fertility preservation

Q1. What fertility preservation options can be offered to this patient?

The patient should be counseled regarding the following options:

a. Ovarian stimulation by antagonist protocol followed by oocyte retrieval and oocyte cryopreservation.

   Oocyte cryopreservation is discussed in detail in the chapter on cryopreservation

   If she is willing for donor semen, IVF followed by embryo cryopreservation can be done.

b. Ovarian tissue cryopreservation prior to chemotherapy later by to be followed by transplantation either in the remaining ovarian tissue, the peritoneal cavity or in the extraperitoneal sites including forearm, abdominal wall and the chest.

c. GnRH agonist therapy along with chemotherapy. This has the advantage of no delay in cancer treatment. Two trials have reported a statistically significant reduction in the incidence of chemotherapy-induced POF in patients receiving GnRH agonist.[12,13]

Case 7

A 35-year-old nulliparous woman with BMI of 35.4 kg/m^2 presented with primary infertility and polymenorrhagia. She has been married for 10 years. Her transvaginal sonography was suggestive of thickened endometrium of 20 mm. Bilateral adnexa were normal. She was taken up for hysteroscopy that revealed multiple polypoid areas. Directed biopsy was taken. Histopathology report revealed adenocarcinoma grade I. MRI of the pelvis revealed thickened endometrium with absence of myometrial invasion.

Q1. What are the criteria for fertility preservation in carcinoma endometrium?

The criteria for fertility preservation in carcinoma endometrium are:

- Age <40 years
- Nulliparous

- Stage IA, grade I adenocarcinoma
- Absence of myometrial invasion and extrauterine spread by imaging study (MRI)
- Absence of a concurrent ovarian neoplasm
- Possessing a strong desire to preserve fertility
- Willing for follow-up

Q2. What are the fertility preservation options for patients with carcinoma endometrium? How would you follow up such patients?

Fertility preserving options for carcinoma endometrium include:

- Megestrol acetate: 40–160 mg/day
- Medroxyprogesterone acetate: 200–600 mg/day
- GnRH analogue (triptorelin, leupride)
- Progesterone containing intrauterine device
- Antiestrogens, aromatase inhibitor

Recurrence risk in patient undergoing fertility preserving management for carcinoma endometrium is 24%. Therefore, follow up is done by histopathological endometrial evaluation and transvaginal ultrasound at 3 to 6 months after initiating progestin therapy.

Key Points

- Fertility preservation options should always be discussed with all women of reproductive age group undergoing cancer treatment.
- Random-start cycles, are as effective as conventional cycles for ovarian stimulation in these patients.
- Oocyte cryopreservation is an option for women without a partner and not willing for donor semen.
- Ovarian tissue cryopreservation followed by transplantation later, is the only available option for fertility preservation in prepubertal girls.

REFERENCES

1. American cancer society. Cancer facts and figures 2015.
2. Lee SJ, Schover LR, Partridge AH, Patrizio P, Patricia P, Wallace WH, Hagerty K, et al. American Society of Clinical Oncology recommendations on fertility preservation in cancer patients: J Clin Oncol 2006; 24:2917–31.

3. Loren AW, Mangu PB, Beck LN, Brennan L, Magdalinski AJ, Partridge AH, et al. Fertility Preservation for Patients With Cancer: American Society of Clinical Oncology Clinical Practice Guideline Update. J Clin Oncol 2013;31: 2500–10.

4. Radon C, Borka A, Homburg R. Female fertility preservation: a fertile future: The Obstetrician and Gynaecologist 2015;17:116–124.

5. Maetto L, Lucia DM, Anderson C, Pescio M, Azim H, Peccatori F, et al. Cancer and fertility preservation: international recommendation from expert meeting. BMC Medicine 2016; 14:1

6. Oktay K, Harvey BE, Partridge AH, Quinn GP, Reinecke J, Taylor HS, et al. Fertility Preservation in Patients With Cancer: ASCO Clinical Practice Guideline Update. J Clin Oncol 2018; 36:1994-2001.

7. Oktay K, Hourvitz A, Sahin G, Oktem O, Safro B, Cil A, et al. Letrozole reduces estrogen and gonadotrophin exposure in women with breast cancer undergoing ovarian stimulation before chemotherapy. J Clin Endocrinol Metab 2006; 91:3885–90.

8. Li F, Turan V, Oktay K. Sphingosine 1 phosphate prevents chemotherapy induced human primordial follicle death. Human Reprod 2014;29:107-113

9. Nishio S, Ushijima K, Fukui A, Fujiyoshi N, Kawano K, Komai K, et al. Fertility preserving treatment for patients with malignant germ cell tumors of the ovary. J Obstet Gynaecol Res 2006;32:416-21

10. Donnez J, Dolmans MM, Demylle D, Jadoul P, Pirard C, Squifflet J. Live birth after orthotopic transplantation of cryopreserved ovarian tissue. Lancet 2004;364:1405-10

11. Oktay K, Economos K, Kan M, Rucinski J, Veeck L, Rosenwaks Z. Endocrine function and oocyte retrieval after autologous transplantation of ovarian cortical strips to the forearm. JAMA 2001;286:1490–3

12. Del Mastro L, Boni L, Michelotti A, Gamucci T, Olmeo N, Gori S, et al. Effect of the gonadotropin-releasing hormone analogue triptorelin on the occurrence of chemotherapy-induced early menopause in premenopausal women with breast cancer: a randomized trial. JAMA 2011; 306:269–76.

13. Moore HCF, Unger JM, Phillips K-A, Boyle F, Hitre E, Porter D, et al. Goserelin for ovarian protection during breast-cancer adjuvant chemotherapy. N Engl J Med 2015;372: 923–32.

Uterine Transplantation

Deepali Dhingra, Anjali Tempe

Introduction

Since the inception of assisted reproductive techniques (ART), majority of causes of infertility can be addressed. Presence of uterine factor infertility (UFI), due to lack of anatomical and functional uterus, usually require women to consider the options of surrogacy or adoption. Strict surrogacy laws and moral and ethical issues limit the option of surrogacy for many women. Uterine transplantation, which was experimental till now, due to technical advances, is being attempted by many from around the globe and could become a future for uterine factor infertility.

Q1. What is uterine factor infertility?

It is inability to carry pregnancy due to anatomical absence of uterus or physiologically non-functional uterus. It affects 3–5% of infertile population. Various causes of UFI are:

- **Absent uterus:**
  - Congenital Müllerian malformations-Mayer-Rokitansky-Küster-Hauser (MRKH) syndrome
  - Previous hysterectomy
- **Non-functional uterus:**
  - Intrauterine adhesions
  - Radiation damage
  - Myoma
  - Uterine malformation other than MRKH
  - Severe adenomyosis

Q2. What is historical view point on uterine transplantation?

Uterine transplantation dates backs to 1966 where fallopian tubes transplantation was tested in dogs.[1] Due to unavailability of effective immune suppression drugs and rapid advancements in field of assisted reproductive techniques, uterine transplantation remained dormant for years. Uterine transplantation research began in 1999, by Brännström et al, which included experiments in many animal species. First ever human uterine transplantation was reported in year 2000 by team in Saudi Arabia.[2] They performed uterine transplantation in 26 year old hystrectomised woman from a living donor who had hysterectomy, but the graft was rejected after 100 days because of thrombosis due to inadequate structure support of the uterus. The second attempt of uterine transplantation was done by Turkey group, which resulted in two pregnancies but ended in miscarriages.[3]

The first successful live birth after uterine transplantation was reported by Swedish group in September 2014, in a group of nine transplanted recipients. In November 2014, two more women gave birth in the same group.

Q3. What are types of donors in uterine transplantation?

Live donor: When uterus is procured from a live donor, timing of transplantation can be set apart. Both donor and recipient are in optimized condition and well prepared to decrease chances of graft rejection. Donors are generally close relative or a family member of the recipient. Donors are thoroughly evaluated for systemic illness, prior history of subfertility, cervical or uterine pre-cancerous

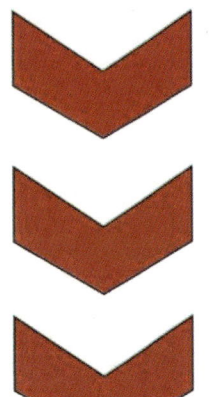

- Appropriate selection of donor and recipient
- Consents and counselling
- In-vitro fertilization for recipient started before uterine transplantation. 6–10 embryos-targeted. Cryopreserved

- Donor surgery: Removal of uterus, internal iliac arteries, distal to the branching of the gluteal artery, as well as the major uterine veins down to, and including parts of the internal iliac veins along with 1–1.5 cm of vagina
- Recipient surgery: Uterus along with vessels is anastomosed with external illiac vessels

- Immunosuppressive drugs to prevent rejection for 1 year
- Embryo transfer attempted after 12 months. If patient concieves, to continue immunosuppression throughout pregnancy. Caeserean section delivery. Followed by hystrectomy after 6 months

Fig. 20.1

lesion or malignancy, human papilloma virus infection, myoma, adenomyosis and intrauterine adhesions. The surgery is long, lasting almost 10 hours. Most time consuming part is isolation of vessels particularly uterine veins.

Deceased donor: The benefit of deceased uterine donation is that there is no surgical risk to the donor, takes shorter time; larger vessel diameter can be procured for anastomoses. The only drawback is long ischemic time, which leads to increased incidence of graft rejection.

Q4. What are the risks associated with uterine transplantation?

Donor risks

- Anesthetic risks
- Ureteric, bladder and bowel injuries
- Prolonged time of surgery leads to thrombotic complications
- Intra-operative blood loss
- Psychological burden

Recipient risks

- Surgical and anesthetic risks
- Graft rejection
- Pregnancies complicated by pre-eclampsia, liver disorders and graft rejection

Q5. What is the procedure of uterine transplantation?

See Fig. 20.1

Q6. What is experience of our country in terms of uterine transplantation?

In May 2017, India's first ever uterine transplant procedure was done in two patients on consecutive days by team of 12 doctors under Dr Shailesh Puntambekar in Galaxy Hospital, Pune. They performed laparoscopic assisted uterus retrieval from donors. Recipient surgery time was four hours. Pregnancies are yet to be reported.

REFERENCES

1. Eraslan S, Hamernik RJ, Hardy JD. Replantation of uterus and ovaries in dogs, with successful pregnancy. Arch Surg 1966;92:9–12.
2. Fageeh W, Raffa H, Jabbad H, Marzouki A. Transplantation of the human uterus. Int J Gynaecol Obstet 2002;76:245–51.
3. Erman Akar M, Ozkan O, Aydinuraz B, Dirican K, Cincik M, Mendilcioglu I et al. Clinical pregnancy after uterus transplantation. Fertil Steril 2013;100:1358–63.
4. Brännström M, Johannesson L, Bokström H, Kvarnström N, Mölne J, Dahm-Kähler P et al. Livebirth after uterus transplantation. Lancet 2015;385:607–616.
5. Puntambekar S, Telang M, Kulkarni P, Puntambekar S, Jadhav S, Panse M, et al. Laparoscopic-Assisted Uterus Retrieval From Live Organ Donors for Uterine Transplant: Our Experience of Two Patients. J Minim Invasive Gynecol 2018;25:622–631.

Endometrial Hyperplasia and Endometrial Cancer

Gauri Gandhi, Anubhuti Rana

Endometrial carcinoma is a common gyneco-logic malignancy with endometrial hyper-plasia being its precursor in majority of cases. A comprehensive understanding of the epidemiology, pathophysiology and management of endometrial carcinoma allows the gyneologists to recognize the women at increased risk and aid in early detection of this cancer.

Case 1

A 54-year-old postmenopausal lady complains of bleeding per vaginum for two months.

Q1. Enumerate the causes of postmeno-pausal bleeding.

The important causes of postmenopausal bleeding are:

A. Non-genital: Diseases of urinary tract such as urethral caruncle, papilloma and carcinoma of bladder can be misleading. Bleeding from hemorrhoids, anal fissure and rectal cancer can also be mistaken for genital tract bleeding.

B. Genital: Can be extra-uterine or uterine.

1. *Extra-uterine causes:*
   a. Vulva: Trauma, vulvitis, malignancy
   b. Vagina: Senile vaginitis, post radiation vaginitis, foreign body such as pessary, malignancy
   c. Cervix: Erosion, cervicitis, polyp, malignancy
   d. Ovary: Hormone producing ovarian tumor such as granulosa and theca cell tumors
   e. Fallopian tube malignancy

2. *Uterine causes:* Endometrial atrophy (60–80%), estrogen replacement therapy (15–25%), endometrial polyps (2–12%), endometrial hyperplasia (5–10%), and endometrial cancer (10%).[1]

Q2. What are the important points to be noted in history and examination for this case?

Any bleeding in postmenopausal women requires a detailed history and a careful clinical examination to rule out malignancy.

The important points to be noted in history are:
- Age
- Present illness: Duration, severity and pattern of bleeding, relation to intercourse, anorexia, weight loss, bladder or bowel symptoms, trauma, foreign body
- Menstrual history: age at menarche, pattern of previous cycles, age at menopause.
- Obstetric history
- Past history: Diabetes, hypertension, pap smear testing, history of breast or colon cancer
- Family history: History of breast, ovarian, endometrial or colon cancer in the family especially in first-degree relatives.
- Drug history: Any history of hormone replacement therapy, tamoxifen, treatment for anovulation, treatment for endometrial hyperplasia.

The important features to be noted in examination are:
- General physical examination: Body mass index (BMI), pallor, lymphadenopathy
- Breast
- Thyroid

- Systemic: Cardiovascular, respiratory
- Abdomen: Mass, ascites, organomegaly
- Local: Any growth or ulcer on vulva, near urethra or anus
- Per speculum (P/S): Cervix and vagina
- Per vaginum (P/V): Size and mobility of uterus, adnexal mass, parametrium
- P/V/R: Rectal mucosa, nodules in pouch of Douglas (POD)

In this case, there is no significant history and the general physical examination is also unremarkable except for BMI of $30 \, kg/m^2$. On P/S examination, cervix and vagina are healthy. On P/V examination, minimal bleeding is seen through os, a firm non-tender mobile anteverted uterus of normal size is present, bilateral fornices are clear. On P/V/R examination, rectal mucosa is free and there are no nodules in POD.

Q3. What will be the next step in work up of this case?

Since the patient has no local cause on examination and bleeding through os is seen, investigations to rule out uterine causes of postmenopausal bleeding should be done.

- Ultrasound pelvis
- Endometrial aspiration and endocervical curettage: The gold standard for diagnosis of endometrial cancer is an office endometrial sampling.

  Also, the following can be done as a part of the routine workup:
- Complete blood count, blood sugar fasting and postprandial, kidney function test. If there is anemia, a detailed work up to be done for it.
- Urine microscopy
- X- ray, ECG
- Pap smear

Q4. Discuss the role of transvaginal sonography (TVS) in a case of postmenopausal bleeding?

TVS has been explored as a technique to visualize the endometrium. It has various roles in evaluation of the endometrium.

- Appropriate as a reasonable alternative to endometrial sampling for work up of initial episode of postmenopausal bleeding. Endometrial thickness of ≤4 mm has a negative predictive value of 99% for endometrial cancer.[2]

  However, it is known that type II endometrial cancers arise in a background of atrophic endometrium (thickness less than 3 mm). Thus, persistent or recurrent uterine bleeding should be evaluated by endometrial sampling regardless of endometrial thickness.[2]
- It can be offered as triage for cases in which office endometrial sampling did not provide adequate tissue for diagnosis.[2]
- An endometrial thickness greater than 4 mm discovered incidentally in a postmenopausal woman without bleeding should not routinely trigger an endometrial sampling, instead an individualized approach based on patient characteristics and risk factors is advised.[2]

Q5. Is there any role of hysteroscopy?

Hysteroscopic guided biopsy may be indicated in the following conditions:
- Cervical stenosis
- Recurrent bleeding after a negative endometrial sampling
- Inadequate specimen

The report of endometrial biopsy reveals endometrial hyperplasia.

Q6. What is the recent classification of endometrial hyperplasia?

The revised 2014 World Health Organization (WHO) classification for endometrial hyperplasia is based upon the presence of cytological atypia, i.e. (i) hyperplasia without atypia and (ii) atypical hyperplasia.[3]

Q7. What is the approach for management of hyperplasia without atypia?

- Observation alone with follow-up endometrial biopsies to ensure disease regression can be considered, especially when identifiable risk factors such as obesity and use of hormone replacement therapy can be reversed.

- Progestogen treatment is indicated in women who fail to regress following observation alone and in symptomatic women with abnormal uterine bleeding.
- Both oral and local intrauterine (levonorgestrel-releasing intrauterine system [LNG-IUS]) can be used and the treatment should be for a minimum of 6 months.
- The LNG-IUS should be used as the first-line medical treatment instead of oral progestogens because it has a higher disease regression rate with a more favorable bleeding profile and fewer adverse effects. Women should be encouraged to retain the LNG-IUS for up to 5 years if fertility is not desired.
- Continuous progestogens that can be used are medroxyprogesterone 10–20 mg/day or norethisterone 10–15 mg/day.
- Endometrial surveillance with outpatient endometrial biopsy is recommended at a minimum of 6-monthly intervals and at least two consecutive 6-monthly negative biopsies should be obtained.[4]

Q8. What are the indications for surgical management in hyperplasia without atypia?

Hysterectomy is indicated in women not wanting to preserve their fertility in the following conditions:[4]

- progression to atypical hyperplasia occurs during follow-up.
- no histological regression of hyperplasia despite 12 months of treatment.
- relapse of endometrial hyperplasia after completing progestogen treatment.
- persistence of bleeding symptoms.
- the woman declines to undergo endometrial surveillance or comply with medical treatment.

- Postmenopausal women requiring surgery should be offered a bilateral salpingo-oophorectomy together with the total hysterectomy.
- For premenopausal women, the decision to remove the ovaries should be individualized; however, bilateral salpingectomy should be considered as this may reduce the risk of a future ovarian malignancy.

Q9. What is the management of atypical hyperplasia?

- Women with atypical hyperplasia should undergo a total hysterectomy because of the risk of underlying malignancy or progression to cancer.
- Bilateral salpingo-oophorectomy should be offered together with hysterectomy in postmenopausal women.
- For premenopausal women, the decision to remove the ovaries should be individualized; however, bilateral salpingectomy should be considered as this may reduce the risk of a future ovarian malignancy.
- Routine lymphadenectomy is not recommended.
- Women wishing to retain their fertility should be counselled about the risks of underlying malignancy and subsequent progression to endometrial cancer.
- First-line treatment with the LNG-IUS should be recommended, with oral progestogens as a second-best alternative. Once fertility is no longer required, hysterectomy should be offered in view of the high risk of disease relapse.[4]

Q10. Is there a role for endometrial ablation in the management of endometrial hyperplasia?

Endometrial ablation is not recommended because complete and persistent endometrial destruction cannot be ensured and intrauterine adhesion formation may preclude endometrial histological surveillance.[4]

Q11. What are the most common risk factors for development of endometrial cancer?

The common risk factors for development of endometrial cancer are as follows:[5]

- Age
- Nulliparity, infertility, early age at menarche, and late age at menopause.
- Prolonged unopposed estrogen exposure is associated with most of the type I endometrial cancers:
  - Estrogen replacement therapy
  - Chronic anovulation (polycystic ovary syndrome)
  - Estrogen-producing tumors
  - Excessive peripheral conversion of androgens to estrone in adipose tissue in obesity
- Endometrial hyperplasia especially atypical
- Use of Tamoxifen, a selective estrogen receptor modulator, acts as an estrogen antagonist in breast tissues and an agonist in bone and endometrial tissues
- Diabetes mellitus
- Hypertension
- Lynch syndrome or hereditary nonpolyposis colon cancer (HNPCC)
- Cowden syndrome

Importantly, the use of combination oral contraceptive pills, depot medroxyprogesterone acetate, and progesterone secreting intrauterine devices reduce the risk of developing endometrial cancer. Smoking has also been associated with a reduced risk.

Case 2

A 60-year-old, obese, hypertensive postmenopausal lady had complaint of postmenopausal bleeding for 6 months. Endometrial sampling reveals moderately differentiated endometrioid adenocarcinoma.

Q1. What are the pathological types of endometrial cancer?

There are two types of endometrial cancer.[1]

- Type I: They are commonly endometrioid, well differentiated, seen in 80% of cases, affecting perimenopausal and obese women, often begin in the background of hyperplastic epithelium. These have a good prognosis.
- Type II: They are commonly high grade, poorly differentiated, seen in 20% of cases, affecting postmenopausal and thin women, begin in the background of atrophic endometrium, poor prognosis.

Q2. What are the common clinical features of endometrial cancer?

It is noted that more than 90% of patients with endometrial cancer present with abnormal peri- or postmenopausal bleeding as the most common symptom. The second common clinical feature is vaginal discharge. A few patients experience pelvic pressure or discomfort from uterine enlargement. Patients who have advanced disease may have malignant cells on pap smear, hematometra and pyometra.[1]

Q3. What is the role of universal screening of endometrial cancer?

There is no cost-effective, appropriate, acceptable test that reduces mortality. Also, as noted above, up to 90% of patients are symptomatic at an early stage itself. Hence, universal screening of endometrial cancer is not recommended.

However, screening may be justified in high risk cases such as:[1]

- Women receiving estrogen replacement therapy without progestins.
- Members of families with HNPCC.

Q4. What preoperative work up would you like to do in this case and elaborate the role of imaging modalities in the diagnosis and metastatic evaluation of newly diagnosed endometrial cancers.

The preoperative work up would include:

- Complete blood count, blood sugar fasting and postprandial, kidney function test.
- Urine microscopy
- X- ray chest, ECG
- Pap smear
- Imaging

Role of imaging modalities in diagnosis and metastatic work up:[5]

- Endometrial cancer is a surgically staged disease. Preoperative assessment of spread is not typically required.
- However, under special situations such as poor surgical candidate due to medical comorbidities or when symptoms suggest possible metastasis to bone or central nervous system, preoperative assessment of metastatic disease may become clinically important.
- TVS – thickness of endometrium more than 4 mm in a postmenopausal lady, polypoidal endometrial mass or fluid in the uterus.
- Magnetic resonance imaging (MRI) – accurate diagnosis of cancer and myometrial invasion in 70–90% of cases.
- Computed tomography (CT) – detects lymph nodes better than MRI, however accuracy of myometrial invasion is inferior.
- Integrated positron emission tomography and computed tomography (PET/CT) scan – evolving technology especially for metastasis.

Q5. Is there any role of tumor markers in this patient?

The measurement of serum CA125 has also been investigated as a means of preoperative evaluation for metastasis, however, its role remains ill defined. A correlation between preoperative CA125 concentrations and extrauterine disease, including lymph node metastasis has been noted.[6] Hence, it can be selectively used in the management of patients who may not be able to undergo comprehensive staging surgery and in those with high-risk endometrial cancer histology, such as papillary serous.[7]

Q6. Describe the staging of endometrial cancer?

The revised 2009 FIGO staging for carcinoma for the endometrium:[8]

IA Tumor confined to the uterus, no or <½ myometrial invasion

IB Tumor confined to the uterus, >½ myometrial invasion

II Cervical stromal invasion, but not beyond uterus

IIIA Tumor invades serosa or adnexa

IIIB Vaginal and/or parametrial involvement

IIIC1 Pelvic node involvement

IIIC2 Para-aortic involvement

IVA Tumor invasion bladder and/or bowel mucosa

IVB Distant metastases including abdominal metastases and/or inguinal lymph nodes

Q7. What is the recommended comprehensive surgical staging for endometrial cancer?

The recommended surgical staging is a procedure that includes total extrafascial hysterectomy with bilateral salpingo-oophorectomy and bilateral pelvic and para-aortic lymph node dissection.[5] Although peritoneal cytology does affect the stage of the disease, it is still to be reported separately as it is an important prognostic factor.[1]

Q8. What additional step is performed in case of papillary serous or clear cell histological types of endometrial cancer?

These are high-grade tumors with an aggressive behavior like advanced ovarian cancer. Hence, omentectomy is also done as a part of surgical staging for them.

Q9. Enumerate the routes of surgery for endometrial cancer.

The routes of surgery for endometrial cancer are:[5]

- **Laparotomy:** By midline vertical incision
- **Laparoscopy:** Compared to laparotomy, although longer operative time is noted in laparoscopy but it has similar rate of intraoperative complications and 5 year survival rate, with the advantages of less postoperative complications and shorter hospital stay.

- **Vaginal hysterectomy:** Selected for women who are elderly, obese, or have extensive comorbid conditions in which the risks associated with surgical staging via an abdominal or laparoscopic approach may outweigh its potential benefit.
- **Robotic:** The benets are similar to those for laparoscopy with the additional advantage that technical prociency is attained more easily with robotic assistance than with conventional laparoscopy.

Q10. What is the type of hysterectomy performed for stages I and II endometrial cancer?

Extra fascial hysterectomy is performed for stage I whereas a modified radical hysterectomy is performed for stage II endometrial cancer.

Q11. What is the surgical management of advanced endometrial cancer (stage III/IV)?

Surgical staging and maximum cytoreductive surgery to achieve optimal debulking is the current approach for advanced endometrial cancer.

Q12. What are the fertility sparing approaches for young women with endometrial cancer? Enlist the criteria for selection of candidates for such an approach.

Fertility-sparing options for the treatment of endometrial cancer are not the standard of care. Progestin preparations are used for this purpose, most common being medroxyprogesterone acetate (MPA) and megestrol acetate. Progestin-releasing intrauterine device (LNG-IUS) can also be used as an acceptable alternative. It is recommended that patients undergo definitive surgical management after the completion of childbearing or if conservative management fails.

The criteria for using fertility sparing approaches are:[9]

- A well-differentiated endometrial carcinoma, grade 1

- No myometrial invasion
- No extrauterine involvement
- Strong desire for sparing fertility
- No contraindications for medical management
- Informed consent of the patient accepting that this is not standard treatment.

Q13. Enumerate the indications for lymphadenectomy in endometrial cancer?

The decision to perform lymphadenectomy is based on the following factors:[1]

- Type of endometrial cancer
- Grade of tumor
- Size of tumor
- Depth of myometrial invasion (determined during surgery)
- Presence of extra-uterine disease (cervical or adnexal involvement)

In cases of stage IA, Grade 1 and 2 disease, lypmphadenectomy may be omitted.

Bilateral pelvic and para-aortic lypmphadenectomy is performed if the patient has non-endometrioid type, grade 3 tumor, evidence of more than 50% myometrial invasion or presence of extra-uterine disease.

In the absence of these factors, bilateral pelvic lymphadenectomy is performed if the tumor size is greater than 2 cm; and para-aortic lymphadenectomy is performed if pelvic nodes are positive for metastasis.

Q14. Describe the role of sentinel node sampling in endometrial cancer.

Sentinel lymph node assessment, which is commonly performed as a standard of care in malignancies such as breast cancer and melanoma, is now being introduced in gynecologic cancers as pelvic lymphadenectomy can be associated with long-term morbidity such as lymphedema.[10] The current role in endometrial cancer in only investigational.

Q15. What are the prognostic factors in patients with endometrial carcinoma?

The most important prognostic factors at diagnosis are: age, stage, histological type, grade, tumor size, myometrial invasion, lymphovascular space invasion, involvement of cervix, involvement of adnexa, hormone receptor status, peritoneal cytology which is to be interpreted only in light of other prognostic factors or extrauterine disease.[1]

Q16. What is the role of adjuvant radiation therapy and adjuvant chemotherapy in management of patients with stage I or II endometrial cancers?

Patients who have FIGO grade 1 or 2 endometrioid carcinomas limited to the inner half of endometrium (IA, G1/2, endometrioid) will not benefit from any additional adjuvant therapy. However, some form of adjuvant therapy has been considered for all others.

Role of adjuvant radiation:
- Adjuvant radiation therapy has been associated with a reduction in loco-regional recurrence but has no impact on overall survival.[11]
- Vaginal brachytherapy has been shown to be equivalent to whole pelvic radiation therapy and is also associated with significantly fewer gastrointestinal toxic effects as well as a better quality of life.[9]

Role of adjuvant chemotherapy: The use of adjuvant chemotherapy for stage I or II endometrial carcinomas is not supported by available evidence.[9]

Q17. What is the role of adjuvant radiation therapy and/or adjuvant chemotherapy in patients with advanced endometrial cancer?

- The role of *radiotherapy* is same as described above for early endometrial cancer.
- The role of *chemotherapy* has expanded from use as palliation in recurrent or inoperable disease to use after cytoreductive surgery.[12]
- The most common chemotherapy regimen used is paclitaxel with carboplatin as it is as effective as other regimens with the advantage of least toxicity.[13]
- Chemotherapy and radiation therapy used in combination may offer superior outcomes

compared to single-modality treatment. This is especially noted in patients with positive para-aortic lymph nodes who received extended field radiation versus treatment with chemotherapy followed by pelvic and para-aortic radiation.

Q18. What is the management for patients who have an incidental diagnosis of endometrial cancer following hysterectomy for another indication?

Women found to have endometrial cancer incidentally after hysterectomy should have their risk of extrauterine disease and potential for disease recurrence evaluated based on age, pathological details of uterine tumor such as histologic type, grade, depth of myometrial invasion, presence of lymphovascular space invasion and tumor size and imaging findings of CT, MRI or PET/CT along with CA-125.

Individualized treatment plans can be based on the findings.

If histopathological findings are endometrioid histology, grade 1 or 2 tumors, small tumor volume, and superficial myometrial invasion, further intervention may not be indicated.

Patients who have intermediate- or high-risk features for extrauterine spread or recurrence, may be considered for comprehensive surgical staging or adjuvant radiation and/or chemotherapy.[9]

Q19. What is the appropriate follow-up for women after treatment of endometrial cancer?

The aim of surveillance following treatment of endometrial cancer is detection of treatable recurrent disease, thereby ensuring improved survival.[13]

- Current guidelines of the National Comprehensive Cancer Network (NCCN) recommend physical examination every 3 to 6 months for 2 years and every 6 months or annually thereafter.
- The role of vaginal cytology and chest radiography during follow up remains controversial. The NCCN recommends

vaginal cytologic evaluation to aid in the detection of cuff recurrence and annual chest radiograph. Society of Gynecologic Oncology (SGO) review on the other hand recommends against these evaluations as most vaginal recurrences are detected with clinical examination alone and chest radiography is of low utility in detecting asymptomatic recurrence.

- The SGO review also recommends that radiologic evaluation such as CT scan of the chest, abdomen and pelvis or PET/CT scans be reserved for assessment in women with suspected recurrent disease
- The utility of serum CA125 assessment is a subject of debate.

Key Points

- Endometrial hyperplasia and endometrial cancer usually manifest as perimenopausal abnormal uterine bleeding or as postmenopausal bleeding.
- Clinical examination and imaging by ultra-sonography or MRI help in suspecting the diagnosis.
- Confirmation of diagnosis is by histopathological assessment of the endometrial tissue obtained by endometrial sampling.
- Endometrial hyperplasia without atypia is managed medically with progesterones while atypical hyperplasia is usually managed with hysterectomy.
- Management of endometrial cancer depends on the stage of the disease. Surgical staging of the disease is done followed by postoperative radiotherapy for advanced disease.

REFERENCES

1. Uterine cancer. In: Berek JS (Ed). Berek & Novak's Gynecology, 14th edition. Philadelphia: Lippincott, Williams & Wilkins; 2007.
2. ACOG Committee Opinion No. 734 Summary: The Role of Transvaginal Ultrasonography in Evaluating the Endometrium of Women With Postmenopausal Bleeding. Obstet Gynecol 2018;131:945-946.
3. Kurman RJ, Carcangiu ML, Herrington CS, Young RH, (Eds). WHO Classification of Tumours of Female Reproductive Organs 4th ed. [Lyon]: IARC; 2014.
4. Gallos ID, Alazzam M, Clark TJ. Management of Endometrial Hyperplasia. RCOG/BSGE Green-top Guideline No. 67. 2016;67:2–30.
5. SGO Clinical Practice Endometrial Cancer Working Group, Burke WM, Orr J, Leitao M, Salom E, Gehrig P, Olawaiye AB,et al. Endometrial cancer: a review and current management strategies: part I.Gynecol Oncol 2014;134:385-92.
6. Hsieh CH, ChangChien CC, Lin H, Huang EY, Huang CC, Lan KC, et al. Can a preoperative CA 125 level be a criterion for full pelvic lymph-adenectomy in surgical staging of endometrial cancer? Gynecol Oncol 2002;86:28-33.
7. Olawaiye AB, Rauh-Hain JA, Withiam-Leitch M, Rueda B, Goodman A, del Carmen MG.Utility of pre-operative serum CA-125 in the management of uterine papillary serous carcinoma. Gynecol Oncol 2008;110:293-8.
8. Mutch DG: The New FIGO staging system for cancers of the vulva, cervix, endometrium, and sarcomas. Gynecol Oncol 115:325-328, 2009.
9. SGO Clinical Practice Endometrial Cancer Working Group, Burke WM, Orr J, Leitao M, Salom E, Gehrig P, Olawaiye AB, et al. Endometrial cancer: a review and current management strategies: part II.Gynecol Oncol 2014;134:39 3-402.
10. Abu-Rustum NR, Alektiar K, Iasonos A, Lev G, Sonoda Y, Aghajanian C, et al. The incidence of symptomatic lower-extremity lymphedema following treatment of uterine corpus malignan-cies: a 12-year experience at Memorial Sloan-Kettering Cancer Center. Gynecol Oncol 2006; 103: 714-8.
11. Straughn JM, Huh WK, Orr JW Jr, Kelly FJ, Roland PY, Gold MA, et al. Stage IC adenocarcinoma of the endometrium: survival comparisons of surgically staged patients with and without adjuvant radiation therapy. Gynecol Oncol 2003; 89:295-300.
12. Barlin JN, Puri I, Bristow RE. Cytoreductive surgery for advanced or recurrent endometrial cancer: a meta-analysis. Gynecol Oncol 2010;118: 14–8.
13. National Comprehensive Cancer Network: NCCN Clinical Practice Guidelines in Oncology -Uterine Neoplasms. Version 2.2016. www.nccn.org

Cervical Cancer

YM Mala, Snigdha Pathak

INTRODUCTION

Carcinoma cervix is one of the common cancers occurring in women all over the world and it has the fourth highest mortality rate among cancers in women.[1] In India, it is the second most common cancer in women aged 15–44 years with 122, 844 new registered cases.[2,3] Carcinoma cervix can be prevented by screening and early treatment of precancerous lesions.

Q1. How will a woman with cervical cancer present in the out patient department?

A typical patient is a multiparous woman between 45 and 55 years who married and delivered her first child at an early age and will present with any of the following complaints:

- Thin, watery, blood tinged vaginal discharge
- Bleeding per vaginum—postcoital or post-menopausal or irregular bleeding
- Discharge per vaginum (characteristically foul smelling)
- Backache/chronic pelvic pain
- Bladder/bowel complaints-dysuria, hematuria, rectal bleeding, obstipation
- Lower limb edema (late stages; lymphatic and venous blockage)
- Anorexia, weight loss.

Q2. How will you examine a woman with suspected cancer cervix on history?

- Per-speculum (P/S) Examination
  - Cervix may show no growth, but bleeds on touch

  - Growth seen on cervix-cauliflower, friable, bleeds heavily
  - Punched out ulcerative growth
  - Barrel shaped cervix
  - Vaginal involvement may be seen
- Per Vaginal (P/V) Examination
  - Cervix will feel hard/friable/ulcerated depending on type of growth
  - Vaginal involvement to be looked for
  - Forniceal involvement
  - Size of uterus (uterus will be enlarged in cases of pyometra)
- Rectovaginal Examination
  - P/V/R: (NOT TO BE MISSED)
  - Parametrial extension
  - Rectal mucosal involvement by tumor

Q2. How do you stage carcinoma cervix?

Staging of cancer cervix is clinical. Investigations which are acceptable for staging are:

- Biopsy to confirm the disease
- Routine radiographs
- Colposcopy
- Cystoscopy, proctosigmoidoscopy
- IVP, barium studies -lower colon and rectum

  USG, MRI, CT, PET scans, laparoscopy are not recommended for staging.

FIGO Staging[4,5]

- **Stage I:** Carcinoma confined to cervix (extension to uterine corpus disregarded)
  - IA: Invasive cancer identified only microscopically (all gross lesions are stage IB).

(Depth of invasion should be <5 mm taken from base of epithelium; lymphovascular space invasion (LVSI) should not alter staging)

- o IA1: Stromal invasion ≤3 mm in depth and ≤7 mm width
- o IA2: Stromal invasion >3 mm and <5mm in depth and ≤7 mm width
- IB: Clinical lesions confined to cervix or preclinical lesions greater than IA
  - o IB1: Clinical lesions <4 cm size
  - o IB2: Clinical lesions >4 cm size
- **Stage II:** Carcinoma extends beyond the uterus but not to pelvic wall or lower third of vagina
  - IIA: Involvement of upper 2/3rd of vagina. No parametrial involvement.
    - o IIA1: Clinically visible lesion <4 cm
    - o IIA2: Clinically visible lesion >4 cm
  - IIB: Parametrial involvement, but not to pelvic side wall
- **Stage III:** Tumor extends to the pelvic wall and/or involves lower 1/3rd of vagina and/or causes hydronephrosis or non-functioning kidney (not attributable to other causes)
  - IIIA: Tumor involves lower 1/3rd of vagina, with no extension to pelvic wall
  - IIIB: Extension to pelvic wall and/or hydronephrosis or non-functioning kidney.
- **Stage IV:** Carcinoma has extended beyond true pelvis or has clinically involved mucosa of bladder or rectum.
  - IVA: Spread to adjacent organs
  - IVB: Spread to distant organs

Q3. What investigations will you get done in a patient with cancer cervix?

Biopsy of the lesion confirms the diagnosis

- Complete blood count, serum chemistry
- Urinanalysis
- Cystoscopy (with biopsy and urine cytology)
- Proctoscopy (with biopsy)
- IVP
- Chest radiography

- Ultrasound abdomen and Pelvis (special emphasis on KUB)—not mandatory for staging
- MRI abdomen and pelvis (preferable to CT scan)—not mandatory for staging.

Q4. Once you have staged the disease, what treatment options are available for each stage of carcinoma cervix?

Stage-wise treatment options include:

- **In situ cancer cervix (Cervical intra-epithelial neoplasia—CIN III/Adeno carci-noma in situ—AIS)**
  - Conization (fertility preserving)
  - Extrafascial hysterectomy (when AIS)
  - Radiotherapy (medically inoperable)
- **Stage IA**
  - Conization (IA1) +/– laparoscopic lym-phadenectomy (IA1 with LVSI)
  - extrafascial hysterectomy (IA1) +/– lymphadenectomy (IA1 with LVSI)
  - modified radical hysterectomy + lym-phadenectomy (IA2)
  - radical trachelectomy + lymphadenec-tomy (IA2; fertility preserving)
  - intracavitary radiation therapy

Note: In stage IA2, risk of nodal metastasis is 6.3%, so lymphadenctomy is always done

- **Stages IB1, IIA**
  - Radical hysterectomy + lymphadenec-tomy + tailored adjuvant therapy
  - Radical trachelectomy + lymphadenec-tomy (fertility preserving)
  - Concurrent chemoradiation
  - Neoadjuvant chemotherapy (role in certain cases)
  - Intensity modulated radiation therapy (IMRT)
- **Stages IB2, IIB, III, IVA**
  - Concurrent chemoradiation (treatment of choice) + High dose rate (HDR) brachy-therapy + pretreatment laparoscopic extraperitoneal lymphadenectomy (as clinically indicated)
  - Radical hysterectomy + lymphadenec-tomy (selected cases of IB2, II a), adjuvant therapy

– Interstitial brachytherapy
– Neoadjuvant chemotherapy (role in certain cases)
- **Stage IVB:** Palliative radiotherapy/chemotherapy
- **Recurrent cervical cancer**
  – No prior radiotherapy—concurrent chemoradiation
  – Prior radiotherapy—pelvic exenteration

Management of Carcinoma Cervix[6,7]

Q5. What are the treatment options for a woman with carcinoma in situ (CINIII/AIS)?

Before therapy is undertaken, invasive disease must be ruled out with the help of colposcopic directed biopsy or cone biopsy.

1. Cone biopsy (cold-knife/laser/loop):
   – Conventional cold knife cone preferred
   – Can be both diagnostic and therapeutic (if margins free on histopathology)
   – Diagnostic in—failure to identify lesion, extension of lesion into endocervical canal, AIS (adenocarcinoma in situ wanting fertility preservation), lack of correlation between pap smear and colposcopic findings.
   – Therapeutic in—CIN-III; AIS (only in patients wanting fertility preservation)
   – Complications—hemorrhage, infection, cervical stenosis, incompetent cervix
2. Extrafascial hysterectomy:
   – Standard for AIS (because AIS is in endocervix and is difficult to completely excise with conization)
   – Not acceptable as first line therapy for squamous cancer in situ; performed when conization not possible or positive margins after conization.
   – Specimen includes pubocervical fascia and 1cm vaginal cuff. (During hysterectomy, clamps are not bounced over cervix, so adjacent parametrium is removed with specimen).
   – Oophorectomy is optional and should be deferred in younger women (ovarian metastasis are rare in cancer cervix)

3. Intracavitary radiotherapy—if medically inoperable.

Case 1

Mrs X, 38-year-old P3L3 , presented to Gynae OPD with complaint of postcoital vaginal bleeding for 4 months. On per speculum examination, cervix looked unhealthy and bled on touch, but no gross lesion was seen. Per vaginal examination was unremarkable. Pap smear showed 'high grade squamous intra epithelial lesion' (HSIL). Colposcopy guided biopsy was taken and reported as moderately differentiated keratinizing squamous cell carcinoma with depth of invasion 3–4 mm.

Impression

Stage IA1 cancer cervix.

Q1. How will you treat a woman with Stage IA cancer cervix diagnosed on histopathology report of biopsy specimen?

Stage IA1
1. Conization alone is sufficient if margins of cone are negative and no LVSI. If LVSI present, then laparoscopic lymphadenectomy also to be done.
2. Extrafascial hysterectomy (previously discussed). Lymphadenectomy to be done if LVSI present.

Stage IA2
1. Modified radical hysterectomy with lymphadenectomy (also called Type II hysterectomy/Wertheim's hysterectomy) Specimen consists of—uterus, cervix, medial half of parametrium, upper 1/3rd of vagina
2. Radical trachelectomy with lymphadenectomy:[8]
   – In IA2 and IB1(<2 cm only) where future fertility is desired
   – Age <40 years
   – Cervix and medial half parametrial tissues removed along with 1 cm vaginal cuff; uterine body and ovaries preserved; lymphadenectomy is done
   – Prophylactic ligature is placed over lower uterine segment (as increased risk

of mid-trimester abortions and prematurity after trachelectomy)
- If intraoperatively more advanced disease
is encountered, procedure is abandoned
- Margins of specimen are assessed at the
time of surgery; if inadequate margins
found, radical hysterectomy is performed.
3. Intracavitary radiation therapy:
- For poor surgical candidates
- When invasion depth <3 mm and no LVSI,
EBRT (external beam radiation therapy)
is not needed and intracavitary radiation
suffices.

Case 2

Mrs Y, 35-year-old lady, P2L2 presented with
complaint of discharge per vaginum for
4 months and heavy menstrual bleeding on and
off for last 1 year. She was examined and on
P/S examination, was found to have an
exophytic cervical growth ~ 2 × 2 cm, friable,
bleeds on touch. On P/V examination same size
hard growth was felt, uterus was bulky, firm,
mobile and fornices and vagina were free. On
P/V/R examination, bilateral parametrium
were free. A biopsy was taken the same visit
and report came out as well differentiated
keratinizing squamous cell carcinoma.

Impression

Stage IB1 cancer cervix

Q1. **What are the treatment options for stage
IB1 and stage IIA of the disease?**

Stage IB1, IIA

1. Radical hysterectomy (Type III) + lymphadenectomy + tailored adjuvant therapy:
- Specimen includes—uterus, cervix, entire
cardinal and uterosacral ligaments, upper
1/3rd of vagina
- Preoperative preparation and opening of
abdomen remains same as for abdominal
hysterectomy
- All peritoneal surfaces and pelvic cavity
assessed for extent of tumor and enlarged
lymph nodes; suspicious lymph nodes
sent for frozen section; if para-aortic
lymph node is found positive for

metastasis on frozen section, surgery
is abandoned in favor of adjuvant
chemoradiation.
- Pelvic lymphadenectomy—common
iliac, external iliac and obturator nodes are
dissected; lateral group of nodes in external iliac chain to be spared to avoid
lymphedema of lower limbs; careful dissection to be done to avoid genitofemoral
nerve injury
- Uterine artery is ligated at its origin (but
superior vesical artery is preserved)
- Ureteric tunnel dissection is done; ureter
is separated from vesicouterine ligament
and traced to its entry into bladder.

*Adjuvant therapy

Post surgery: Given to patients with risk of
tumor recurrence

Two classes of recurrence risk:

- Intermediate risk—large tumor size, LVSI,
deep stromal invasion (greater than 1/3rd
stromal depth)—candidates for postoperative External beam radiotherapy (EBRT)[9].
- High risk—positive margins, positive para-
metria, positive lymph nodes—candidates
for postoperative concurrent chemoradiation.
- Extended field radiation—when paraaortic
nodes involved. Drawback is that toxic effects are more in extended field radiation
than with pelvic radiation alone.

Other treatment options

2. Radical Trachelectomy + Lymphadenectomy
- In IB1 (<2 cm) when fertility preservation
required
3. Concurrent chemoradiation (discussed
later)—in patients with larger tumors
concurrent chemoradiation is preferable to
surgery as adjuvant radiation might be
required after surgery for larger tumors
and dual modality treatment has greater
complications than single modality.
4. Neoadjuvant chemotherapy (NACT):
- To convert conventional chemoradiation
candidates into candidates for radical
surgery

- Platinum based compounds used for 3 cycles followed by evaluation for surgery.
- EORTC 55994 trial is ongoing in patients of stage IB2, IIA2, IIB cervical cancer, comparing primary chemoradiation with NACT + adjuvant surgery, and it may help in further defining role of NACT in this group.

5. Intensity modulated radiation therapy (IMRT):
   - Radiation is targeted at tumor site while sparing neighbouring tissue
   - Decreased radiation toxicity

Case 3

Mrs Z, P6L6 60-year-old lady was referred from surgery department to gynae outpatient clinic for the complaint of vaginal discharge. She gave history of foul smelling discharge P/V for several years and on asking, revealed history of postmenopausal bleeding P/V on and off. She also complained of loss of appetite since last 1 year. There were no urinary or bowel complaints. On P/S examination, cervix was replaced by a large cauliflower growth ~5 × 4 cm, which was friable and bled on touch. On P/V examination same hard growth was felt, uterus was anteverted, 8 weeks size, bilateral fornices appeared involved. On P/V/R examination, bilateral parametrium were involved just short of lateral pelvic wall. On cervical biopsy -moderately differentiated non-keratinizing squamous cell cancer. An ultrasound was done to determine the reason was uterine enlargement and ~150 cc uterine collection was detected.

Impression: Stage IIB Cancer Cervix with hematometra/pyometra

Q1. What is the first thing to be done in this patient before treatment for Ca Cervix can begin?

Pyometra drainage: Any treatment for cervical cancer can begin only after hematometra/pyometra drainage as it can act as a source of infection during the treatment. Cervix can be dilated and left as such for pyometra to drain or an intrauterine Foley's catheter can be inserted to allow for drainage. After it is ascertained that uterine cavity is empty, the woman can go for chemoradiation.

Q2. What is the treatment for locally advanced cancer cervix (Stage IB2, IIB, III, IVA)?

Concurrent chemoradiation is the first line treatment.

1. **Radiotherapy**
   - Only modality that can be used in all stages of disease including palliation.
   - Localized disease—brachytherapy (intra-cavitary).
   - Widespread disease—teletherapy/External beam radiotherapy (EBRT).
   - Para aortic nodes–extended field radiation/Intensity Modulated Radiation Therapy (IMRT).
   - Usually EBRT followed by 1 or 2 cycles of brachytherapy is the standard treatment.
   - Although low-dose rate (LDR) brachy-therapy, typically with cesium Cs 137 (137Cs), has been the traditional approach, the use of high-dose rate (HDR) therapy, typically with iridium Ir 192 provides the advantage of eliminating radiation exposure to medical personnel, a shorter treatment time, patient convenience, and improved outpatient management.[10]

2. **Concurrent chemoradiation**
   - Platinum based chemotherapy sensitises tumor cells prior to radiation exposure.
   - Many trials have been undertaken which show significant survival benefit of combining chemosensitisation with radiotherapy.[11,12]
   - Nowadays concurrent chemoradiation is the standard of care.
   - Common regimen is—cisplatin 40 mg/m^2 weekly for 6 weeks along with concurrent EBRT in divided doses, generally 3 times/week) followed by 2 cycles of brachytherapy.

3. **Lymph node management**
   - If postoperative EBRT is planned following surgery, extraperitoneal lymph node sampling is associated with fewer radiation-induced complications than a transperitoneal approach.[13]
   - The resection of macroscopically involved pelvic nodes may improve rates of local control with postoperative radiation therapy.[14]

4. **Interstitial brachytherapy**

   For patients who complete EBRT and have bulky cervical disease such that standard brachytherapy cannot be placed anatomically, interstitial brachytherapy has been used to deliver adequate tumoricidal doses with an acceptable toxicity profile.[15]

5. **NACT (as discussed earlier)**

 Key Points

- Carcinoma cervix can be prevented by screening and early treatment of precancerous lesions.
- Biopsy of the lesion confirms the diagnosis (punch/ cone/ endocervical currettage/colposcopy guided (when no visible lesion).
- Pelvic and para-aortic lymphadenectomy provides prognostic information.
- Radical hysterectomy should be avoided in patients who are likely to require adjuvant therapy.
- In women with cancer cervix (Stage I to IIA) at high risk of requiring post-op radiotherapy, ovaries should be transposed to paracolic gutters at the time of hysterectomy.

REFERENCES

1. International Agency for Research on Cancer. GLOBOCAN 2012: estimated cancer incidence, mortality and prevalence worldwide in 2012.
2. ICO Information Centre on HPV and cancer (Summary Report 2014-08-22). Human Papillomavirus and Related Diseases in India. 2014
3. Singh GK, Azuine RE, Siahpush M. Global inequalities in cervical cancer incidence and mortality are linked to deprivation, low socioeconomic status and human development. Int J MCH and AIDS. 2012;1:17-30.
4. FIGO Committee on Gynecologic Oncology: FIGO staging for carcinoma of the vulva, cervix, and corpus uteri. Int J Gynecol Obstet. 2014; 125:97-8.
5. DiSaia PJ, Creasman WT, Mannel RS, McMeekin DS, Mutch DG. Clinical Gynecologic Oncology E-Book. Elsevier Health Sciences; 2017 Feb 4.
5. Berek JS. Berek and Novak's Gynaecology, 15th edition. 2011.
6. Jones III HW, Rock JA. TeLinde's Operative Gynaecology, 11th edition 2015.
7. Raju SK, Papadopoulos AJ, Montalto SA, Coutts M, Culora G, Kodampur M, et al. Fertility-sparing surgery for early cervical cancer-approach to less radical surgery. Int J Gynecol Cancer 2012; 22: 311-7.
8. Sedlis A, Bundy BN, Rotman MZ, Lentz SS, Muderspach LI, Zaino RJ.. A randomized trial of pelvic radiation therapy versus no further therapy in selected patients with stage IB carci-noma of the cervix after radical hysterectomy and pelvic lymphadenectomy: A Gynecologic Oncology Group Study. Gynecol Oncol 1999;73:177-83.
10. Nag S, Erickson B, Thomadsen B, Orton C, Demanes JD, Petereit D.The American Brachytherapy Society recommendations for high-dose-rate brachytherapy for carcinoma of the cervix. Int J RadiatOncolBiol Phys 2000;48: 201-11.
11. Whitney CW, Sause W, Bundy BN, Malfetano JH, Hannigan EV, Fowler WC Jret al.Randomized comparison of fluorouracil plus cisplatin versus hydroxyurea as an adjunct to radiation therapy in stage IIB-IVA carcinoma of the cervix with negative para-aortic lymph nodes: a Gynecologic Oncology Group and Southwest Oncology Group study. J Clin Oncol 1999;17:1339-48.
12. Thomas GM. Improved treatment for cervical cancer--concurrent chemotherapy and radiotherapy. N Engl J Med 1999;340:1198-200.
13. Weiser EB, Bundy BN, Hoskins WJ, Heller PB, Whittington RR, DiSaia PJ,et al.Extraperitoneal versus transperitoneal selective paraaortic lymphadenectomy in the pre-treatment surgical staging of advanced cervical carcinoma (a Gynecologic Oncology Group study). Gynecol Oncol 1989;33:283-9.
14. Downey GO, Potish RA, Adcock LL, Prem KA, Twiggs LB. Pretreatment surgical staging in cervical carcinoma: therapeutic efficacy of pelvic lymph node resection. Am J Obstet Gyne-col 1989; 160:1055-61
15. Pinn-Bingham M, Puthawala AA, Syed AM, Sharma A, Disaia P, Berman M, et al. Out-comes of high-dose-rate interstitial brachytherapy in the treatment of locally advanced cervical cancer: long-term results. Int J RadiatOncolBiol Phys 2013;85:714-20.

23 | Malignant Ovarian Tumors

Latika Sahu, Tarang Preet Kaur, Reetu Yadav

Ovarian malignancies are among the commonly occurring gynecological malignancies. The management varies depending on the histological type of tumor and the age of the patient. A detailed workup including the tumor markers and imaging studies is required before proceeding to treatment. This is discussed with the help of some clinical case scenarios in this chapter.

Case 1

Mrs X, 60-year-old postmenopausal lady, presented with lump abdomen for last 6 months, loss of appetite, flatulence and weight loss for last 3 months. She had no significant past and family history. She had two live issues, both were vaginal deliveries and her last child birth was 30 years back. She had a tubectomy done 25 years back.

On physical examination, she was cachectic with body mass index (BMI) of 22 kg/m², edema of legs and prominent leg veins. Other general examination findings were unremarkable.

On abdominal examination, a mass was palpable in the hypogastric and both iliac regions measuring 20 × 18 cm, firm to solid consistency, irregular surface, irregular margins, restricted mobility, non-tender, lower limit could be reached with difficulty and ascites was detected. Liver and spleen were not palpable. On local examination, no significant finding was detected. On bimanual examination, a large abdominal mass was made out

with restricted mobility. Uterus was felt separate from the mass. Bilateral fornices were full and same mass could be palpated. On per rectal examination, rectal mucosa was free and lower abdominal mass was felt (Fig. 23.1).

Q1. What is the provisional diagnosis on the basis of history and clinical examination?

A 60-year-old para 2, postmenopausal woman with lump lower abdomen probably ovarian tumor, possibily malignant in nature.

Q2. What are the differential diagnoses for this case?

This mass could be:
- Large tubo-ovarian mass
- Abdominal tuberculosis
- Peritoneal tumor
- Gastrointestinal tumor
- Retroperitoneal tumor like lymphoma, lipoma, etc.

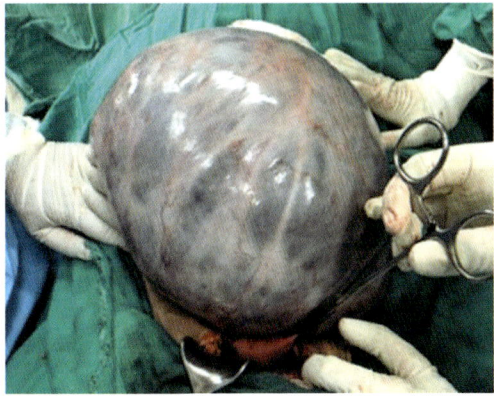

Fig. 23.1: Mucinous cystadenocarcinoma

Q3. What investigations will you ask for?

The investigations will include:[1]

- Routine investigations such as ABO, Rh factor, complete blood count (CBC), liver function tests (LFT), kidney function test (KFT), serum electrolyte (SE), Urine analysis, Blood sugar, Chest X-ray, ECG, occult blood in stool.
- Tumor markers—CA-125, CEA.
- Ultrasound and CT scan of pelvis and abdomen.
- Gastrointestinal evaluation—endoscopy, colonoscopy.

Biopsy or FNAC—if planned for neoadjuvant chemotherapy (NACT).

Investigation reports of this patient:

CBC, LFT, KFT, SE = within normal limits

Blood sugar fasting/post prandial = 118/140 mg/dL

CA-125 = 300 U/mL, **CEA** = 10 ng/mL

CXR/ECG—no abnormality detected

Occult blood in stool—negative

USG: 20 × 18 cm solid cystic mass arising from right adnexa. Papillary projections seen. Increased blood flow on Doppler. Right and left ovary not visualized separately.

CT scan: A large right abdominopelvic solid cystic lesion measuring 20 × 18 cm occupying the entire pelvis and lower abdomen suggestive of mitotic etiology. Left ovary not visualized.

Upper and lower gastrointestinal endoscopy: Normal study.

Q4. What are the points suggestive of malignant ovarian tumor in this case?

The points suggestive of malignancy are:

History

Postmenopausal status for 15 years and short duration of symptoms

Physical examination

- Cachectic appearance
- Edema of legs, prominent leg veins

Abdominal examination

- *Mass*: Firm to solid, irregular margins, irregular surface, restricted mobility, nontender
- *Ascites*

Bimanual examination

- Uterus is felt separate from the mass, bilateral fornices are full and mass is palpable.
- Restricted mobility of mass.

Investigations

USG, CT scan findings.

Q5. What is the stage of disease for this patient?

Staging for ovarian tumor is done surgically (Table 23.1)[2]

Q6. What are the various scoring systems available for estimating the risk of malignancy in an ovarian tumor?

Various clinical and ultrasound-based prediction models and scoring systems have been developed to support the diagnosis, these are:

1. *Risk of malignancy index (RMI)[3,4,5]:* It includes menopausal status (M), serum CA 125, and USG features (U) (Table 23.2)
   [sensitivity = 70%, specificity = 90%]
   USG score includes: Multilocular cyst, solid areas, bilateral cyst, ascites and intra-abdominal metastasis.
   CA 125 in u/mL
   Menopausal status: Pre-menopausal or post-menopausal
   - RMI (1, 2, 3) = U × M × CA 125 level
     Total score of > 200 used as a cut-off for malignancy
   - RMI 4: U × CA 125 × M × S
     Here, S = Largest diameter of the mass, which is

     Score 1 = mass <7 cm
         2 = mass ≥7 cm

     Cut-off >450 used for malignancy for RMI 4.

2. *IOTA simple ultrasound based rules[6]:* It is entirely based on ultrasound parameters. (Table 23.3).
   [Sensitivity = 95 %, specificity = 91%.]

Table 23.1: Ovarian cancer staging FIGO classification 2014

Stage I. Limited to ovaries	IA: Limited to one ovary IB: Limited to both ovaries IC: Limited to one or both ovaries with one of the following: IC 1: Surgical spill IC 2: Capsule ruptured before surgery or tumor on ovarian surface IC 3: Malignant cells in ascites or peritoneal washings
Stage II. Pelvic extension	IIA: Extension/implants on uterus or fallopian tube IIB: Extension/implants on other pelvic tissues
Stage III. Abdominal extension ±Regional lymph nodes involvement	IIIA: Positive RPLN ± microscopic metastasis beyond pelvis IIIA 1: Positive RPLN only (i) metastasis ≤ 10 mm (ii) metastasis >10 mm IIIA 2: Microscopic, extra pelvic, peritoneal involvement ± positive RPLN IIIB: Macroscopic, extra pelvic, peritoneal metastasis ≤ 2 cm ± positive RPLN. **[Includes extension to liver/ spleen capsule]** IIIC: Macroscopic, extra pelvic, peritoneal metastasis > 2 cm ± positive RPLN. **[Includes extension to liver/ spleen capsule]**
Stage IV. Distal metastasis outside peritoneal cavity	IVA: Pleural effusion with positive cytology IVB: Metastasis to liver/spleen parenchyma, extra-abdominal organs including inguinal lymph nodes and lymph nodes outside of the abdominal cavity

Table 23.2: Different RMI variant scores

RMI variant	USG score (U) Characteristic	Score	Menopausal status (m) Characteristic	Score
RMI 1	No feature present 1 feature present 2>/features present	0 1 3	Pre-menopausal Postmenopausal	1 3
RMI 2	≤1 feature present ≥2 features present	1 4	Pre-menopausal Postmenopausal	1 4
RMI 3	≤1 feature present ≥2 features present	1 3	Premenopausal Postmenopausal	1 3
RMI 4	0–1 feature ≥2 features	1 4	Premenopausal Postmenopausal	1 4

Table 23.3: IOTA simple USG model

B-rule (benign)	M-rule (malignant)
B1. Unilocular cysts	M1. Irregular solid tumor
B2. Presence of solid components with largest diameter < 7mm	M2. At least four papillary structures
B3. Presence of acoustic shadows	M3. Presence of ascites
B4. Smooth multi-locular tumor with largest diameter < 100 mm	M4. Irregular multilocular solid tumor with largest diameter ≥10 mm
B5. No blood flow on color Doppler	M5. Very strong blood flow on color Doppler

If one or more B features present in absence of M feature: Benign

And vice versa for malignant.

If both B and M features or none of B and M features: Inconclusive.

3. *IOTA LR2 model (logistic regression model)[7]:* It includes both clinical and ultrasound features. Six variables are used to estimate the probability of malignancy:

a. Age (in years)

b. Presence of ascites (yes = 1/no = 0)

c. Presence of blood flow in papillary projection (yes = 1/no = 0)

d. Max. diameter of sold component (capped at 50 mm) yes = 1/no = 0

e. Irregular internal cyst wall (yes = 1/no = 0)

f. Presence of acoustic shadow (yes = 1/no = 0)

Probability of malignancy = 1/1 exp (–z)

Z = –5.3718 + 0.0354a + 1.6159b + 1.1768c + 0.0697d + 0.9586e – 2.9486f

Cut-off: >/= 0.1 used to predict the malignancy.

Risk of malignancy calculated by IOTA online application which predict, risk of malignancy as well as stage and risk of metastasis in percent.

4. *ADNEX (assessment of different neoplasia in the adnexa)[8]:* It predicts not only whether a mass is malignant or not but also to a certain extent the type of malignancy.

It includes 9 variables:

a. Age (years)

b. CA125 (u/mL)

c. Type of centre where treated (oncology centre/other hospital)

d. Max diameter of lesion (mm)

e. Proportion of solid tissue (%)

f. No. of papillary projection (0/1/2/3/>3)

g. More than 10 cyst locules (yes/no)

h. Acoustic shadow (yes/no)

i. Ascites (yes/no)

Other methods:

• Risk of ovarian malignancy algorithm (ROMA)

Calculates numerical score for assessing risk of ovarian cancer based on human epididymis protein (HE4), CA 125 levels and patient's menopausal status.

FDA approved, NCCN guideline does not recommend it.

• Risk of ovarian cancer algorithm (ROCA)

Serial CA 125 measurements drawn at regular intervals are plotted and slope obtained is used to assess the risk of ovarian cancer.

• Ova 1 panel

Measures serum levels of 5 biomarkers: Apolipoprotein A1, beta-2 macroglobulin, CA-125, transthyretin, transferrin. A score is generated using multivariate index assay algorithm. Score of 5 in premenopausal woman and 4.4 in postmenopausal women is considered to be at high risk of malignancy.[9]

• *Ova Sure test:* Measures levels of six biomarkers—CA-125, osteopontin, insulin-like growth factor II, leptin, prolactin, macrophage inhibitory factor.

Q7. What is the assessment of risk of malignancy by risk assessment models for this case?

The risk assessment according to different models is:

1. RMI (1): US feature (U) × menopausal status (M) × CA 125 = 3 × 3 × 300 = 2700.

RMI >200

Suggestive of malignant lesion.

2. IOTA simple ultrasound-based rules: Findings M1, M2, M3, M4, M5

Suggestive of malignant lesion.

3. IOTA LR2 (logistic regression model):

Probability of malignancy = 1/1 exp (–z)

Z = –5.3718 + 0.0354a (age) + 1.6159b (presence of ascites) +1.1768c (presence of blood flow in papillary projection) + 0.0697d (max. diameter of solid component capped at 50 mm + 0.9586e (irregular internal cyst wall) –2.9486f (presence of acoustic shadow)

Probability of malignancy = 0.9744

Cut off ≥ = 0.1 used to predict malignancy

Suggestive of malignant lesion.
[online site for risk calculation: http://gin-onc-calculators.com/iota.php.]
4. ADNEX model (assessment of different neoplasia in the adnexa):
[online site for risk calculation: www.iotagroup.org/adnexmodel/site% 20 iota.html]
IOTA—ADNEX model
After entering all values:

Patient specific risk	Relative risk (%)	Baseline risk	
Chance of benign tumor	1.2	0	68.2%
Risk of malignancy	98.8	3.1	31.8 %
• Risk borderline	39.9	6.3	6.3 %
• Risk stage I ovarian cancer	11.5	1.5	7.5 %
• Risk stage II–IV ovarian cancer	42.2	3	14.1 %
• Risk metastatic cancer to the adnexa	5.2	1.3	4.0 %
Suggestive of malignant lesion.			

Q8. What are current recommendations regarding screening of ovarian cancer?

The screening recommendations are:
- *ACOG*: No routine screening strategy for ovarian cancer is recommended in general population as positive predictive value of these tests is not sufficient for detecting early ovarian cancer[9].
- *American cancer society*[10]:
  - Low risk women: Screening not recommended
  - High risk women: Offer combination of pelvic exam, CA-125, TVS.

Screening is mainly done by[1]:
- Symptoms
  New and frequent symptoms (>12 days/month) such as bloating, pelvic or abdominal pain, early satiety, difficulty in eating and urinary symptoms such as urgency or frequency.
  Not very sensitive or specific for early stage cancer.

- Biomarkers
  - CA-125 levels—low sensitivity and specificity.
    Only 85 % of women with ovarian cancer have raised CA-125.
    Only 50 % of women with early stage ovarian cancer have raised CA-125.
    It can be elevated in several benign conditions (PID, fibroid, endometriosis, etc.) and other malignant conditions (breast, lung, pancreas, colon).
  - HE4 protein—similar sensitivity to CA-125 when compared to healthy controls. More sensitive to rule out benign gynecologic diseases.
  - Other available markers—CA 19-9, CA 15-3, CA 72-4, CEA, lysophosphatidic acid, sFas, mesothelin, haptoglobin-alpha, bikunin, OVX1.
- *TVS*: Low positive predictive value when used alone in general population.
- *Multimodal screening*: CA 125 with TVS: Higher positive predictive value and specificity than either investigation alone.

Q9. What are the risk factors for ovarian cancer?

The risk factors are:[11]
- Age: 56–60 years for epithelial ovarian cancer—Over 80% of ovarian cancers are found in postmenopausal women
- White race
- Diet: Animal fat (red meat, whole milk or cheese)
- Nulliparity or older age at first pregnancy (>35 years)
- Infertility
- History of endometrial or breast cancer
- Ovarian stimulation for IVF—low malignant potential (LMP) tumors
- Smoking (mucinous carcinoma)
- Family history of ovarian, breast, endometrial or colon cancer
  - Hereditary familial ovarian cancer—10% of all newly diagnosed cases
    One first degree relative—5 % lifetime risk
    Two first degree relatives—7 % lifetime risk

– Familial ovarian cancer—includes three autosomal dominant syndromes

  i. Site-specific ovarian cancer

  ii. Breast-ovarian cancer:
    BRCA1—lifetime risk of 25–60%
    BRCA2—lifetime risk of 15–25%

  iii. HNPCC or Lynch syndrome II—12% lifetime risk of ovarian cancer

• Hormone replacement therapy (HRT)—5 years of use of estrogen only HRT increases risk by 22 %

• Oral contraceptive pills (OCPs), pregnancy, breastfeeding, tubal ligation and hysterectomy reduce risk.

Q10. What are the various types of epithelial tumors and their incidences?

Each of the following type is further classified as benign, borderline or malignant[12] (Table 23.4).

Q11. Outline the management for this patient.

The primary treatment for all epithelial ovarian cancer is appropriate surgical staging and debulking surgery. Postoperative chemotherapy is given depending upon the stage and histopathological grade of the tumor (HPE report).

For this patient primary surgical staging was done.

Q12. What are the principles of surgery in ovarian cancer?

The general principles are:[1]

• Preferably gynecologic oncologist should perform the surgery.

• Open laparotomy with midline incision. If necessary, intraoperative frozen section to be done.

• Surgeon should describe in their operative notes the extent of the disease, residual disease after debulking, mention the type of resection—complete or incomplete (maximum diameter of the lesion left and number of lesions).

• Achieve maximum cytoreduction of the disease during primary surgery. For patients planned for intraperitoneal (IP) therapy, IP catheter placement may be done.
(Refer to further reading).

Table 23.4: Different types of epithelial ovarian cancer		
Type	*HPE resemblance*	*Incidence*
Serous	Fallopian tube lining	75–80%
Mucinous	Endocervical epithelium	8-10%
Endometrioid	Endometrial lining	6%
Clear cell	Vaginal mucosa	3%
Transitonal cell/Brenner	Bladder	<1%
Mixed	—	
Undifferentiated	—	

Table 23.5: Epithelial ovarian cancer: 5 year survival rates			
Stage	*5-year survival (%)*	*Stage*	*5-year survival (%)*
IA	94	IIC	57
IB	91	IIIA	45
IC	80	IIIB	39
IIA	76	IIIC	35
IIB	67	IV	18

Q13. What is the final staging of this patient after HPE?

Her HPE shows:

Right ovarian tissue: Mucinous cystadeno-carcinoma, grade 2.

Left ovarian tissue: No evidence of malignancy.

Uterus: Normal endometrial tissue seen.

Ascitic fluid: Positive for malignant cells.

Omental tissue: No evidence of malignancy seen.

Pelvic, para-aortic, obturator lymph nodes: Normal lymphoid tissue seen.

Final staging: Stage IC 3.

Q14. What is the role of postoperative chemotherapy?[1]

Stage-wise recommendations for postoperative chemotherapy (Table 23.6)

Recent Cochrane review in 2015 has shown prolonged survival in early stage epithelial ovarian cancer (EOC) in the patient who received platinum-based chemotherapy (high quality evidence). However, in women with low and intermediate risk early stage disease, benefits from adjuvant chemotherapy should be weighed against adverse effects taking into account of individual factors.[13]

Recommended Regimens

Stage 1

1. Day 1: Paclitaxel, 175 mg/m² over 3 hours intravenous infusion followed by carboplatin, dosed at an area under curve (AUC) of 5 to 6 intravenous over 1 hour—given every 3 weeks for 6 cycles.
2. Carboplatin AUC 5 plus pegylated liposomal doxorubicin 30 mg/m²—every 4 weeks for 6 cycles.

   According to Cochrane review 2013, pegylated doxorubicin (PLD)/carboplatin can be considered as first-line alternative to paclitaxel/carboplatin for EOC. PLD/carboplatin regimen was associated with increased delay of doses due to high incidence of anemia and low platelet counts but has low risk of alopecia and neurotoxicity. There are no survival benefits associated with the alternating triplet regimen of paclitaxel/carboplatin (high quality evidence).[14]

Table 23.6: Indications for postoperative chemotherapy	
Epithelial ovarian cancer	Stage IA or IB: Grade 1. Observation (Chemotherapy is not recommended) Grade 2. Observation or Intravenous (IV) platinum-based therapy, 3–6 cycles Stage 1A/B. Grade 3 and Stage IC (grade 1, 2, 3)—IV platinum-based therapy, 3–6 cycles Stage II–IV. Platinum-based chemotherapy, 6 cycles
Malignant sex cord-stromal tumors	Stage I: Low risk: Observe High risk: Observe or platinum-based chemotherapy (Ruptured Stage IC or poorly differentiated stage I) Stage II–IV. Platinum based chemotherapy or RT for limited disease
Malignant germ cell tumors	Immature teratoma, Stage I. Grade 1: Observe Stage I. Grade 2 or 3: Chemotherapy (BEP regimen) Stage II–IV. Chemotherapy (BEP regimen) Dysgerminoma, Stage I. Any grade: Observe Stage II–IV. Chemotherapy (BEP regimen) Embryonal tumor Endodermal sinus tumor chemotherapy (BEP regimen)

3. Day 1: Docetaxel, 60–75 mg/m^2 IV infusion followed by carboplatin AUC 5 to 6 IV over 1 hour every 3 weeks for 6 cycles. Side effect—neutropenia.

Stage II–IV

Intravenous regimens (Table 23.7)

In 2013, Cochrane review concluded that interferon did not improve overall survival or progression free survival compared to observation alone in postsurgical patients of advanced ovarian cancer who had received first-line chemotherapy.[15]

Intraperitoneal:

Day 1: Paclitaxel 135 mg/m^2 continuous IV infusion over 3 or 24 hours

Day 2: Cisplatin 75 to 100 mg/m^2 IP

Day 8: Paclitaxel 60 mg/m^2 IP

Repeat above cycle every 3 weeks for 6 cycles

Maintenance chemotherapy: According to Cochrane review 2013, there is insufficient data to prove that the use of platinum agents, doxorubicin or paclitaxel as maintenance chemotherapy is more effective than observation alone (moderate quality of evidence).[16]

Q15. What is the role of intraperitoneal chemotherapy in ovarian malignancy?

Chemosensitivity of ovarian tissue and its location on the peritoneal surface makes it an efficient target for IP therapy. It increases anticancer effect and decreases systemic adverse effects of IV therapy.

Indication:

- Patients with stage III cancer with optimally debulked (<1 cm) disease/completely resected disease (R0).
- Optimally debulked/completely resected (R0) stage II disease.
- It is not recommended for stage I or IV disease.

Advantage: A Cochrane review in 2016 compared the effectiveness of postoperative

Table 23.7: Various chemotherapeutic regimens for epithelial ovarian cancer	
Regimen	*Side effect*
1. Day 1: Paclitaxel, 175 mg/m^2 over 3 hours intravenous infusion followed by carboplatin, dosed at an area under curve (AUC) of 5 to 6 intravenous over 1 hour—given every 3 weeks for 6 cycles.	Sensory peripheral neuropathy
2. Dose dense paclitaxel, 80 mg/m^2 IV over 1 hour on day 1, 8 and 15 followed by carboplatin AUC 5 to 6 IV over 1 hour on day 1—given every 3 weeks for 6 cycles.	Anemia, decreased quality of life
3. Weekly regimen: Paclitaxel 60 mg/m^2 over 1 hour plus carboplatin AUC 2 IV over 30 min—given weekly for 18 weeks. Considered for elderly patients or poor PS patients as per phase 3 MITO-7 trial	Fewer side effects, better quality of life
4. Day 1: Docetaxel, 60–75 mg/m^2 IV infusion followed by carboplatin AUC 5 to 6 IV over 1 hour—every 3 weeks for 6 cycles.	Neutropenia
5. Carboplatin AUC 5 plus pegylated liposomal doxorubicin 30 mg/m^2—every 4 weeks for 6 cycles.	
6. Bevacizumab containing regimens per ICON-7 and GOG-218 • Paclitaxel 175 mg/m^2 IV over 3 hours followed by carbolplatin AUC 5–6 IV over 1 hour and bevacizumab 7.5 mg/kg IV over 30–90 minutes on day 1—every 3 weeks for 5–6 cycles. Continue bevacizumab for 12 additional cycles. • Paclitaxel 175 mg/m^2 IV over 3 hours followed by carboplatin AUC 6 IV over 1 hour–day 1—repeat every 3 cycles for 6 cycles. Starting day 1 of cycle 2, give bevacizumab 15 mg/kg IV over 30–90 minutes every 3 weeks for up to 22 cycles.	

intraperitoneal versus intravenous chemotherapy for EOC of any stage. It concluded that overall survival and progression-free survival was increased in patients who received IP therapy. Less systemic adverse effects were observed.[17]

Disadvantage: Toxic events, catheter related complications such as blockage, infection, abdominal pain, nausea, dehydration, vomiting which prevents completion of all 6 cycles.

Q16. What is the role of neoadjuvant chemotherapy (NACT) in ovarian cancer?[1]

NACT refers to the use of drugs to reduce the tumor burden before cancer surgery.[1]

Indication: Bulky stage III to IV disease which are considered unlikely to be completely cytoreduced to R0. It should be assessed by gynecologic oncologist. It is not recommended for tumor apparently confined to ovary.

Cochrane review in 2012 concluded that NACT could be an alternative to primary debulking surgery (PDS) particularly in stage IIIc and IV, whereas PDS is the standard primary treatment for stage IIIa and IIIb ovarian cancer. Resectability, age, histology, and stage should be taken into account for selecting patients with bulky disease for NACT (moderate level evidence).[18]

Regimens used: Standard intravenous regimens as described before.

First line: Intravenous taxane/carboplatin and liposomal doxorubicin/carboplatin regimens.

IV/IP regimen may be used after NACT and Interval debulking surgery (IDS).

Prerequisite:

Histologic confirmation of ovarian cancer—Core biopsy is preferred; FNAC, paracentesis CA-125:CEA ratio is also helpful.

Advantage: Fewer complications compared to primary upfront surgery in stage IV disease.

Appropriate alternative for patients with poor general condition prohibiting surgery.

Disadvantage: Lower overall survival compared to initial surgery in patients with potentially resectable tumor.

Q16. What are the prognostic factors and prognosis of EOC?

The prognostic factors are:[1]

* *Stage:*
  5-year survival correlates directly with the stage of tumor (American Cancer Society, 2010) Refer to Table 23.5
* *Grade:*
  – Based on architecture, mitotic index, nuclear atypia
  Grade 1—well differentiated
  Grade 2—moderatley differentiated
  Grade 3—poorly differentiate
  – Grade of tumor is an important prognostic factor particularly in early stage disease.
* *Histology of tumor:*
  – Each epithelial tumor is subtyped as benign, malignant or LMP.
  – Clear cell—poorest prognosis
  – Endometrioid—better prognosis than serous type.
* *Residual disease after initial debulking surgery*
  – Patients with R0 resection have the greatest survival advantage.
* *Age of the patient:* Patients younger than 65 years at the time of diagnosis have nearly twice the 5-year survival rate (57%) as compared to women older than 65 years (28%).

Q18. What is the role of radiotherapy in ovarian cancer?

There is limited role of radiotherapy in ovarian cancers[1]:

   a. Whole abdomen radiation therapy—rarely used.

   b. Palliative localized RT—in recurrent cancer for symptom control.

Disadvantage: Vaginal stenosis leading to impaired sexual function.

Q19. What is the management of recurrent disease.

Following scenarios are encountered[1]:

a. *Raised CA-125 with no prior chemotherapy or clinical relapse with no prior chemotherapy:* Perform relevant investigations and consider primary treatment as needed.

b. *Serially rising CA-125 with prior chemotherapy:* Perform relevant investigations and
   - Observe and treat when there is clinical relapse (Category 2A).
   - Provide treatment immediately as for recurrent disease (described below) category 2B.
   - Enroll patient under clinical trial. (Category 2A)

c. *Clinical relapse with prior chemotherapy:* Perform relevant investigations and treat as recurrence.
   - Persistent disease on primary chemotherapy/relapse <6 month after chemotherapy completion (platinum resistant disease)/stage 2–4 with partial response/progression following recurrence for chemotherapy—clinical trial or supportive care or recurrence therapy as described below.
   - Relapse after 6 months of chemotherapy completion:
     - In case of clinical relapse, consider cytoreductive surgery/clinical trial/platinum-based chemotherapy/different chemotherapy/supportive care.
     - In case of biochemical relapse, consider delaying treatment until clinical relapse/clinical trial/platinum-based chemotherapy/supportive care.

Therapies for recurrent EOC:
- *Platinum sensitive disease:* Carboplatin/gemcitabine, carboplatin/gemcitabine/bevacizumab, carboplatin/liposomal doxorubicin, carboplatin/paclitaxel, cisplatin/gemcitabine, carboplatin/paclitaxel/gemcitabine
- *Platinum resistant disease:* Docetaxel, Etoposide, Gemcitabine, Liposomal doxorubicin, Topotecan, Bevacizumab, Pazopanib

Cochrane review 2013: For platinum-sensitive relapsed EOC, Pegylated doxorubicin/carboplatin can be considered as first-line treatment as it is better tolerated than paclitaxel/carboplatin (high quality evidence). However, there is insufficient evidence to prove its role in platinum-resistant relapsed EOC either alone or in combination with other agents.[14]

- *Targeted therapy:* Bevacizumab, Olaparib, Rucaparib

  PARP (Poly ADP-ribose polymerase) inhibitors—these drugs prevent DNA repair of cancer cells once chemotherapy damages it. Common side effects include fatigue and anemia.

  - Olaparib: Approved by FDA and NCCN for single-agent recurrence therapy for advanced ovarian cancer who have BRCA mutation, are platinum sensitive and have received 3 or more lines of chemotherapy. It has also been approved as maintenance therapy for women who have received 2 or more lines of chemotherapy.[19]
  - Rucaparib: FDA and NCCN panel recommend it as single-agent recurrence therapy for patients who have received 2 or more lines of chemotherapy. It works in both platinum sensitive and resistant patients.[20,21]
  - Niraparib: Approved as maintenance therapy for platinum sensitive patients who have received 2 or more lines of platinum-based therapy or complete or partial response to new recurrent therapy.[22,23]
  - According to Cochrane review 2015, Progression free survival in women with recurrent platinum-sensitive disease improves but further research is needed to prove its role in platinum-resistant disease (moderate quality evidence).[24]

- *Hormonal therapy:* Aromatase inhibitors (anastrozole, exemestane, letrozole), Leuprolide, megestrol, tamoxifen.
- *Radiation therapy:* Palliative localized radiotherapy.
- *Antigen specific active immunotherapy:* Antibody therapy targeting CA-125 should

not be included in standard treatment due to lack of high quality evidence.

- Epidermal growth factor receptor (EGFR) inhibitor (pertuzumab) may be beneficial in addition to conventional chemotherapy for treatment of platinum-resistant ovarian cancer. Cochrane review in 2011 concluded that before EGFR inhibitors are introduced as first- or second-line treatment of ovarian cancer, further RCTS are required[25] (low quality evidence).

- *LHRH agonist:* Cochrane review in 2016 did not find enough evidence on the safety and effectiveness of LHRH agonists in the treatment of platinum-refractory and platinum-resistant EOC (low quality evidence).[26]

Case 2

Ms Z, 16-year-old girl, presented with complaint of abdominal distention over 4 months and heaviness in lower abdomen for 2 months. She had no other significant past or family history. She attained menarche at 10 years of age and had periods at 2–3 months interval with soakage of 1–2 pads/day. On physical examination, patient was of normal built; there was no cervical lymph node enlargement. Development of breasts was Tanner stage 4 and pubic hair was Tanner stage 3. The abdomen was distended, a mass was palpable in the umbilical, hypogastric and bilateral iliac region measuring 20 × 15 cm. It was of tense cystic consistency, smooth surface, smooth margins, restricted mobility, non-tender and its lower limit could be reached with difficulty. There was no ascites. Liver and spleen were not palpable. On bimanual examination, a large abdominal mass was made out with restricted mobility. Uterus was felt separate from the mass. Bilateral fornices were full and same mass was palpated. On per rectal examination, rectal mucosa was free and a lower abdominal mass with firm to hard consistency was felt. (Figs 23.2 and 23.3).

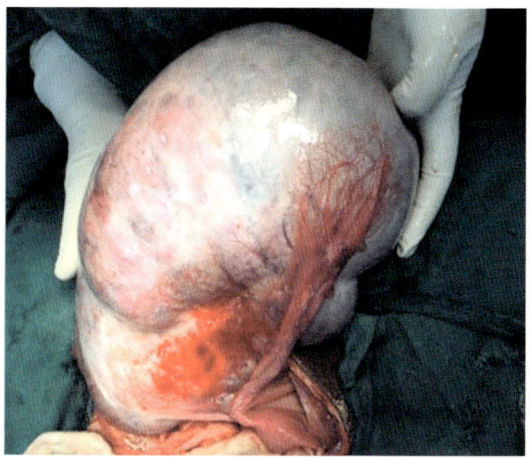

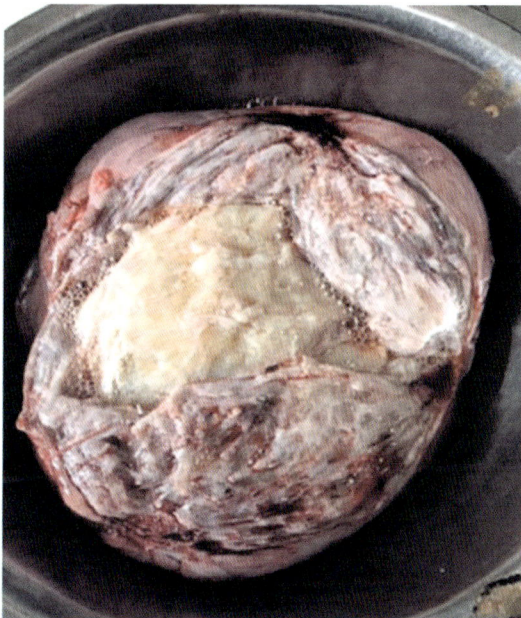

Figs 23.2 and 23.3: Dysgerminoma of ovary

USG: 20 × 15 cm solid cystic mass arising from left adnexa. Right and left ovary not visualized separately. Papillary projections were seen. Increased blood flow was observed on Doppler.

CT scan: A large left abdominopelvic solid cystic lesion measuring 20 × 15 cm occupying entire pelvis and lower abdomen suggestive of mitotic etiology. Left ovary was not visualized.

Tumor markers: AFP/HCG/CA-125— Normal.

Q1. What is the likely diagnosis?

Adolescent girl with adnexal mass-likely malignant ovarian tumor.

Q2. What are the types of germ cell tumors (GCT) and their management[1]?

Origin: Primordial germ cells of ovary

Characteristics: Aggressive, mostly unilateral and if treated early, mostly curable.

Incidence: 20% of all ovarian tumors

2–3% of these tumors are malignant

70% of ovarian masses before 20 years age are germ cell tumors and 1/3rd of these are malignant.

Types:
- *Dysgerminoma*: Most common malignant tumor
- Endodermal sinus tumor (Yolk sac tumor)
- Embryonal carcinoma
- Polyembryoma
- Choriocarcinoma
- Teratoma
  - Benign/mature/cystic (dermoid)—most common germ cell tumor
  - Immature—solid
- Mixed germ cell

Clinical features:
- Acute pelvic pain—stretching of ovarian capsule, necrosis, hemorrhage or torsion.
- Abdominal distension
- Abnormal vaginal bleeding
- Pressure symptoms due to mass

Treatment:
- *Surgery:* Primary treatment for all stages
  - Fertility desired: Fertility sparing surgery and comprehensive staging for all stages. Unilateral oophorectomy along with comprehensive staging. Contralateral ovary should be grossly checked and biopsy is taken in case of suspicion.
  - Fertility not desired: Complete surgical staging
- *Adjuvant treatment:*

- Stage I Dysgerminoma or stage I grade 1 immature teratoma—observe
- Any stage embryonal tumor or any stage endodermal sinus tumor or Stage II–IV Dysgerminoma or Stage I, grade 2 or 3 or Stage II–IV immature teratoma—chemotherapy

Primary chemotherapy for GCT:

BEP (Bleomycin, Etoposide, Cisplatin)
- Bleomycin 30 units per week. Daily for days 1–5.
- Etoposide at 100 mg/m^2 and cisplatin 20 mg/m^2.
- Repeat every 21 days
- 3 cycles—good risk (category 2B), 4 cycles for poor risk

Etoposide/Carboplatin:
- Selected patients with stage IB–III dysgerminoma for whom minimal toxicity is critical, 3 cycles of carboplatin/etoposide can be used.
- Day 1—carboplatin 400 mg/m^2
- Day 1, 2, 3—etoposide 120 mg/m^2
- Repeat every 4 weeks
- 3 cycles given

Radiation therapy (RT):
- Very sensitive to RT.
- Rarely used as first line therapy due to loss of fertility.

Prognosis:
- *Stage Ia:* 5-year survival is >95%
- *Advanced stage after adjuvant chemotherapy:* 5-year survival rate of 85–90%.
- *Higher chances of recurrence:* Masses larger than 10–15 cm diameter, <20 years age, increased mitosis, anaplasia and medullary pattern in HPE.

Recurrence therapies:
- *Potentially curative*: High dose chemotherapy TIP (paclitaxel, ifosfamide, cisplatin)
- *Palliative therapy*: Cisplatin/etoposide, docetaxel, docetaxel/carboplatin, paclitaxel, paclitaxel/ifosfamide, VeIP (vinblastine,

ifosfamide, cisplatin), VAC (vincristine, dactinomycin, cyclophosphamide), TIP.

Q3. What are the types of sex cord stromal tumor and what is their management?

The essential features of sex cord stromal tumors are enumerated below:[1]

Origin: Sex cord and mesenchyme of embryonic gonad.

Incidence: 5–8% of all ovarian tumors

Characteristics: Many are hormonally active—Granulosa cell and theca cell tumors secrete estrogen; Sertoli and leydig cell tumors secrete androgens.

Types:

- Granulosa-stromal cell tumors – Granulosa cell, Thecoma, Fibroma, Unclassified
- Androblastomas: Sertoli cell tumor, Leydig cell tumor
- Gynandroblastoma
- Sex cord tumor

Treatment

Surgery

Primary treatment

- For stage IA/IC if fertility desired: Fertility sparing surgery and comprehensive staging.
- All others: Complete surgical staging

Adjuvant treatment

Primary chemotherapy—BEP regimen

- Stage I: Low risk—observe
- Stage I: High risk (ruptured stage IC or poorly differentiated) (category 2B)
  - Intermediate risk (heterologous elements)
- Stage II–IV: Platinum-based chemotherapy (category 2B) or RT for limited disease (Category 2B)
- Relapse: Clinical trial, secondary cytoreductive surgery, recurrence therapy.

Radiotherapy: Only for palliative use for isolated pelvic recurrences

Follow-up:

- *Physical examination*: Every 2–4 months for 2 years and then every 6 monthly.
- *Serum tumor markers*: Every 2–4 monthly for 2 years and then every 6 monthly.
- *Imaging studies*: No supportive data.

Prognosis

- Granulosa cell tumors have tendency to recur, even as late as 30 years after primary tumor.

  10-year and 20-year survival rates are 90% and 75% respectively.
- *Sertoli-Leydig cell tumor*: 5-year survival is 70–90%.

Recurrence therapies: Docetaxel, paclitaxel, paclitaxel/ifosfamide, paclitaxel/carboplatin, VAC, Aromatase inhibitors (anastrazole, letrozole), leuprolide acetate (for granulosa cell tumors), Bevacizumab, palliative localized RT.

Q5. What is the role of frozen section in ovarian tumor?

Cochrane review in 2016 evaluated the use of intraoperative frozen section analysis for diagnosis of early stage ovarian cancer in suspicious pelvic masses. It included 38 retrospective studies involving 11, 181 participants. The final diagnosis the same in 94% and 99% of the benign or invasive cancer frozen section reports respectively. For those with borderline tumor diagnosis on frozen section, 21% of the final diagnosis came out to be invasive cancer.[27]

Further Reading

Readers can go through the chapter written by same author in book "Evidence based Clinical Gynecology" Editors Kumar D, Tempe A, 2017 Jaypee, Chapter 30 ovarian cancer, for Risk-Reducing Salpingo-Oophorectomy (RRSO) Protocol, treatment protocol, principles of surgical staging and cytoreduction, second look surgery, follow up after treatment, prognosis of epithelial ovarian cancer.

Key Points

- In young patient with ovarian mass germ cell tumors should be suspected.
- In postmenopausal women with ovarian mass epithelial ovarian cancer should be suspected.
- Staging laparotomy and upfront surgery is the recommended treatment of choice in any type of ovarian cancer.
- NACT followed by interval debulking surgery has a role in some clinically inoperable cases.
- Postoperative chemotherapy has a definite role in improving 5-year survival rate in most of the cases.
- Follow up of all the ovarian cancer patients is essential.

REFERENCES

1. NCCN Guidelines for Patients® | Ovarian Cancer [Internet]. [cited 2018 Jun 17]. Available from: https://www.nccn.org/patients/guidelines/ovarian/index.html
2. Prat J; FIGO Committee on Gynecologic Oncology. Staging classification for cancer of the ovary, fallopian tube, and peritoneum. Int J Gynaecol Obstet 2014;124:1–5.
3. Royal College of Obstetrician and Gynaecologist. The management of ovarian cyst in postmenopausal women. Green top guideline no 34, July 2016.
4. Karimi-Zarchi M, Mojaver SP, Rouhi M, Hekmatimoghaddam SH, Moghaddam RN, Yazdian-Anari P, et al. Diagnostic Value of the Risk of Malignancy Index (RMI) for Detection of Pelvic Malignancies Compared with Pathology. Electron Physician 2015; 7:1505–10.
5. Yavuzcan A, Caglar M, Ozgu E, Ustun Y, Dilbaz S, Ozdemir I, et al. Should cut-off values of the risk of malignancy index be changed for evaluation of adnexal masses in Asian and Pacific populations? Asian Pac J Cancer Prev 2013; 14:5455–9.
6. Timmerman D, Van Calster B, Testa A, Savelli L, Fischerova D, Froyman W, et al. Predicting the risk of malignancy in adnexal masses based on the Simple Rules from the International Ovarian Tumor Analysis group. Am J Obstet Gynecol 2016; 214:424–437.
7. Testa A, Kaijser J, Wynants L, Fischerova D, Van Holsbeke C, Franchi D, et al. Strategies to diagnose ovarian cancer: new evidence from phase 3 of the multicentre international IOTA study. Br J Cancer 2014; 111:680–8.

8. Van Calster B, Van Hoorde K, Valentin L, Testa AC, Fischerova D, Van Holsbeke C, et al. International Ovarian Tumour Analysis Group. Evaluating the risk of ovarian cancer before surgery using the ADNEX model to differentiate between benign, borderline, early and advanced stage invasive, and secondary metastatic tumours: prospective multicentre diagnostic study. BMJ 2014;349:g5920.
9. ACOG Statement on FDA Safety Communication on Ovarian Cancer Screening Tests - ACOG [Internet]. [cited 2018 Jun 17]. Available from: https://www.acog.org/About-ACOG/News-Room/Statements/2016/ACOG-Statement-on-FDA-Safety-Communication-on-Ovarian-Cancer-Screening-Tests
10. US Preventive Services Task Force, Grossman DC, Curry SJ, Owens DK, Barry MJ, Davidson KW, Doubeni CA, et al. Screening for Ovarian Cancer: US Preventive Services Task Force Recommendation Statement. JAMA 2018;319:588–594.
11. Chappelear A. Risk Factors and Symptoms: Johns Hopkins Ovarian Cancer Center [Internet]. [cited 2018 Jun 17]. Available from: https://www.hopkinsmedicine.org/kimmel_cancer_ center/centers/ovarian/about/risk_factors.html
12. Berek JS, Longacre TA, Freidlander M (Eds). Ovarian, fallopian tube and peritoneal cancer. In Berek JS, Berek and Novaks Gynecology. 15th ed. New Delhi: Wolter Kluwer Lippincott Williams and Wilkins; 2012. p 1350–1409.
13. Lawrie TA, Winter-Roach BA, Heus P, Kitchener HC. Adjuvant (post-surgery) chemotherapy for early stage epithelial ovarian cancer. Cochrane Database Syst Rev 2015;(12):CD004706.
14. Lawrie TA, Bryant A, Cameron A, Gray E, Morrison J. Pegylated liposomal doxorubicin for relapsed epithelial ovarian cancer. Cochrane Database Syst Rev 2013;(7):CD006910.
15. Lawal AO, Musekiwa A, Grobler L. Interferon after surgery for women with advanced (Stage II-IV) epithelial ovarian cancer. Cochrane Database Syst Rev 2013;(6):CD009620.
16. Mei L, Chen H, Wei DM, Fang F, Liu GJ, Xie HY, et al. Maintenance chemotherapy for ovarian cancer. Cochrane Database Syst Rev 2013;(6): CD007414.
17. Jaaback K, Johnson N, Lawrie TA. Intraperitoneal chemotherapy for the initial management of primary epithelial ovarian cancer. Cochrane Database Syst Rev. 2016;(1):CD005340.
18. Morrison J, Haldar K, Kehoe S, Lawrie TA. Chemotherapy versus surgery for initial

treatment in advanced ovarian epithelial cancer. Cochrane Database Syst Rev 2012;(8):CD005343.

19. Kim G, Ison G, McKee AE, Zhang H, Tang S, Gwise T, et al. FDA Approval Summary: Olaparib Monotherapy in Patients with Deleterious Germline BRCA-Mutated Advanced Ovarian Cancer Treated with Three or More Lines of Chemotherapy. Clin Cancer Res 2015;21:4257–61.

20. Swisher EM, Lin KK, Oza AM, Scott CL, Giordano H, Sun J, et al. Rucaparib in relapsed, platinum-sensitive high-grade ovarian carcinoma (ARIEL2 Part 1): an international, multicentre, open-label, phase 2 trial. Lancet Oncol 2017;18:75–87.

21. Balasubramaniam S, Beaver JA, Horton S, Fernandes LL, Tang S, Horne HN, et al. FDA Approval Summary: Rucaparib for the Treatment of Patients with Deleterious BRCA Mutation-Associated Advanced Ovarian Cancer. Clin Cancer Res Off J Am Assoc Cancer Res 2017; 23:7165–70.

22. Mirza MR, Monk BJ, Herrstedt J, Oza AM, Mahner S, Redondo A, et al. Niraparib Maintenance Therapy in Platinum-Sensitive, Recurrent Ovarian Cancer. N Engl J Med 2016;375:2154–64.

23. Scott LJ. Niraparib: First Global Approval. Drugs. 2017;77:1029–1034.

24. Wiggans AJ, Cass GK, Bryant A, Lawrie TA, Morrison J. Poly(ADP-ribose) polymerase (PARP) inhibitors for the treatment of ovarian cancer. Cochrane Database Syst Rev 2015;(5):CD007929.

25. Haldar K, Gaitskell K, Bryant A, Nicum S, Kehoe S, Morrison J. Epidermal growth factor receptor blockers for the treatment of ovarian cancer. Cochrane Database Syst Rev 2011;(10):CD007927.

26. Wuntakal R, Seshadri S, Montes A, Lane G. Luteinising hormone releasing hormone (LHRH) agonists for the treatment of relapsed epithelial ovarian cancer. Cochrane Database Syst Rev 2016; CD011322.

27. Ratnavelu ND, Brown AP, Mallett S, Scholten RJ, Patel A, Founta C, et al. Intraoperative frozen section analysis for the diagnosis of early stage ovarian cancer in suspicious pelvic masses. Cochrane Database Syst Rev 2016;3:CD010360.

24 | Carcinoma Vulva

Shakun Tyagi, Aashima Aron

Carcinoma vulva accounts for 4% of gyneco-logical malignancies.[1] It is usually diagnosed late because the patient does not seek medical attention or due to delay in biopsy for confir-mation by treating doctor.

The peak age of developing cancer vulva has bimodal distribution. Carcinoma vulva in young women is caused by human papilloma-virus (HPV). In older postmenopausal women (65–75 years) vulvar cancer occurs in associa-tion with chronic vulvar dystrophies like lichen-sclerosis.[2]

WHO histological classification (2014) of tumor of the vulva is depicted in Appendix A24.1.

Case 1

Mrs X, 45 years old P2L2 lady presented to the gynae outpatient clinic with chief complaints of itching, irritation and depigmentation with growth over the vulva for 6 months.

History of Presenting Illness

Patient was apparently well 6 months back, when she developed persistent vulvar itching. It was accompanied with depigmentation and raised lesion in the vulva region. There was no history of discharge or bleeding from vulva or vagina. No history of groin mass. No history of dysuria. Patient has no history of diabetes mellitus.

Patient suspected extra-marital relations in husband

No history of HIV/AIDS or immuno-suppressive therapy.

No history of screening, HPV immunization for cancer cervix or receiving treatment for vulva/vaginal/cervical pre-neoplastic or neoplastic lesion.

No history of cigarette smoking, alcohol consumption, diabetes and hypertension.

Menstrual History

Menstrual cycles: regular, 4–5 days of bleeding with 28–30 days cycle, normal flow. No history of dysmenorrhea.

Obstetric History

P2L2 married for 16 years. All normal vaginal deliveries. Last child birth 12 years back.

Past History

No history of hypertension, tuberculosis, thyroid disorder

Examination

General Physical Examination

Patient was conscious, oriented and sitting comfortably. Average built.

Height = 154 cm, weight = 46 kg, BMI = 19.40 kg/m^2, vitals stable.

No pallor, icterus, cyanosis. Orodental hygiene well maintained. No thyromegaly. No peripheral lymphadenopathy. Bilateral breast normal. No clubbing and pedal edema.

Systemic Examination

Respiratory, cardiovascular system and abdominal examination: No abnormality detected.

Local Examination (Fig. 24.1)

Inspection: Irregular exophytic growth of about 4 × 3 cm present over the labia minora and labia majora on the left side associated with depigmentation. Irregular raised lesion about 1 × 2 cm over right labia minora

Palpation: Local temperature not raised, 4 × 3 cm growth present over the labia minora and labia majora with irregular raised surface, base appears indurated, non-tender, not fixed to the underlying bone. No inguinal or femoral lymph node palpable.

Speculum examination: Cervix-cervicitis present, vagina-healthy. No abnormal discharge or bleeding.

Vaginal examination: Cervix firm, regular, pointing downward. Uterus anteverted, normal size. Bilateral fornices free, non-tender

Q1. What is your differential diagnosis?

The differential diagnosis include:
  i. Carcinoma vulva
 ii. Tuberculosis of vulva
iii. Condyloma acuminata

Q2. How will you confirm the diagnosis?

The diagnosis is confirmed by performing vulvar biopsy. A wedge biopsy or a punch biopsy using Keyes punch biopsy instrument can be taken under local or regional anesthesia. The biopsy should be taken from the interface between normal and abnormal epithelium and

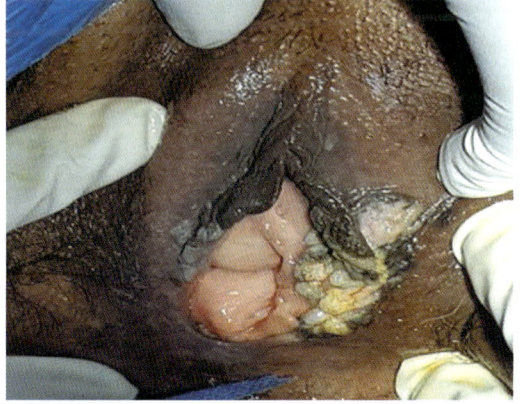

Fig. 24.1

should be of at least 4 mm depth from skin surface to include sufficient underlying dermis to assess for micro-invasion.[4]

Q3. What precautions will you take during transport of vulvar biopsy?

An accurate description of the site and appearance of the gross lesion and the type of biopsy (excisional or diagnostic) should be mentioned. Large radical resection specimen should be pinned out on corkboard. The specimen can also be oriented by means of marker sutures. In case of frozen section, it should be kept moist with normal saline, and sent as fresh tissue to the pathology department as early as possible.

Q4. What is the role of vulvar cytology?

The use of exfoliative cytology using scalpel scrapings or Dacron swabs in women with pre-existing vulvar disease has shown variable results. Hence, vulvar cytology cannot be used as a substitute for diagnostic biopsy of suspicious lesions.[4]

Q 5. What are the predisposing risk factors?

The risk factors for vulvar carcinoma include[5]:

  i. **Human papilloma virus (HPV):** HPV can lead to both VIN and invasive vulvar cancer (basaloid or warty type). HPV DNA is documented in 89% of VIN3, 86% of warty or basaloid type carcinoma vulva and in <10% of keratinizing type of carcinoma of the vulva.[6] HPV 16 and 33 are the common subtypes.[7]

 ii. **Vulvar intraepithelial neoplasia (VIN):** There is 9% progression rate of high grade VIN (VIN3) to vulvar cancer in untreated cases, over 12–96 months.[8] VIN is found adjacent to basaloid/warty type of vulvar carcinoma in more than 80% of cases. 10% to 20% of vulvar carcinoma in situ lesion harbour an occult invasive component.[9,10]

iii. **Vulvar dystrophies:** Itch-scratch cycle associated with lichen sclerosus is a risk factor for keratinizing carcinoma. In keratinizing carcinoma, associated lichen sclerosus is found in >80% of patients.[11,12]

iv. **Cervical intraepithelial neoplasia (CIN)** and cervical cancer are other pathologies associated with vulvar cancer due to common etiology of HPV. Susceptibility of the cervical, vaginal and vulvar epithelium is referred to as a field effect, which is more common in immunocompromised patients (HIV/AIDS or organ transplant recipients) and tobacco users.

v. **HIV/AIDS** (immunosuppression) or Immunosuppressant therapy.

vi. **Other risk factors** for vulvar cancer includes cigarette smoking, alcohol consumption and north European ancestry.[13]

Diabetes mellitus, obesity, hypertension and arteriosclerosis are the associated features seen in patients with vulvar cancer because of increased incidence of these diseases associated with aging.

This patient's husband had multiple sexual partners increasing the risk of HPV infections, which is a risk factor for carcinoma vulva.

Q6. Histopathological report of left vulvar lesion of the patient: Keratinizing squamous cell carcinoma with >1 mm of stromal invasion. HPR report of excison biopsy of right side vulvar lesion: Dysplasia without invasion with negative margins. How will you stage the malignancy?

As the growth of the vulva is >2 cm in size, does not involve adjacent perineal structures and no lymph nodes are palpable, it appears to be carcinoma vulva stage IB as per revised FIGO surgico-pathological staging (2009)[14] (Appendix A24.2).

Q7. Once diagnosis is made, how will you further manage the patient?

Following investigations should be done:

i. To rule out associated CIN, VIN, vaginal intraepithelial neoplasia (VAIN), surrounding vulvar dystrophies and other genital malignancies-Pap smear, HPV testing, colposcopy of cervix and vagina, vulvoscopy for lesion at other site on the vulva.

ii. Imaging-CT/MRI scan of abdomen, pelvis and groin to see the extent of tumor, involvement of lymphnodes and resectability of the tumor in advance cases and treatment planning.[15] Pelvic MRI can be considered in surgical and radiation treatment planning. Whole body PET/CT or chest/abdominal/pelvic CT is considered for T2 or larger tumours or if metastasis is suspected. Indications include:

• Bulky vulvar tumour (≥4 cm or close to critical structures)
• Vaginal, urethral or anal involvement
• Delay in presentation or treatment
• Pelvic, abdominal or pulmonary symptoms

iii. Additional investigations that may be performed in large and locally advanced lesions:

• Cystourethroscopy
• Intravenous pyelography
• Proctosigmoidoscopy

iv. Routine preoperative investigations

Q8. What is the route of spread of vulvar cancer?

Vulvar cancer is spread by the following routes:

i. **Direct extension:** To involve adjacent structures such as urethra, vagina and anus.

ii. **Lymphatic spread:** Figure 24.2 shows the lymphatic spread from vulva to locoregional lymph nodes.

• Lymphatic spread to regional inguinal and femoral lymph nodes. Initially spread is to the inguinal lymph nodes located between Camper fascia and fascia lata. From the superficial groin nodes, the tumor spreads to the deep femoral nodes. Metastases to the femoral nodes without involvement of inguinal nodes has been reported.[16]

• From the inguinal-femoral nodes, the cancer spreads to the pelvic nodes (external iliac group). The pelvic nodes are essentially never involved with

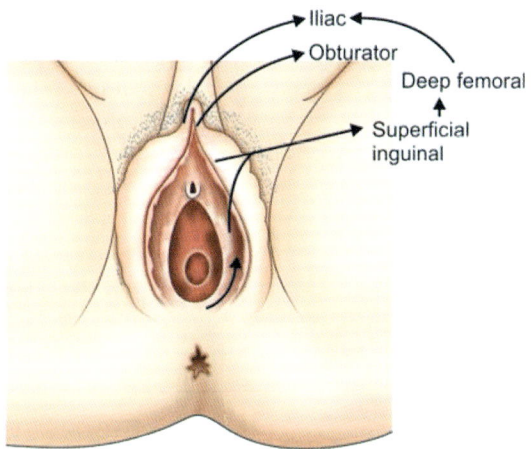

Iliac
Obturator
Deep femoral
Superficial inguinal

Fig. 24.2: Lymphatic spread of vulvar cancer

metastatic disease when inguinal nodes are uninvolved.[17] The overall incidence of inguinal-femoral nodal metastases is 32% and metastases to pelvic nodes occur in about 12%.[18]

- Lymphatic drainage from the clitoris, anterior labia minora and perineum is bilateral.

- The larger the tumor, the greater the chances of inguinal and pelvic node metastases. In T1 lesion (<2 cm in diameter), the incidence of lymph node metastasis was 21%, while it was 45% with T2 lesion (>2 cm in diameter).[19] Patients with stage III and stage IV lesion have 53% and 90% incidence of inguinal node metastases respectively.[20]

iii. **Hematogenous spread:** To distant sites including lung, liver and bones. Hematogenous spread is uncommon in the initial presentation and encountered more frequently in the recurrent vulvar cancer in 8% of patients.[21]

Q9. What is the management for this patient?

In this 45 years old woman with lateralized stage IB vulvar cancer, radical local excision or modified radical vulvectomy with ipsilateral inguinofemoral lymphadenectomy will be planned.

- The primary tumor should be resected with a 1 cm margin of normal tissue and dissection is carried up to the deep perineal fascia of the urogenital diaphragm.[22]

- In a primary vulvar tumour i.e. ≤4 cm located 2 cm or more from the vulvar midline and with clinically negative inguinofemoral lymph nodes, ipsilateral inguino femoral lymphadenectomy or sentinel lymph nodes biopsy is appropriate[23] as lymphatic cross-over is less likely in lateral tumor. Superficial inguinal as well as deep femoral nodes should be removed as superficial inguinal node dissection alone is associated with higher rate of groin node recurrence.[24]

The ipsilateral inguinal lymph nodes are sent for frozen section. If nodes are positive, then contralateral inguinal lymphadenectomy or adjuvant radiotherapy of the contralateral groin is needed. If nodes are negative, then no further dissection or radiotherapy is needed.[25]

Q10. What is sentinel node biopsy for carcinoma vulva?

Sentinel lymph node biopsy is done by identifying the sentinel lymph node by lymphatic mapping using the isosulfan blue dye or technetium 99 m labelled nanocolloid. Lymphoscintigraphy is done preoperative and intraoperatively to identify nodes with metastases. If the sentinel lymph node is negative for malignancy, then the other nodes in the basin will be negative. Thus, precluding the need for full nodal dissection. The eligibility criteria for sentinel lymph node biopsy include:

i. Primary squamous vulvar cancers

ii. Cancers measuring less than 4 cm in maximum dimension

iii. Macroscopic unifocal cancers

iv. No clinical or radiological evidence to suspect lymph node metastasis

v. No known safety issues for the use of patent blue dye and/or technetium—99

vi. Informed patient consent and acceptance of close follow-up (recommended 2-monthly in the first year)

vii. No previous vulvar surgery that may have impacted lymphatic flow to the inguinal region.

Radio colloid 99mTc (technetium) and isosulfan or methylene blue are inserted around the lesion before operation. Subsequently, a hand held gamma detection device is used to identify the injected radio colloid in the sentinel lymph nodes. Isosulfan blue dye 1% (3–4 cc) is injected intradermally within 15–30 minutes of starting the procedure. The dye is injected peritumorally using 4 points injection technique at 2, 5, 7, 10 o' clock position. Naked eye visualization can be done in case of these dyes.

- If the sentinel node is positive, a full inguinofemoral lymphadenectomy and/or postoperative radiation therapy to affected groin is recommended. If ipsilateral sentinel lymph node is positive, then contralateral groin should be evaluated surgically and/or treated with radiotherapy.
- If the sentinel lymph nodes identified by mapping are histologically negative, no further treatment is indicated.[26]
- If a sentinel lymph node cannot be identified, then complete inguinofemoral lymphadenectomy should be done.

However, 2.3% rate of groin recurrence has been shown in patients with negative sentinel lymph nodes.

Q11. What are the steps of radical vulvectomy?

The lymph node dissection is performed first followed by vulvectomy.

Inguino-femoral lymph node dissection: An 8 cm incision is made parallel to the inguinal ligament two finger breadths (4 cm) beneath the inguinal ligament and 4 cm lateral to the pubic tubercle. The incision is carried down through the camper fascia and skin flaps dissected superiorly and inferiorly, allowing access to the fat pad containing the superficial nodes. The dissection is carried superiorly to inguinal ligament, inferiorly to a point 2 cm proximal to the opening of the Hunter canal, laterally to the

sartorius muscle and medially to the adductor longus muscle fascia. This facilitates identification of the cribriform fascia and with optimal traction on the lymphovascular fat bundle of the inguinal area, all the inguinal and femoral nodes can be removed. Figure 24.3 depicts the femoral triangle.

Closed suction drain are placed in the groin dissection and skin incision is closed by running delayed absorbable suture.

Vulvectomy

i. The mons pubis is incised anteriorly extending medially to the genitocrural fold and posteriorly midway between anus and posterior fourchette. A bloodless space is dissected between vulvar fat and subcutaneous tissue of the thigh. The tissue is transected and ligated at the level of fascia of thigh.

ii. Posterior dissection is performed sharply. The clitoris and its suspensory ligament are clamped, divided and ligated at its inferior attachment to the pubic bone. The ischiocavernosus muscle is clamped, divided and ligated, as laterally as possible. The pudendal artery and vein are ligated bilaterally.

iii. The vaginal mucosal incision is completed, separating the vagina from the specimen. The perineal defect is closed with vertical

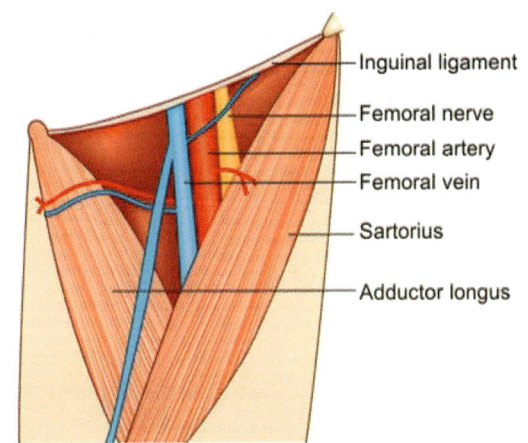

Fig. 24.3: The femoral triangle

Inguinal ligament
Femoral nerve
Femoral artery
Femoral vein
Sartorius
Adductor longus

mattress 2-0 delayed absorbable sutures. If the defect is too large for primary closure, intra-position of a split-thickness skin graft or rhomboid or rotational flaps can be used.

Q12. What are the complications of this surgery?

The postoperative complication may be early or late.

Early complications

i. **Wound breakdown:** It occurs in more than 50% of patients. Groin wound infection, necrosis and breakdown is seen in about 53–85% patients having en bloc excision, is reduced to about 44% with triple excision technique. Routine prophylactic antibiotics, removing lessor amount of skin, decreasing the undermining of skin flaps and use of closed suction drainage have reduced the incidence of wound breakdown.

ii. **Lymphedema of the lower extremities:** Lymphedema seen in 28–39% of patients is much more common in patients who undergo inguinal and pelvic lymphadenectomy.[27] Low dose prophylactic antibiotic therapy after lymphadenectomy and use of elastic support during the first postoperative year has reduced the incidence of lymphedema. Sparing of the saphenous vein reduces the incidence of chronic lymphedema with similar recurrence rate in patients undergoing complete resection versus preservation of saphenous vein.

iii. **Femoral nerve injury:** It is a complication of inguinofemoral lymphadenectomy. This complication can be prevented by avoiding dissection on the lateral side of the femoral artery.

iv. **Femoral vessel rupture:** Severe postoperative hemorrhage from femoral vessel rupture is seen in 1–2% of patients. Coverage of the vessel by transposition of the Sartorius muscle can prevent this complication.

v. **Urinary tract infection**

vi. **Thromboembolism:** Deep vein thrombosis and pulmonary embolism may occur due to immobilization.

vii. **Osteitis pubis:** Occurs if the periosteum is traumatized. Extensive use of cautery on the periosteum should be avoided. Treatment includes bed rest and non-steroidal anti-inflammatory drugs.

Late complications

i. Chronic lymphedema

ii. Recurrent lymphadenitis or cellulitis of leg

iii. Dyspareunia: Due to introital stenosis. Modified radical vulvectomy with preservation of the anterior vulvar structures help maintains sexual functions.

iv. Urinary and fecal incontinence

v. Rectocele

vi. Femoral hernia

vii. Pubic osteomyelitis and rectovaginal fistula.

viii. Psychosexual complications

Q13. How can you improve surgical outcome?

The recent modifications in surgical management include individualization of treatment for patients with invasive disease by:

i. **Modified radical vulvectomy/wide radical resection:** Modified radical vulvectomy includes anterior, posterior hemivulvectomy or lateral vulvectomy with clitoral sparing. Wide local resection includes resection of the primary tumor with a 1 cm margin of normal tissue and to carry the dissection up to the deep perineal fascia of urogenital diaphragm.

ii. Use of separate incisions for groin dissection and vulvectomy to improve wound healing (Fig. 24.3)

iii. Omission of groin dissection for patients with stage IA disease and no risk factor

iv. Omission of contralateral groin dissection in patients with lateral lesion <2 cm in size and negative ipsilateral nodes.[28]

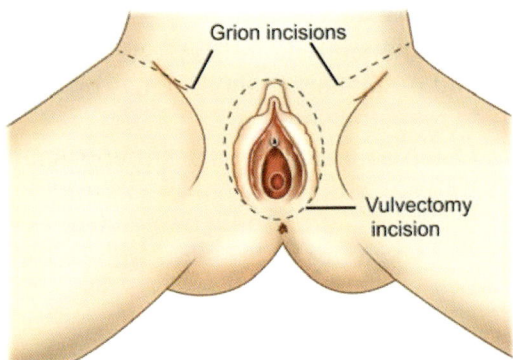

Fig. 24.3: Triple incision technique

v. Elimination of routine pelvic lympha-denectomy if inguinofemoral nodes are negative

vi. Use of preoperative radiation to eliminate the need for exenteration in patients with advanced disease.

vii. Use of postoperative radiation to decrease the incidence of groin recurrence.

Q14. How will you follow up the patient?

A life-long follow up is needed after treatment of carcinoma vulva, i.e. every three months for the first year, six monthly for the second year and yearly thereafter. The follow up aims to detect local recurrence, recurrence in groin nodes, distant metastases or a new primary vulvar tumor. Surveillance for associated cervical or vaginal malignancies is also done. Complications as a result of surgery or radiotherapy are addressed.

Q15. What is the role of chemoradiation?

Role of Radiotherapy

Adjuvant postoperative radiotherapy (following initial surgery): Absolute indications of postoperative radiotherapy include:

- Gross node metastases (complete replacement of node with tumour)
- Extra capsular extension in any node
- 2 or more lymph nodes involved with microscopic metastases or 1 lymph node with more than 2 mm metastases
- Close or positive margins

Relative indications include:

- Depth of invasion >5 mm
- Presence of lymphovascular invasion

Postoperative adjuvant treatment should be initiated after adequate healing is achieved i.e. 6–8 weeks. The radiation field should include the vulva, inguinofemoral, external iliac and internal iliac lymph nodes. Treatment should be based on three-dimensional planning using high quality CT or MRI images. Adequate dosing is accomplished using 3D conformal approach or Intensity Modulated Radiation Therapy (IMRT). Combined photon and electron techniques are used to treat the regional nodes.

Target issue should be treated once daily, 5 days per week. The dose of radiation is determined by the initial extent of regional disease. After a groin dissection with microscopic metastases, 50 Gy in 1.8–2 Gy fractions is given. If there are multiple positive nodes or if there is extra capsular spread dose of 60 Gy is given. Gross residual disease requires 60–70 Gy to achieve high probability of regional disease control.

The estimated 2 years survival rate was 68% for the patients who received radiotherapy and 54% for pelvic node resection group. Radiotherapy resulted in reduction in groin failure from 24% in patients who underwent only surgery to 5% in patients who received postoperative radiotherapy.[29]

Neoadjuvant radiotherapy/primary therapy in locally advanced disease: Radiotherapy, with or without chemotherapy, is increasingly used in the management of locally advanced vulvar cancer. Neoadjuvant radiotherapy has advantages over exenterative surgery such as high probability of bladder and/or rectal preservation, low primary mortality and morbidity, downstaging the initial tumor bulk to limit the morbidity associated with extensive surgery.[30,31]

The initial radiation treatment field includes the pelvis, inguinal nodes and the primary site. A prophylactic dose of 45–50 Gy is delivered. Areas of gross disease are boosted by a second phase by electrons, conformal radiotherapy or brachytherapy with a total dose of 65 Gy. Surgery is performed 4–6 weeks after completion of external beam radio-therapy, as radiotherapy impairs the wound healing.[20]

Secondary therapy/palliation in recurrent/ metastatic disease.

Role of Chemotherapy

Neoadjuvant chemotherapy: It is used in locally advanced vulvar cancer with anorectal, urethral or bladder involvement which require extensive surgery. Vulvar cancer responds to chemotherapy to a variable extent and in some cases surgery is possible after chemotherapy because of reduced tumor mass. Bleomycin, cisplatin and 5-flurouracil have been used for neoadjuvant chemotherapy.

Adjuvant chemotherapy: Usually radiotherapy is used as adjuvant treatment in vulvar cancer and only one study has focused on adjuvant chemotherapy. It concluded that radical surgery followed by chemotherapy in patients with multiple lymph nodes metastases is a feasible strategy however further studies are required.

Q16. What are the new developments in medical management of cancer vulva?

Newer biological agents have been identified in the treatment of cancer vulva. Gefitinib and erlotinib are oral reversible tyrosine kinase inhibitors. By inhibiting the tyrosine kinase, they prevent Epidermal Growth Factor Receptors from stimulating the uncontrolled growth of cells that contribute to tumor growth. These agents may prove useful in women not fit for aggressive chemotherapy in vulvar cancer.[32]

Key Points

- Early detection by biopsy by keeping high level of suspicion is paramount.
- Screening for vaginal and cervical cancer in HPV related cases must be done.

- Individualization of treatment depending on stage of the disease and patient profile to reduce surgical morbidity and optimize outcome.
- Sentinel lymph node sampling may be used to avoid inguino-femoral lymphadenectomy if inguinal sentinel lymph node is negative and avoid pelvic lymphadenectomy in case of negative Cloquet's lymph node.
- Modified radical vulvectomy has reduced both acute and chronic complications of surgery.
- Cancer vulva patients require lifelong follow up to detect recurrence as well as development of Carcinoma cervix and vagina
- For detailed stage wise treatment of carcinoma vulva NCCN guidelines at www.nccn.org may be referred to.

REFERENCES

1. Siegel R, Ward E, Brawley O. Cancer's statistics, 2011. CA Cancer J Clin 2011;61:212–36.
2. Beller U, Quinn MA, Benedet JL. Carcinoma of the vulva. FIGO 26th Annual Report on the results of treatment in Gynaecological Cancer. Int J Gynaecol Obstet 2006;95: 57–527.
3. Kurman RJ, Carcangiu ML, Herrington CM, Young RH. Tumour of the Vulva, In: Kurman RJ, Carcangiu ML, Herrington CM, Young RH, WHO classification of tumour of female reproductive organ. 4th ed. Lyon, International Agency for Research on cancer, 2014;230
4. RCOG: Guidelines for the Diagnosis and Management of Vulval Carcinoma; 2014
5. Madsen BS, Jensen HL, Ven JL. Risk factors for invasive squamous cell carcinoma of the vulva and vagina - Population based case-control study in Denmark. Int J Cancer 2008;122:2827–34.
6. Trimble CL, Hildesheim A, Brinton LA, Shah KV, Kurman RJ. Heterogeneous etiology of squamous carcinoma of the vulva. Obstet Gynecol 1996; 87:59–64.
7. Insinga RP, Liaw KL, Johnson LG, Madeleine MM. A systematic review of the prevalence and attribution of human papilloma virus types among cervical, vaginal and vulvar precancers and cancers in the United States. Cancer Epidemiol Biomarkers Prev 2008;17:1611–22.
8. van Seters M, van Beurden M, de Craen AJ. Is the assumed natural history of vulvar intraepithelial neoplasia III based on enough evidence? A systematic review of 3322 published patients. Gynecol Oncol 2005;97:645–51.
9. Hording U, Junge J, Poulsen H, Lundvall F. Vulvar intraepithelial neoplasia III: A viral disease of

undetermined progressive potential. Gynecol Oncol 1995;56:276–9.

10. Modesitt SC, Waters AB, Walton L, Fowler WC Jr, Van Le L. Vulvar intraepithelial neoplasia III: occult cancer and the impact of margin status on recurrence. Obstet Gynecol 1998;92:962–6.

11. Kurman RJ, Toki T, Schiffman MH. Basaloid and warty carcinomas of the vulva: distinctive types of squamous cell carcinoma frequently associated with human papillomaviruses. Am J Surg Pathol 1993; 17:133–45.

12. Vilmer C, Cavelier-Balloy B, Nogues C, Trassard M, Le Doussal V. Analysis of alterations adjacent to invasive vulvar carcinoma and their relationships with the associated carcinoma. Eur J Gynaecol Oncol 1998:19:25–31.

13. Brinton LA, Nasco PC, Mallin K, Baptiste MS, Wilbanks GD, Richart RM. Case-control study of cancer of the vulva. Obstet Gynecol 1990:75: 859–66.

14. FIGO committee on Gynecologic Oncology. Revised FIGO staging for carcinoma of the vulva, cervix and endometrium. Int J Gynecol Obstet 2009;105:103–4.

15. Viswanathan C, Kirschner K, Truong M, Balachandran A, Devine C, Bhosale P. Multi-modality imaging of vulvar cancer: Staging, Therapeutic response and complications. American Journal of Roentgenology 2013; 6:200. Available from https://doi.org/10.2214/AJR 12. 9714 accessed on 23.6.18

16. Chu J, Tamimi HK, Figge DC. Femoral node metastasis with negative superficial inguinal nodes in early vulvar cancer. Am J Obstet Gynecol 1981;140:37–9.

17. Curry SL, Wharton JT, Rutledge F. Positive lymph nodes in the vulvar squamous carcinoma. Gynecol Oncol 1980; 9:63–69.

18. Levenback C, Burke TW, Morris M, Malpica A, Lucas KR, Gershenson DM. Potential applications of intraoperative lymphatic mapping in vulvar cancer. Gynecol Oncol 1995; 59:216–20.

19. Hopkins MP, Morley GW. Pelvic exenteration for the treatment of vulvar cancer. Cancer 1992; 70:2835–8.

20. Malfetano J, Piver MS, Tsukada Y. Stage III and IV squamous cell carcinoma of the vulva. Gynecol Oncol 1986; 23:192–8.

21. Maggino T, Landoni F, Sartori E, Zola P, Gadducci A, Alessi C, et al. Patterns of recurrence in patients with squamous cell carcinoma of the vulva: a multicenter CTF study. Cancer 2000; 89:116–22.

22. Herzog TJ. Invasive Cancer of the Vulva. In: Disaia PJ, Creasman WT, Mannel RS, Mcmeekin DS, Mutch DG. Clinical Gynecologic Oncology, 9 th ed. Philadelphia, Elsevier, 2017; 190–216.

23. Watson M, Saraiya M, Ahmed F, Cardinez CJ, Reichman ME, Weir HK, et al. Using population-based cancer registry data to assess the burden of human papillomavirus-associated cancers in the United States: overview of methods. Cancer 2008; 113:2841–54.

24. Sedlis A, Homesley H, Bundy BN, Marshall R, Yordan E, Hacker N, et al. Positive groin lymph nodes in superficial squamous cell vulvar cancer. A Gynecologic Oncology Group Study. Am J Obstet Gynecol 1987;156:1159–64.

25. Te Grootenhuis NC, van der Zee AG, van Doorn HC, van der Velden J, Vergote I, Zanagnolo V, et al. Sentinel nodes in vulvar cancer: Long-term follow-up of the GROningen INternational Study on Sentinel nodes in Vulvar cancer (GROINSS-V) I. Gynecol Oncol 2016; 140:8–14.

26. Oonk MH, van Hemel BM, Hollema H, de Hullu JA, Ansink AC, Vergote I, et al. Size of sentinel-node metastasis and chances of non-sentinel-node involvement and survival in early stage vulvar cancer: results from GROINSS-V, a multicentre observational study. Lancet Oncol 2010; 11: 646–52.

27. Gaarenstroom KN, Kenter GG, Trimbos JB, Agous I, Amant F, Peters AA, et al. Postoperative complications after vulvectomy and inguinofemoral lymphadenectomy using separate groin incisions. Int J Gynecol Cancer 2003; 13:522–27.

28. Homesley HD, Bundy BN, Sedlis A, Yordan E, Berek JS, Jahshan A, et al. Prognostic factors for groin node metastasis in squamous cell carcinoma of the vulva (a Gynecologic Oncology Group study). Gynecol Oncol 1993;49:279–83.

29. Homesley HD, Bundy BN, Sedlis A, Adcock L. Radiation therapy versus pelvic node resection for carcinoma of the vulva with positive groin nodes. Obstet Gynecol 1986;68:733–40.

30. Russell AH, Mesic JB, Scudder SA, Rosenberg PJ, Smith LH, Kinney WK, et al. Synchronous radiation and cytotoxic chemotherapy for locally advanced or recurrent squamous cancer of the vulva. Gynecol Oncol 1992;47:14–20.

31. GS Montana, GM Thomas, DH Moore, Saxer A, Mangan CE, Lentz SS, et al. Preoperative chemo-radiation for carcinoma of the vulva with N2/N3 nodes: a Gynecology Oncology Group study. Int J Radiat Oncol Biol Phys 2000; 48:1007–13.

32. Henson ES, Gibson SB. Surviving cell death through epidermal growth factor (EGF) signal transduction pathways: implications for cancer therapy. Cell Signal 2006;18:2089–97.

Appendix A24.1: WHO classification of tumor of the vulva

Epithelial tumours

Squamous cell tumours and precursors

Squamous intraepithelial lesions

Low-grade squamous intraepithelial
lesion   8077/0

High-grade squamouw intraepithelial
lesion   8077/2

Differentiated-type vulvar intraepithelial
neoplasia   8071/2*

Squamous cell carcinoma   8070/3

Keratinizing   8071/3

Non-keratinizing   8072/3

Basaloid   8083/3

Warty   8051/3

Verrucous   8051/3

Basal cell carcinoma   8090/3

Benign squamous lesions

Condyloma acuminatum

Vestibular papilloma   8052/0

Seborrheic keratosis

Keratoacanthoma

Giandular tumours

Paget disease   8542/3

Tumours arising from Bartholin and
other specialized anogenital glands

Bartholin gland carcinomas

Adenocarcinoma   8140/3

Squamous cell carcinoma   8070/3

Adenosquamous carcinoma   8560/3

Adenoid cystic carcinoma   8200/3

Transitional cell carcinoma   8120/3

Adenocarcinoma of other types

Adenocarcinoma of sweat gland type   8140/3

Adenocarcinoma of intestinal type   8140/3

Benign tumours and cysts

Papillary hidradenoma   8405/0

Mixed tumour   8940/0

Fibroadenoma   9010/0

Adenoma   8140/0

Adenomyoma   8932/0

Bartholin gland cyst

Nodular Bartholin gland hyperplasia

Other vestibular gland cysts

Other cysts

Neuroendocrine tumours

High-grade neuroendocrine carcinoma

Small cell neuroendocrine carcinoma   8041/3

Large cell neuroendocrine carcinoma   8013/3

Merkel cell tumour   8247/3

Neuroectodermal tumours

Ewing sarcoma   9364/3

Soft tissue tumours

Benign tumours

Lipoma   8850/0

Fibroepithelial stromal polyp

Superficial angiomyxoma   8841/0*

Superficial myofibroblastoma   8825/0

Cellular angiofibroma   9160/0

Angiomyofibroblastoma   8826/0

Aggressive angiomyxoma   8841/0*

Leiomyoma   8890/0

Granular cell tumour   9580/0

Other benign tumours

Malignant tumours

Rhabdomyosarcoma

Embryonal   8910/3

Alveolar   8920/3

Leiomyosarcoma   8890/3

Epithelioid sarcoma   8804/3

Alveolar soft part sarcoma   9581/3

Other sarcomas

Liposarcoma   8850/3

Malignant peripheral nerve sheath tumour 9540/3

Kaposi sarcoma   9140/3

Fibrosarcoma   8810/3

Dermatofibrosarcoma protuberans   8832/1*

Malanocytic tumours

Melanocytic naevi

Congenital melanocytic naevus   8761/0

Acquired melanocytic naevus   8720/0

Blue naevus   8780/0

Atypical melanocytic naevus of genital type 8720/0

Dysplastic melanocytic naevus   8728/0

Malignant melanoma   8720/3

Germ cell tumours

Yolk sac tumour

Lymphoid and myeloid tumours

Lymphomas

Myeloid neoplasms

Secondary tumours

---

aThe morphology codes are from the Internal Classificationof Disease for Oncology (ICD-O) {575A]. Behaviour is coded /0 for benign tumours, /1 for unspecified, Borderline or uncertain behaviour, /2 for carcinoma in situ and grade III intraepithelial neoplasia and /3 for malignant tumours; bThe classification is modified from the previous WHO classification of tumours {1906A},

*These new coded were by the IARC/WHO Committee for ICD-O in 2013.

Appendix 2: FIGO Staging of Carcinoma Vulva, 2009

Stage I	Tumour confined to the vulva
IA	Lesions ≤2 cm size, confined to vulva/ perineum and with stromal invasion <1 mm and no nodal metastasis.
IB	Lesions >2 cm size or with stromal invasion >1 mm, confined to vulva/ perineum and no nodal metastasis.
Stage II	Tumor of any size with extension to adjacent perineal structures (1/3 lower urethra, 1/3 lower vagina, anus) with negative nodes.
Stage III	Tumor of any size with or without extension to adjacent perineal structures (1/3 lower urethra, 1/3 lower vagina, anus) with positive inguinofemoral lymph nodes
IIIA	1 lymph node ≥5 mm or 1–2 lymph nodes <5 mm
IIIB	2 or more lymph nodes ≥5 mm; 3 or more lymph nodes <5 mm
III C	Positive node with extracapsular spread
Stage IV	Tumor invades other regional (2/3 upper urethra 2/3 upper vagina) or distant structures.
IVA	Tumor invades any of the following: • Upper urethral and/or vaginal mucosa, bladder mucosa, rectal mucosa or fixed to pelvic bone, or • Fixed or ulcerated inguinofemoral lymph nodes.
IVB	Any distant metastases including pelvic lymph nodes

Depth of invasion is defined as the measurement of the tumour from the epithelial stromal junction of the adjacent most superficial dermal papilla to the deepest point of invasion.

25 Gestational Trophoblastic Neoplasia

Vijay Zutshi, Sana Tiwari

Gestational trophoblastic disease (GTD) is a spectrum of abnormal growth and proliferation of the trophoblasts. It encompasses a group of conditions like hyadatidiform mole, invasive mole, choriocarcinoma, placental site trophoblastic tumor (PSTT) and epithelioid trophoblastic tumor (ETT).

The incidence of gestational trophoblastic neoplasia (GTN) is 1 in 5000 to 50,000. Invasive mole constitutes 15% of all GTN, choriocarcinoma 3% and PSTT 1%.

Persistent trophoblastic disease (PTD) is persistence of trophoblastic activity following evacuation of molar pregnancy 50%. However, 25% can occur after abortion or ectopic and a few occur after normal pregnancy. Due to the continuing presence of the trophoblastic layer, this abnormal conceptus can continue to grow in the uterus or ectopically.

Case 1

A 26-years-old primigravida had uterine evacuation done for hyadatidiform mole four months back. During her follow up human chorionic gonadotropin (βhCG) was plateauing. Her β hCG values were: 2305 IU/L (Day-14); 2227 IU/L (Day-28); 2124 IU/L (Day-42). She had no other complaints.

Q1. What is your diagnosis?

Persistent trophoblastic disease following evacuation of molar pregnancy.

Q2. What is the criteria for diagnosis of postmolar GTN?

There is "FIGO diagnostic criteria" for post molar GTN depending on levels of β hCG on follow up.[2]

- 4 or more values of plateaued β hCG over at least 3 weeks time.
- A rise of β hCG >10% for >3 values over at least 2 weeks time.

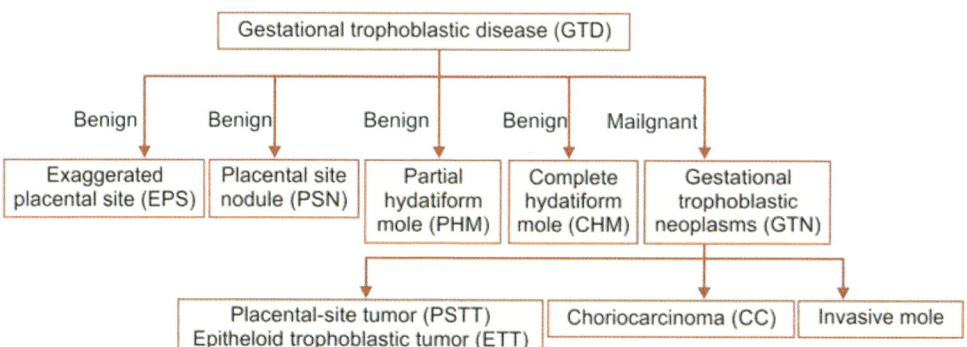

Fig. 25.1: WHO classification[1]

- Histological diagnosis of choriocarcinoma.
- Persistence of β hCG beyond 6 months of mole evacuation.

Q3. What are the usual clinical features of PTD?

The clinical features with which the patient presents depends on the site of the primary tumor and the secondary deposits:

- Patient can be asymptomatic
- Irregular vaginal bleeding
- Amenorrhea with history of repeated dilatation and curettage (D&Cs).
- If metastatic lesion is there:
  - Lung—cough, breathlessness, hemoptysis
  - Cerebral—headache, convulsions
  - Liver—epigastric pain, jaundice
  - Vagina—nodules, hemorrhage

Q4. What are the risk factors for GTN?

The risk factors are:

- β hCG titres >1,00,000 IU/L
- Excessive uterine enlargement
- Presence of theca lutein cyst 6 cm or more in diameter.

In this case

- β hCG titre was 1,20,000 IU/L
- The size of uterus was more than the period of gestation with no theca lutein cyst.

Q5. What is to be done after diagnosis of PTD?

Patient has to be worked up and WHO Prognostic scoring has to be done (Table 25.1).

Q6. What all investigations are required for work up of GTN?

The work up involves:

- Detailed history and physical examination
- Chest X-ray if not done earlier
- Complete blood count (CBC), Liver function test (LFT), Kidney function test (KFT), Serum electrolyte (SE), Thyroid stimulating hormone (TSH)
- Ultrasonography (USG) whole abdomen and pelvis
- Computed tomography (CT) of head/chest if indicated.

Q7. How to do WHO prognostic scoring?

Low risk <6   High risk ≥7
In this case, score was 5: $0 + 0 + 0 + 4 + 1 + 0 + 0$

Q8. How is chemotherapy given?

Based on scoring:

- Women with scores ≤6 (low risk) are treated with single-agent chemotherapeutic agent.
- Women with scores ≥7 (high risk) are treated with multi-agent chemotherapy, which includes combinations of methotrexate, dactinomycin, etoposide, cyclophosphamide and vincristine.

Q9. In Case 1 what further management will be done?

Case 1 had WHO prognostic scoring of <6 (low risk). Hence, single agent chemotherapy should be advised.

Table 25.1: Modified WHO prognostic scoring system as adapted by FIGO (2000)[3]				
Prognostic factors	*Score*			
	0	*1*	*2*	*4*
Age	<40	>40	—	—
Antecedent gestation	Mole	Abortion	Term	—
Interval (months)	<4	4–6	7–12	>13
Pretreatment serum hCG (mIU/mL)	$<10^3$	10^3 to $<10^4$	10^4 to $<10^5$	$>10^5$
Largest tumor size (including uterus)(cm)	<3	3 to 4	>5	—
Site of metastases	Lung, pelvis	spleen, kidney	GIT, lung	Brain
Number of metastases	—	1–4	5–8	>8
Previous failed chemotherapy	—	—	Single drug	>2

Q10. What are the different chemotherapeutic drug regimens used in low risk patients?

The regimens involve either single drug or a combination of drugs.

a. *Single agent:*

i. Methotrexate alternating with folinic acid

Methotrexate (MTX)	1 mg/kg IM on Day 1, 3, 5, 7
Calcium folinate (folinic acid)	0.1 mg/kg IM on Day 2, 4, 6, 8

*The courses are repeated at interval of 7 days.

ii. Actinomycin D   10–12 µg/kg IV daily for 5 days.

*The course is repeated at interval of 14 days.

b. *Combination regimen:*

MAC Protocol

Methotrexate (MTX)	1 mg/kg IM on Day 1, 3, 5, 7
Calcium folinate (folinic acid)	0.1 mg/kg IM on Day 2, 4, 6, 8
Actinomycin D	10–12 µg/kg IV daily for 5 days
Cyclophosphamide	3 mg/kg IV daily for 5 days

*The course is repeated at interval of 2 weeks.

Q11. What do you understand by adequate fall of β hCG?

Adequate fall is defined as fall in β hCG level by 1 log within 18 days after completion of first treatment cycle.

Q12. What are the indications for change in chemotherapy?

These are:
- Side effects of chemotherapeutic agents as enumerated below:
  - Thrombocytopenia
  - Neutropenia
  - Hepatotoxicity
  - Mouth sores
  - Nausea and vomiting
- Adequate fall of β hCG not achieved.

Q13. How do you follow up these patients?

The patient is followed up with weekly β hCG.

Follow up of Case 1
Required six cycles of chemotherapy for β hCG to normalize and two more cycles were given following a normal report.

Q14. How is follow up done after giving chemotherapy?

β hCG is done weekly till the value is negative for 3 consecutive weeks.

↓

Monthly for 6 months

↓

6 monthly for 2 years

Q15. What advice is given regarding next pregnancy?

- Women should be advised not to conceive until their follow-up is complete.[4]
- Women who receive chemotherapy are advised not to conceive for 1 year after completion of treatment.
- Women who conceive are advised to get an early USG. After 6 weeks of delivery they are followed up with β hCG levels to rule out persistent trophoblastic disease.

Q16. Which different contraceptives can be advised during follow up?

- Barrier methods are safe to use.
- Oral contraceptives can be used after normalization of β hCG.
- Intrauterine device is not recommended due to risk of uterine perforation.

Case 2

A 25-years-old woman presented to hospital with complaint of heaviness in lower abdomen and irregular vaginal bleeding. She did not remember her last menstrual period (LMP) as she was lactating. On general physical examination she was conscious with stable vitals. The systemic examination was normal.

On per abdominal examination an abdomino-pelvic mass corresponding to 14 weeks gravid uterus was felt which was firm, mobile, non tender. On per speculum examination cervix and vagina were healthy. On pervaginal examination uterus corresponded to 12 weeks, mobile, non-tender. On rectovaginal examination rectal mucosa was free and same mass was felt.

Q1. How will you proceed further in this case?

Urine pregnancy test (UPT) will be done to rule out pregnancy.

In this case UPT was positive and USG pelvis showed size of uterus 12 × 10 × 4 cm with normal bilateral adenexa. A 10 × 6 × 9 cm heterogenous mass with anechoic foci was present in posterior myometrium with increased vascularity that was indenting endometrium.

Q2. What do you suspect in this case?

One must rule out GTN/Missed abortion in such situations.

Q3. What has to be done to settle the diagnosis?

Serum β hCG
In this case β hCG was 1,20,000IU/L.

Q4. What is the final diagnosis for Case 2?
GTN

Q5. What is to be done next?

WHO prognostic scoring has to be done.

Case 2 had a total score of 10 that falls in high risk.

Q6. What treatment will be given to Case 2?

High risk cases require multiagent regimen like EMA-CO and EMA-EP. EMACO is most effective.

Q7. What is EMACO regimen?
See Table 25.2

Follow up of Case 1
Required five courses of EMA-CO for β hCG to normalize. After this cycle her β hCG was normal <2IU/L. She received 2 more cycles of EMACO after normalization of her β hCG.

Table 25.2: EMA-CO regime

Day	Drug	Dose
EMA-CO		
1	Etoposide	100 mg/m² by infusion in 200 mL saline over 30 min
	ActD	0.5 mg IV 100 mg/m² IV followed by
	MTX	200 mg/m² by infusion over 12 h
2	Etoposide	100 mg/m² by infusion in 200 mL saline over 30 min
	ActD	0, 5 mg IV
	Folinic acid	15 mg IM or PO every 12 h for 4 doses starting 24 hours after start of MTX
8	Cyclophosphamide	600 mg/m² by infusion in saline over 30 min
	Vincristine	1 mg/m² IV

Q8. What are other multiagent regimens available?

The other regimens are
- EMA-EP
- Vincristine, Bleomycin, Cisplatin (VBP).

Q9. What investigations are required prior to each cycle of chemotherapy?

- Complete blood count
- Liver function test
- Kidney function test
- Chest X-ray to be repeated if there is plateauing or rise in β hCG level.

Q10. When should chemotherapy not be given?

If:
- WBC <3000/mm³
- Polymorpholeucocytes <1500/mm³
- Platelet counts <1,00,000/mm³
- Significant rise in LFT, KFT.

Q11. Why do we give one to two more courses of chemotherapy after normalization of β hCG?

More courses are given because 10^2–10^3 trobhoblastic cells are quiescent and are circulating in blood. There is a risk of relapse due to these quiescent cells in 6–10% patients. To prevent recurrence from the same, additional chemotherapy courses are given.

Q12. What is the cure rate of GTN?

The cure rate for women with a score ≤6 is almost 100%; and for women with a score ≥7 is 95%.

Case 3

A 40-year-old woman, para 3, presented in emergency with complaint of irregular vaginal bleeding for two months. She had undergone molar evacuation 6 months back. Her β hCG was showing a rising trend. Based on WHO Prognostic scoring she was a "High Risk" patient and therefore received EMACO multiagent drug therapy. After receiving 5 cycles of chemotherapy there was inadequate fall of β hCG. USG whole abdomen and pelvis was done which revealed a solitary lesion in the endometrial cavity. Medical oncologist reviewed the case and advised for hysterectomy after counseling the patient. Total abdominal hysterectomy with bilateral salpingectomy was done in view of a solitary nodule and inadequate response to chemotherapy. After hysterectomy she required 3 more cycles of EMACO following which her β hCG normalized. Further 2 more courses of chemotherapy were given after normalization of serum β hCG.

Q1. What are the indications of hysterectomy?

Hysterectomy is needed in the following circumstances:

- Placental site trophoblastic tumor
- Intractable vaginal bleeding
- Localized lesion in uterus resistant to chemotherapy
- Uterine perforation during curettage.

Q2. What are the indications for other types of surgery in GTN?

Apart from total hysterectomy other surgical procedures that may be required are:

- Thoracotomy—in cases of pulmonary metastasis in drug resistant cases.

- Craniotomy—to control bleeding or to give acute decompression in cases with intracranial metastasis.
- Hepatic resection—to control acute bleeding or to excise resistant focus in liver.

Q3. What are the indications for radiotherapy in GTN?

- Brain metastasis—whole brain radiation therapy, intrathecal high dose methotrexate.
- Liver metastasis—whole liver radiation.

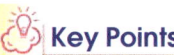 **Key Points**

- High index of suspicion for GTN should be kept in mind for reproductive age group women presenting with abnormal vaginal bleeding.
- The unique thing about GTN is that tissue is not required for diagnosis.
- Serum β hCG is very good marker for diagnosis and follow up.
- GTN has a good prognosis as compared to other gynecological malignancies provided it is diagnosed well in time and treated adequately.
- Surgical intervention may be required occasionally.

REFERENCES

1. F T Stevens, N Katzorke, C Tempfer, U Kreimer, GI Bizjak, MC Fleisch, TN Fehm Geburtshilfe Frauenheilkd. Gestational Trophoblastic Disorders: An Update in 2015.2015;75:1043–50.
2. Richter CE, Schwartz PE Clinical Aspects of Gestational Trophoblastic Disease. In: Hui P. (eds) Gestational Trophoblastic Disease. Current Clinical Pathology. Springer, New York, NY. 2012.
3. FIGO Oncology Committee. FIGO staging for gestational trophoblastic neoplasia. Int J Gynaecol Obstet 2002;77:285–7.
4. Newlands ES. Presentation and management of persistent gestational trophoblastic disease and gestational trophoblastic tumours in the UK. In: Hancock BW, Newlands ES, Berkowitz RS, Cole LA, editors. Gestational Trophoblastic Disease. 3rd ed. London: International Society for the Study of Trophoblastic Disease; 2003.

26 Radiotherapy in Gynecologic Cancers

Aditi Aggarwal, Arun Kumar Rathi, Savita Arora, Kishore Singh

Radiotherapy is the modality used to treat cancers and some benign conditions using radiation (photons or X rays). This is an age-old modality that is delivered either as teletherapy (*TELE* means far in Latin; where radiation source is placed at a distance from the patient) or brachytherapy (*brachy* means short in Latin; where radiation source is placed close to or inside the patient).

Teletherapy was traditionally delivered using cobalt 60 machine (Fig. 26.1A) and is being gradually replaced by linear accelerators (Fig. 26.1B). A linear accelerator uses either electrons or X-rays which are produced by accelerating electrons to a high speed and made to strike a target. There are a number of accessories in the teletherapy machine to modify the radiation beam to get the desired dose distribution in target tissues. All these techniques have been developed with the sole aim to deliver maximal desired radiation dose to the target and minimal dose to surrounding normal structures, namely organs at risk (OARs)

Brachytherapy is delivered using specially designed applicators selected according to the site being treated. Brachytherapy is an essential component of treatment for patients with carcinoma cervix. HDR (High Dose Rate) brachytherapy machine with remote after-loading facility uses Iridium 192 as the radioactive isotope (Fig. 26.2).

The most commonly used applicator for treatment of cervical cancers is the Fletcher Suit Williamson applicator which has a central tandem that goes inside the uterine cavity and two vaginal ovoids that rest in the vaginal fornices (Fig. 26.3). Apart from this metal applicator, CT-MRI compatible applicator is also available (Fig. 26.3). Interstitial brachytherapy is delivered by placing the needles or plastic tubes into the disease using either the

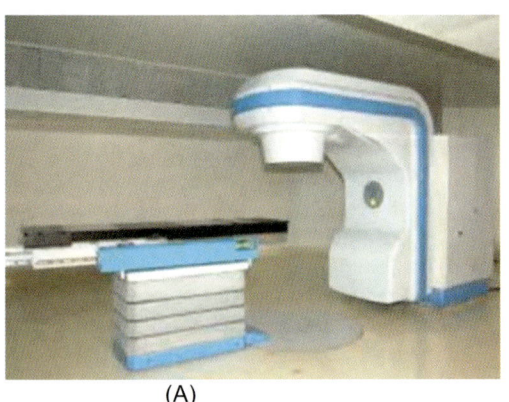

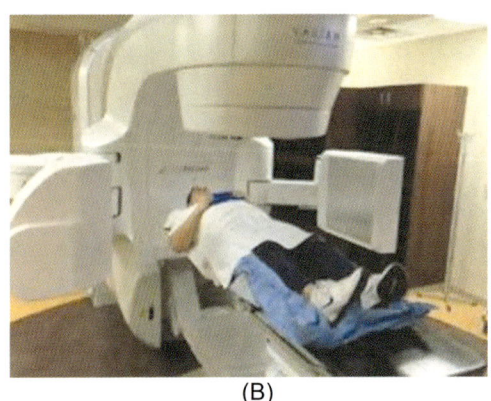

(A) (B)

Fig. 26.1: (A) Cobalt 60 machine and (B) A modern linear accelerator with arms for image verification

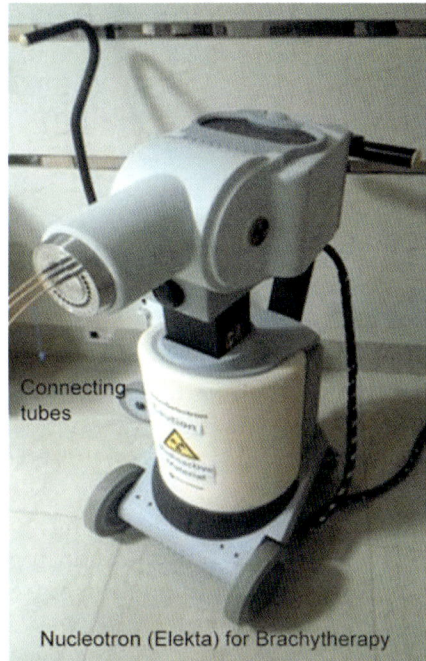

Fig. 26.2: A brachytherapy machine from Elekta-Nucleotron uses Iridium 192 radioactive source

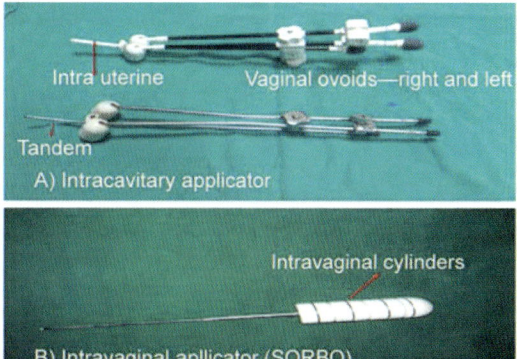

A) Intracavitary applicator

B) Intravaginal apllicator (SORBO)

Fig. 26.3: Applicators for intracavitary brachytherapy—CT-MRI compatible (above) and metallic (below). The central tandem is the intrauterine tandem and the two ovoids fit in the right and left lateral vaginal fornices

template (MUPIT) (Fig. 26.4) or by free hand technique. This is done in case of extensive disease or in vault recurrences. Vault/vaginal brachytherapy in adjuvant setting is delivered using a vaginal applicator (SORBO) using a central tandem with cylinders that rest in the vagina. This is done as an outpatient procedure.

Gynecological cancers constitute a majority of cancers in developing countries like India, especially cervical cancer. The other gynecological cancers are endometrial cancer, vaginal, vulvar and ovarian cancers.

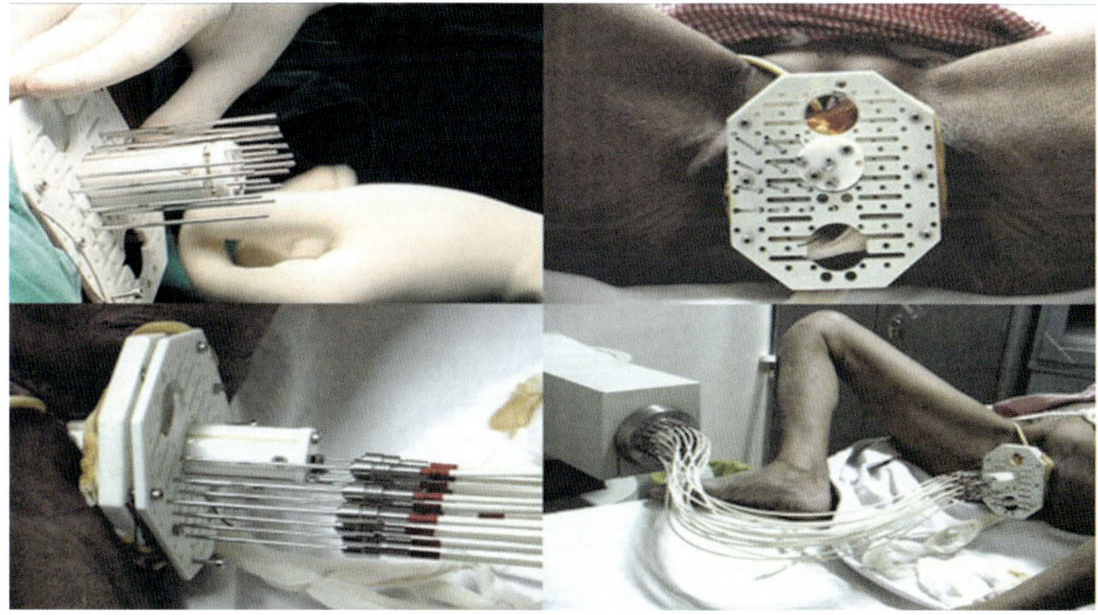

Fig. 26.4: A MUPIT (Martinez Universal Perineal Interstitial Template) applicator for carcinoma cervix patient

Cervical cancer is the second most common cancer in women in the country after breast cancer, and still the commonest in rural populations with an overall incidence of around 20 cases per 1,00,000 population as per GLOBACON 2012 data.[1]

Radical radiotherapy is radiotherapy delivered as a primary modality to treat the disease and the dose delivered is around 80–85 Gy low dose rate (LDR) equivalent. External beam radiotherapy is delivered conventionally at 1.8–2 Gy/fraction with five fractions a week, from Monday to Friday. *Neoadjuvant* is the term used for treatment delivered prior to definitive treatment and *adjuvant* for treatment delivered after it.

This chapter aims to discuss the role of radiotherapy and practical aspects in the management of gynecological cancers. This will be discussed in a case based manner describing the clinical scenario followed by appropriate management for that patient.

CERVICAL CANCER

Case 1

A 55-year-old postmenopausal lady with no comorbidities presents with complaints of vaginal bleeding with associated foul smelling discharge for four months. She also complains of backache and burning sensation during micturition. On examination, there is a large ulceroproliferative growth of 5.5 × 6 × 3 cm at the cervix occupying all fornices. Bilateral parametrium and vagina are free from disease. Biopsy from the growth is suggestive of moderately differentiated squamous cell carcinoma. MRI pelvis shows a hyperintense signal on T_2-weighted images in cervix with extension to lower uterine segment with no vaginal or parametrial extension. The fat planes with bladder and rectum are well maintained. There are also sub centimetric bilateral internal iliac lymph nodes, with no hydroureteronephrosis.

Q.1 Discuss the management for this case.

She has carcinoma cervix FIGO (2009) stage IB2 as per clinical examination. As per AJCC staging, the stage is T1b2 N0 M0 (IB2).

Management

The most appropriate treatment for her would be Definitive Radiotherapy concomitant with cisplatin based weekly chemotherapy. Patients with disease more than 4 cm in size have a high likelihood of being treated with adjuvant radiotherapy after primary surgery and thus upfront chemoradiation for such patients is recommended.[2]

The ideal treatment for cervical cancer patients (disease IB2, IIA2 and beyond) is definitive or radical chemoradiation.[3,4] Radiotherapy comprises external beam radiotherapy to a total dose of 45–50.4 Gy/25–28 fractions/5–5.5 weeks along with weekly platinum-based intravenous chemotherapy and then brachytherapy to complete the total dose to point A to 80–85 Gy LDR (Low Dose Rate) equivalent.[5]

Brachytherapy is either intracavitary or interstitial radiotherapy depending on the response of disease after teletherapy. This is delivered in a fractionated manner at 7–8 Gy/fractions for two to three times to complete the total treatment within 8 weeks time.[5]

Case 2

A 45-year-old lady, hypertensive, presents to the Gynecology outpatient clinic after simple hysterectomy done for abnormal uterine bleeding at her native place. On examination, there is an ulcerative lesion at the cervical stump/vault of dimensions 3 × 3 × 2 cm involving upper 2 cm of vagina with medial parametrium involved on left side. Biopsy from growth reveals a poorly differentiated squamous cell carcinoma with MRI pelvis suggestive of hyperintense signal on T_2-weighted images at residual cervical stump with medial parametrial infiltration on left side. Fat planes with bladder and rectum are well defined with sub centimetric pelvic lymph nodes and mild hydroureteronephrosis on left side.

Q.1   Discuss the management of this case.

She is a case of carcinoma vault/cervical stump stage IIIB (in view of hydroureteronephrosis) (as per FIGO 2009).

Management

She would be treated with radical intent with radiochemotherapy with external beam radiotherapy delivered to the pelvis (nodes+ primary disease) to a dose of 45–50 Gy/25–28 fractions/5–5.3 weeks concomitant with weekly cisplatin chemotherapy. After external beam radiotherapy and response assessment, she should receive radiotherapy by interstitial brachytherapy to the vault to complete a total dose of around 80–85 Gy LDR equivalent to residual disease after external beam radiotherapy. This should be completed in a total time of 8 weeks from start of radiotherapy.

Case 3

A 47-year-old woman P2 L2, is diagnosed with squamous cell carcinoma on routine PAP screening. Speculum examination shows a small unhealthy area on the cervix at 3 o'clock to 7 o'clock position with no involvement of vaginal fornices or parametrium or lower third vagina. MRI pelvis is suggestive of small signal heterogeneity on T_2-weighted images in the cervix not going beyond it. There is no pelvic lymphadenopathy or hydroureteronephrosis. She was managed with radical hysterectomy. Surgical histopathology is suggestive of squamous cell carcinoma of cervix 2 × 2 × 2 cm with deep stromal invasion. Lower uterine segment, adnexa, bilateral parametrium are free, vaginal cut margins are also free. Out of 12 pelvic lymph nodes dissected, 3 are positive with no perinodal extension (PNE). There is no lymphovascular space invasion (LVSI) or perineural invasion (PNI).

Q1.   Discuss her further management.

This patient is a postoperative case of carcinoma cervix stage pT1b1pN1cM0.

Management

She falls in the high-risk group for locoregional recurrence in view of nodal positivity and hence should be treated with adjuvant radiotherapy to pelvis to a dose of 45–50 Gy/25–28 fractions/5–5.3 weeks concurrent with weekly intravenous cisplatin 40 mg/m² after confirming normal laboratory parameters. Thereafter she should receive vaginal brachytherapy to treat the vault and upper third of vagina to a dose of 30 Gy LDR equivalent in order to decrease the incidence of local recurrence.

Indications for adjuvant radiotherapy for carcinoma cervix is decided by the Sedlis criteria which consist of tumor size (≤/>4 cm), depth of stromal invasion (≤/>50%), and LVSI. Patients having two or more of the above features benefit from addition of adjuvant radiotherapy alone after surgery in terms of risk of recurrence and progression free survival.[6] For early stage disease with pelvic node positivity, parametrial involvement or margin positivity, concurrent weekly platinum based chemotherapy is added along with radiotherapy. This has been shown to increase the progression free survival (PFS) and also has an impact on overall survival (OS).[6]

Case 4

A 65-year-old lady presents to Gynaecology outpatient clinic with chief complaint of vaginal bleeding. She looks pale and her haemoglobin is 5 g%. Local examination reveals a growth occupying the whole of cervix. Parametrial involvement cannot be assessed completely due to bleeding. She is bleeding profusely, not controlled with conservative management. On CT pelvis there is a large soft tissue density at cervix, involving the lower uterine segment with bilateral parametrial infiltration up to lateral pelvic wall. The fat planes were lost between the soft tissue and bladder anteriorly and rectum posteriorly. There were enlarged external iliac, common iliac and para-aortic lymph nodes, the largest was 2.2 × 1.5 cm at left common iliac level. Histology is proven as poorly differentiated squamous cell carcinoma.

Q.1   How will you manage her?

She is clinically stage IIIB as per FIGO staging, and T3bN1M1 (Stage IV) in view of para-aortic lymph nodal enlargement.

Management

The treatment of choice for such patients is definitive radiochemotherapy after ruling out bladder rectal infiltration with help of cystoscopy and proctoscopy. However, due to vaginal bleeding not controlled with conservative management, she would be initially managed with **hemostatic radiotherapy** given to control bleeding in a dose of 5 Gy/single fraction to the primary disease. Thereafter on complete local examination, if proven to be IIIB (not IVA as per FIGO), she would be treated with radical radiotherapy with concurrent weekly intravenous cisplatin.[8] Before starting radiation, her haemoglobin needs to be built to around 10 g%. Kidney function tests (KFT) have to be monitored closely. Radiation portal would be designed so as to cover para-aortic nodes up to a dose of 45–50 Gy/25–28 fractions/5–5.3 weeks. Pelvis would be treated with external beam radiotherapy to the same doses as for radical treatment.

The same patient if proven to be stage IVA on cystoscopy and proctoscopy with biopsy confirmation shall be first treated with neo-adjuvant chemotherapy for 2–3 cycles followed by a repeat assessment of response on imaging and cysto-/proctoscopy. This should be done with due consent and discussion with the patient as the chances of fistula formation remain even with chemotherapy. If regression of disease occurs with no fistula formation, she can be taken for radical chemoradiotherapy in the same way as above.

ENDOMETRIAL CANCER

Case 5

A 65-year-old postmenopausal, diabetic and hypertensive lady presents to the Gynecology outpatient clinic with complaints of post-menopausal bleeding for last one year associated with passage of clots. There are no urinary or rectal complaints. She gives no history of fever, weight loss or anorexia. On investigation, her USG pelvis reveals endometrial thickening of around 2 cm with a mass involving the postero-lateral wall of uterus and cervical isthmus. Contrast enhanced MRI pelvis shows a heterogeneously enhancing mass involving the postero-lateral wall of uterus reaching up to serosa with cervical isthmus involvement. There is no significant pelvic lymphadenopathy.

She undergoes a total abdominal hysterectomy with bilateral pelvic lymphadenectomy. Surgical pathology reveals a tumor of size 4 × 3.5 × 2 cm, Endometrial adenocarcinoma (ADCA), grade II, invading more than half of myometrium, no cervical stromal invasion, with no LVSI/perineural invasion (PNI). The vaginal cut margin is 2 cm away from tumor distally and circumferential margin is 1 cm. Bilateral adnexa and parametrium are free. Out of 30 lymph nodes dissected, all are negative.

Q1.   What should be her further management?

As per the risk stratification for adjuvant treatment of carcinoma endometrium, she falls in intermediate risk group in view of grade II, stage Ib.

Management

Vaginal brachytherapy alone is the recommended treatment for such patients in order to reduce the incidence of vault and vaginal recurrences from 15% to <5%. Vaginal brachytherapy reduces the local recurrences and has an impact on disease-free survival, with no impact on overall survival. Radiotherapy is done after complete wound healing by giving a dose of 7 Gy, 2 fractions delivered at one-week gap to the vault and upper half to one-third of vagina prescribed at a distance of 0.5 cm from the mucosa.

Adjuvant treatment for endometrial cancers depends on a number of surgico-pathological features including T stage, depth of myometrial invasion (MMI) >50% or not, Grade of tumor (PORTEC), LVSI (ESMO), tumor size >2 cm (MAYO group). Also patient's age >60 years is a high-risk feature as per GOG-99. These factors are considered differently as per different treatment groups. Table 26.1 shows the risk stratification and the adjuvant treatment for the corresponding groups based on PORTEC (Table 26.1).

Patients who are node positive or margin positive require combination treatment. The role of chemotherapy for endometrial carcinoma is under investigation and yet not established. It is given for advanced—stage III and metastatic disease.[13,14]

CARCINOMA VAGINA

Case 6

A 55-year-old woman P4L4 presents to the Gynecology outpatient clinic with complaints of vaginal discharge and occasional spotting. She also complains of low back pain with burning sensation during micturition. There is associated weight loss of around 6 kg in last four months and decreased appetite. On examination she has an infiltrative lesion in right lateral wall of vagina extending 3 cm from introitus to the cervix, from 6 o'clock to 11 o'clock position. On palpation, this lesion is felt to be separate from the cervix with infiltration of paravaginal and parametrial tissues on the right up to medial half, left parametrium is free from disease. On MRI pelvis there is same lesion in right lateral wall of vagina with involvement of the right parametrium in medial half, not up to lateral pelvic wall. Also, there are a few external iliac and inguinal nodes, largest in inguinal area of 2 × 2 cm with a necrotic centre. On biopsy the lesion is a moderately differentiated squamous cell carcinoma and fine needle aspiration cytology (FNAC) from the node is positive. Metastatic workup including chest X-ray is nomal.

Q1. What should be the management plan for this patient?

She is a case of carcinoma vagina stage T2N1M0, stage III as per TNM staging.

Management

A complete mapping of disease is essential before starting the treatment. Appropriate treatment for her would be radical radiotherapy concurrent with platinum-based chemotherapy to a dose of 50 Gy/25 fractions/5 weeks to the pelvis including vagina, pelvic and inguinal nodes followed by interstitial brachytherapy to deliver a total dose of 80–85 Gy (LDR equivalent) to the residual disease after external beam radiotherapy.[15] Inguinal nodes are boosted to a total dose of 60–66 Gy by external beam radiotherapy.

Table 26.1: Risk stratification for adjuvant treatment of endometrial cancers (PORTEC)		
Risk Group	Characteristics	Adjuvant treatment
Low risk	Endometrioid ADCA, Stage IA, Gr1, 2 No LVSI, Age <60 years	Observation [9]
Intermediate risk	Endometrioid ADCA, Stage IA Gr3; Ib Gr1, 2 II Gr1, 2, 3 with <50% MMI II Gr1, 2 with >50% MMI, without LVSI	Vaginal Brachytherapy alone [10–12] (60 Gy LDR Equivalent)
High risk	Endometrioid ADCA, IB Gr3; II Gr3, >50% MMI, Clear cell carcinoma, Uterine Papillary Serous, Stage III, IV	Pelvic Radiotherapy (50 Gy/25 fractions/5 weeks) + Vaginal Brachytherapy (30 Gy LDR Equivalent)

CARCINOMA VULVA

Case 7

A 60-year-old lady, diabetic, P4 L4 presents with chief complaints of vulval itching with redness for last 4 months. She also reports burning sensation during micturition but no bowel complaints, anorexia or weight loss. On examination of the genitals, there is a proliferative growth of size 4 × 3 × 2.5 cm on labia minora on right side reaching up to distal urethra with sub centimetric palpable inguinal lymph nodes on right side. Biopsy is suggestive of a moderately differentiated squamous cell carcinoma. CT pelvis shows a hypodense lesion with heterogenous contrast enhancement in the labia of size 4 × 3 × 3 cm involving the urethra with bilateral inguinal lymphadenopathy, largest 1.5 × 1 cm on right side.

Q1. How should this case be managed?

She is a case of carcinoma vulva stage T3N1 (III) as per FIGO 2009 and AJCC staging.

Management

In view of urethral involvement, organ preservation can be achieved with appropriate local control with radical radiotherapy along with chemotherapy. Surgery for her would be too extensive and psychosexually disturbing. Radiotherapy is given concurrently with weekly platinum-based chemotherapy to the primary disease, inguinal and pelvic nodes to a dose of 45–50 Gy/25–28 fractions/5–5.3 weeks. This is followed by brachytherapy boost to the residual disease using interstitial brachytherapy.[16] Skin and mucosal reactions are monitored weekly as this area is predisposed to reactions. The treatment fields are large, but treatment is well tolerated and can be completed in time with appropriate planning and review. In all patients with lesions larger than 4 cm, centrally placed, poorly differentiated, LVSI positive, bilateral inguinal nodes have to be treated electively. For cases with involvement of inguinal lymph nodes, pelvic nodes are to be irradiated electively.

REFERENCES

1. Sreedevi A, Javed R, Dinesh A. Epidemiology of cervical cancer with special focus on India. Int J Womens Health 2015;7:405-14.
2. Gupta S, Maheshwari A, Parab P, Mahantshetty U, Hawaldar R, Sastri Chopra S, et al. Neoadjuvant Chemotherapy Followed by Radical Surgery Versus Concomitant Chemotherapy and Radiotherapy in Patients With Stage IB2, IIA, or IIB Squamous Cervical Cancer: A Randomized Controlled Trial. J Clin Oncol 2018;36:1548-55.
3. Chemoradiotherapy for Cervical Cancer Meta-Analysis Collaboration. Reducing uncertainties about the effects of chemoradiotherapy for cervical cancer: a systematic review and meta-analysis of individual patient data from 18 randomized trials. J Clin Oncol 2008;26:5802-12.
4. Shrivastava S, Mahantshetty U, Engineer R, Chopra S, Hawaldar R, Hande V, et al. Gynecologic Disease Management Group. Cisplatin Chemoradiotherapy vs Radiotherapy in FIGO Stage IIIB Squamous Cell Carcinoma of the Uterine Cervix: A Randomized Clinical Trial. JAMA Oncol 2018;4:506-513.
5. Mazeron R, Fokdal LU, Kirchheiner K, Georg P, Jastaniyah N, Šegedin B, et al. Dose-volume effect relationships for late rectal morbidity in patients treated with chemoradiation and MRI-guided adaptive brachytherapy for locally advanced cervical cancer: Results from the prospective multicenter EMBRACE study. Radiother Oncol J Eur Soc Ther Radiol Oncol 2016;120:412–9.
6. Rotman M, Sedlis A, Piedmonte MR, Bundy B, Lentz SS, Muderspach LI, et al. A phase III randomized trial of postoperative pelvic irradiation in Stage IB cervical carcinoma with poor prognostic features: follow-up of a gynecologic oncology group study. Int J Radiat Oncol Biol Phys 2006;65:169–76.
7. Peters WA, Liu PY, Barrett RJ, Stock RJ, Monk BJ, Berek JS, et al. Concurrent chemotherapy and pelvic radiation therapy compared with pelvic radiation therapy alone as adjuvant therapy after radical surgery in high-risk early-stage cancer of the cervix. J Clin Oncol Off J Am Soc Clin Oncol 2000;18:1606–13.
8. Small W, Winter K, Levenback C, Iyer R, Gaffney D, Asbell S, et al. Extended-field irradiation and intracavitary brachytherapy combined with cisplatin chemotherapy for cervical cancer with positive para-aortic or high common iliac lymph nodes: results of ARM 1 of RTOG 0116. Int J Radiat Oncol Biol Phys 2007;68:1081–7.

9. Creutzberg CL, van Putten WL, Koper PC, Lybeert ML, Jobsen JJ, Wárlám-Rodenhuis CC, et al. Surgery and postoperative radiotherapy versus surgery alone for patients with stage-1 endometrial carcinoma: multicentre randomised trial. The Lancet 2000;355:1404–11.

10. Keys HM, Roberts JA, Brunetto VL, Zaino RJ, Spirtos NM, Bloss JD, et al. A phase III trial of surgery with or without adjunctive external pelvic radiation therapy in intermediate risk endometrial adenocarcinoma: a Gynecologic Oncology Group study. Gynecol Oncol 2004;92:744–51.

11. ASTEC/EN.5 Study Group, Blake P, Swart AM, Orton J, Kitchener H, Whelan T, Lukka H, et al. Adjuvant external beam radiotherapy in the treatment of endometrial cancer (MRC ASTEC and NCIC CTG EN.5 randomised trials): pooled trial results, systematic review, and meta-analysis. Lancet 2009;373:137-46.

12. Nout RA, Smit VT, Putter H, Jürgenliemk-Schulz IM, Jobsen JJ, Lutgens LC, et al; PORTEC Study Group. Vaginal brachytherapy versus pelvic external beam radiotherapy for patients with endometrial cancer of high-intermediate risk (PORTEC-2): an open-label, non-inferiority, randomized trial. Lancet 2010;375:816-23.

13. Hogberg T, Signorelli M, de Oliveira CF, Fossati R, Lissoni AA, Sorbe B, et al. Sequential adjuvant chemotherapy and radiotherapy in endometrial cancer—results from two randomised studies. Eur J Cancer 2010;46:2422-31.

14. Humber CE, Tierney JF, Symonds RP, Collingwood M, Kirwan J, Williams C, et al. Chemotherapy for advanced, recurrent or metastatic endometrial cancer: a systematic review of Cochrane collaboration. Ann Oncol 2007;18:409-20.

15. Samant R, Lau B, EC, Le T, Tam T. Primary vaginal cancer treated with concurrent chemoradiation using Cis-platinum. Int J Radiat Oncol Biol Phys 2007;69:746–50.

16. Han SC, Kim DH, Higgins SA, Carcangiu ML, Kacinski BM. Chemoradiation as primary or adjuvant treatment for locally advanced carcinoma of the vulva. Int J Radiat Oncol Biol Phys 2000;47:1235–44.

Care of Patients Receiving Chemotherapy and Radiotherapy for Gynecologic Cancers

Narayan Adhikari, Kishore Singh

Chemotherapy and radiotherapy are integral part of management of gynecologic cancers. While these treatments effectively kill the cancerous cells, exposure of other body tissues to these gives rise to unwanted side effects. Management of these side effects adds another dimension to the care of women receiving chemotherapy and radiotherapy.

Case 1

A 42-year-old patient with carcinoma cervix stage IIIB undergoing chemoradiotherapy presents with diarrhea. She has history of eating roadside Chinese food and drinking fruit juice one day prior to presentation.

Q1. How will you manage such a case?

Diarrhea during chemoradiotherapy is mainly due to pelvic irradiation in such cases. Acute radiation enteritis can be seen in up to 70% of patients, depending on treatment and predisposing factors.[1] The concurrent chemotherapy regimen of weekly Cisplatin may be a less frequent cause of diarrhea. The chemotherapeutic drugs notorious for causing diarrhoea are Irinotecan, 5-Fluorouracil (bolus) or fluoropyrimidines combination regimens.[2] She also has a history of eating street food one day prior to presentation so infective cause of acute gastroenteritis or food poisoning should also be kept in mind during her management. After proper history taking, covering points like presence of fever, dehydration, frequency and consistency of stools, onset and duration of diarrhea, associated symptoms, abdominal pain and cramping, associated bleeding, weakness, medications profile and dietary profile, the diarrhea should be classified as uncomplicated versus complicated. Grading of diarrhea for the patients on chemoradiation is done according to the (a) Common Terminology Criteria for Adverse Events (CTCAE) for chemotherapy induced diarrhea and (b) Radiation Therapy Oncology Group (RTOG) criteria for radiotherapy induced diarrhea. Routine blood investigations are done to see associated neutropenia or neutrophilia, electrolytes and kidney function tests for dehydration and dyselectrolytemia. Any patient with CTC grade 3 or 4 or grade 1 or 2 diarrhea with cramping, nausea, vomiting, decreased performance status, fever, sepsis, neutropenia, frank bleeding, dehydration, etc. is considered complicated diarrhea and should be hospitalized. Uncomplicated grade 1 or 2 diarrhea can be managed on OPD basis. All patients with diarrhea should be started on rehydration therapy. For grade 2 or higher diarrhea, cytotoxic treatment with chemotherapy or radiotherapy may be held back until symptoms are resolved. The patient should be managed in multidisciplinary setting with consultation from oncologist and internist. For uncomplicated cytotoxic treatment induced diarrhea, administer loperamide 4 mg stat followed by 2 mg after each loose stools (maximum 8 tablets per day). Loperamide may cause dangerous prolongation of illness in patients with bloody or inflammatory diarrhea and, therefore, should be restricted to patients with non-bloody stool. If diarrhea does not resolve after 12–24 hours, add antibiotics. Antibiotics may be started upfront when diarrhea is suspected to be infective in nature. Any persistent diarrhoea should be managed like complicated diarrhoea and stool tested for blood, fecal leucocytes, infectious agents *Clostridium difficile*, Salmonella, *E. coli*, Campylobacter, etc. and treatment should be tailored accordingly. Octreotide subcutaneous (100–150 microgram TID) or intravenous (20–50 microgram per hour) may be started for complicated or persistent diarrhoea. Other agents like probiotics, racecadotril, opioids can be supplemented subsequently in case of persistent diarrhea.[2] Rehydration must be continued for all the patients.

Good hygiene, handwashing, safe food preparation, and access to clean water are key factors in preventing infective diarrheal illness and should be advised to all patients under-going cytotoxic treatment with chemoradio-therapy.[3] Patient should also be advised to avoid eating street food, raw fruits and vegetables, drinking fruit juices as they are prone to neutropenia and infection during cytotoxic treatment.

Case 2

A 60-year-old woman with carcinoma ovary living in a tropical climate developed fever and generalized weakness. She was receiving chemotherapy with Paclitaxel and Carboplatin, and hand received third cycle days back.

Q1. How will you manage this case?

Myelosuppression is one of the common side effects of most of the chemotherapeutic regimen. This leads to neutropenia. The nadir period is around 10–14 days but drugs like procarbazine cause delayed neutropenia. Even radiotherapy can cause neutropenia when large areas of pelvis and vertebrae are irradiated. Patients are generally reviewed in second week of chemotherapy to check nadir counts. *Afebrile neutropenia* can be managed on OPD basis with proper counselling for neutropenic precautions and barrier nursing like use of masks, maintenance of sanitary

habits like washing hands, use of sanitizers, staying away from sick and infected people, maintaining oral hygiene, avoiding raw fruits and vegetables, fruit juices, etc. This counselling should also be done for inpatients who are undergoing management of febrile neutro-penia. Patient presenting with fever during nadir period should be evaluated for febrile neutropenia. Complete blood count is done. *Febrile neutropenia* is defined as single oral temperature >38.3° Celsius (101° Fahrenheit) or 38° Celsius (100.4° Fahrenheit sustained over an hour) and absolute neutrophil counts less than 500 cells/mm³ or expected to decrease to <500 cells/mm³ during next 48 hours. If her counts are normal, other causes of fever should be evaluated. If she has grade IV neutropenia with fever, physical examination for catheters, skin lesions, examination of oropharynx, paranasal sinuses, perineal and genitourinary region, etc. should be carried out to look for focus of neutropenic sepsis. Investigations like complete blood count, liver and kidney function tests, coagulation profile, chest X-ray, blood, urine, sputum, stool cultures, culture from skin lesions, catheters, etc. should be done. Markers like procalcitonin and C-reactive protein (CRP) may have some utility to evaluate response during treatment. Risk scoring of febrile neutropenia can be done with Multinational Association for Supportive Care in Cancer (MASCC) Risk Index. Points from 0–20 are considered high risk, whereas 21–26 points are considered low risk. Empirical broad spectrum oral antibiotics active against *Pseudomonas aeruginosa* should be started after the blood culture sample is withdrawn. This can be either monotherapy or dual therapy if prolonged neutropenia or other high-risk features are there. The specific antibiotic may be started after the culture and sensitivity reports. One may follow the guidelines for management of febrile neutropenia. Low risk patients should be considered for early discharge with oral antibiotics. Patients not responding to broad spectrum antibiotics should be given gram positive cover and antifungals according to the guidelines.[4]

Case 3

A 53-year-old woman with carcinoma ovary has absolute neutrophil count of 1200/mm^3 without fever. She insists on getting admitted.

Q1. What should be your advice for her?

Afebrile neutropenia can be managed on OPD basis with proper counselling for neutropenic precautions and barrier nursing as mentioned above. There is not much role of therapeutic granulocyte colony stimulating factor (GCSF) in afebrile neutropenia. ASCO states that its use can be considered in high risk cases of febrile neutropenia.[5] Rampant chemoprophylaxis for afebrile neutropenia should be avoided to prevent development of resistant strains. Unnecessary hospital admission for such patients may increase chance of nosocomial infections and should be discouraged.

Case 4

A 45-year-old patient with carcinoma ovary has done extensive internet research about her chemotherapy and asks you to give GCSF with her chemotherapy.

Q1. How will you counsel her?

Primary prophylaxis of GCSF should be considered when the risk of neutropenia in the given chemotherapeutic agent is more than 20%. Other factors may be considered like age >65 years, previous chemotherapy or radiotherapy, pre-existing neutropenia, bone marrow infiltration by malignancy, poor performance status, no antibiotic prophylaxis, dose dense chemotherapy, standard dose with curative intent, etc.

Secondary prophylaxis with GSCF is considered when there is febrile neutropenia complication in previous cycle. It reduces the risk of febrile neutropenia by 50%. It also avoids treatment delay and chemotherapy dose reduction. But for chemotherapy with low risk of neutropenia and no other indications, routine use of GCSF should be discouraged.[5]

Case 5

A 54-year-old patient with endometrial cancer reciving chemotherapy develops oral mucositis.

Q1. How do you counsel and treat her?

Oral mucositis is a common complication of cancer chemotherapy. It begins 5–10 days after the initiation of chemotherapy and lasts for 7–14 days. Chemotherapy-induced oral mucositis causes the mucosal lining of the mouth to atrophy and break down, forming ulcers. Oral decontamination using antibacterial and antifungal rinses should be advised. Topical and systemic pain management, such as 2% viscous lidocaine, magic mouthwash preparations, and topical morphine solution may be considered. Prophylaxis, such as ice-chip cryotherapy or Palifermin (keratinocyte growth factor, FDA approved for mucositis prevention in hematopoietic cell transplantation) may also be considered.[6] Patients should be counselled for proper maintenance of oral hygiene as they are predisposed to neutropenia during chemotherapy and mucositis, if infected, may increase the risk of neutropenic sepsis. Neutropenic precautions and barrier nursing should be advised to every patient. Nutrition should also be taken care of as mucositis may lead to poor oral intake and in turn increase other complications.

Case 6

A 20-year-old patient with germ cell tumor of ovary is on BEP chemotherapy. She presents to the casualty with diarrhea, vomiting and generalised weakness. On blood investigations, she has deranged electrolytes.

Q1. How will you manage her?

Cisplatin is a highly emetogenic drug. Excessive vomiting and diarrhea can lead to loss of electrolytes and dyselectrolytemia. Severe deficiency of electrolytes can cause many complications. So it is important to prevent vomiting and maintain electrolyte balance. Antiemetics like 5HT3 antagonists, steroids and prokinetics are prescribed during and after chemotherapy to prevent chemotherapy related nausea and vomiting. Neurokinin 1 receptor and Substance P antagonists like aprepitant are used for patients receiving highly emetogenic chemotherapy regimens.[7] Once the patient develops excessive nausea and vomiting, care must be given to control vomiting and the electrolyte imbalance should be simultaneously corrected. Severe dyselectrolytemia should be corrected with the help of internal medicine or critical care specialist after admitting the patient.

Case 7

A 27-year-old woman with invasive mole on methotrexate develops derangement of liver enzymes. She is very apprehensive and asks your to stop chemotherapy and instead treat her with removal of uterus.

Q1. How do you counsel her?

The dose of methotrexate used for treatment of low risk invasive mole is low and does not cause severe complications like kidney or liver failure. Mild derangement of liver enzymes can happen which are self-restored or restored after ursodeoxycholic acid tablet administration.[8] Proper hydration and alternate day leucovorin rescue prevent development of such side effects. Radical cure of invasive mole is possible without aggressive surgical approach which is reserved for resistant case.

Case 8

A 70-year-old patient with carcinoma vulva is undergoing radiotherapy. She develops moist desquamation of skin in perineal region.

Q1. How will you manage her?

Radiation-induced dermatitis is a common complication of pelvic radiotherapy for gynecologic cancers. The severity of dermatitis is graded from grade I for hyperpigmentation and dry desquamation, grade II for moist erythema and desquamation, grade III for confluent moist desquamation and ulceration and grade IV for hemorrhage and necrosis. Grade I dermatitis does not need intervention and occurs in almost every patient. So they should be counselled not to be apprehensive about it. Grade II onwards, application of wet saline dressing can help in quick healing and relief from pain and burning sensation. Local topical antibiotics may be applied to prevent infection. Grade III and IV reactions may warrant withholding of radiation for some time until it starts healing. General skin care measures for patients undergoing radiation therapy include:

- Keeping the irradiated area clean and dry
- Washing with lukewarm water and mild soap (synthetic soaps are preferable)
- Using unscented, lanolin-free, water-based moisturizers
- Avoiding skin irritants such as perfumes and alcohol-based lotions
- Wearing loose-fitting clothes to avoid friction injuries
- Avoiding corn starch or baby powder in skin folds
- Avoiding sun exposure

Evidence from a limited number of randomized trials does not support the use of aloe vera, trolamine (triethanolamine), sucralfate, or hyaluronic acid for the prevention of radiation dermatitis. Topical steroids can be used to prevent severe radiation dermatitis and they also help in reducing discomfort and itching. Low- to medium-potency topical corticosteroids such as mometasone furoate 0.1% or hydrocortisone 1% cream can be applied to the treatment field once or twice daily, after each radiotherapy session. No cream should be applied before radiotherapy session as it may make a layer and produce bolus effect further increasing skin reactions.[9]

Case 9

A 57-year-old patient (weight 55 kg) has carcinoma cervix with hydroureteronephrosis. She comes to you with deranged creatinine of 1.5 mg/dL. She is due for her cisplatin injection.

Q1. How do you manage her?

Her creatinine clearance according to Cockcroft Gault equation is 35.9 mL/min. Cisplatin is not given when serum creatinine is above 1.5 mg/dL. The cause of deranged kidney function test is to be evaluated like dehydration, obstructive uropathy, medical renal disease, diabetic nephropathy, hypertensive nephropathy, etc. In case of carcinoma cervix with hydro-ureteronephrosis, the cause is generally obstructive uropathy. It may be addressed surgically with percutaneous nephrostomy (PCN).[10] Sometimes start of radiation itself may relieve mild obstruction and kidney functions can be restored. Multidisciplinary approach should be used to address obstructive uropathy. Injection cisplatin should be avoided in deranged kidney functions.

Case 10

A 47-year-old female patient of carcinoma of fallopian tube on chemotherapy presents to you with low platelet counts.

Q1. How will you manage her?

First of all, the complete blood counts with peripheral smear has to be done and thrombocytopenia should be graded. Uncomplicated grade 1 and 2 thrombocytopenia may not need active interruption accept withholding the treatment till the platelet counts become normal. For grade 1 or 2 thrombocytopenia, treatment is typically delayed for 1 or 2 weeks, but significant thrombocytopenia (<50,000/μL) may also require chemotherapy dose reductions. Platelet transfusions have been shown to be the most effective rapid treatment for patients with severe thrombocytopenia.[11] The American Society of Clinical Oncology recommends a platelet threshold of 10,000/μL for platelet transfusion among patients receiving chemotherapy for solid tumors. A higher threshold is recommended for patients with localised bleeding or necrotic tumors.[12] Single donor platelet transfusion is better than random donor platelet as it contains higher platelet concentration. Different thrombopoietic agents are being investigated like thrombopoietin, cytokines-IL-1, IL-3, IL-6, IL-11, etc. but only IL11 is approved by FDA for chemotherapy-induced thrombocytopenia (CIT).[11] *Carica papaya* leaf extract, a natural platelet booster has been shown to increase platelet counts in dengue hemorrhagic fever with low platelet counts and is also being investigated for CIT.[13]

REFERENCES

1. Radiation-Induced Enteritis: Incidence, Mechanisms, and Management | Cancer Network [Internet]. [cited 2018 Jul 23]. Available from: http://www.cancernetwork.com/palliative-and-supportive-care/radiation-induced-enteritis-incidence-mechanisms-and-management.

2. Stein A, Voigt W, Jordan K. Chemotherapy-induced diarrhea: pathophysiology, frequency and guideline-based management. Ther Adv Med Oncol 2010;2:51–63.

3. Barr W, Smith A. Acute Diarrhea in Adults. Am Fam Physician 2014;89:180–9.

4. de Naurois J, Novitzky-Basso I, Gill MJ, Marti FM, Cullen MH, Roila F. Management of febrile neutropenia: ESMO Clinical Practice Guidelines. Ann Oncol 2010; 21(suppl. 5):v252–6.

5. Smith TJ, Bohlke K, Lyman GH, Carson KR, Crawford J, Cross SJ, et al. Recommendations for the Use of WBC Growth Factors: American Society of Clinical Oncology Clinical Practice Guideline Update. J Clin Oncol 2015;33:3199–212.

6. Lalla RV, Bowen J, Barasch A, Elting L, Epstein J, Keefe DM, et al. MASCC/ISOO clinical practice guidelines for the management of mucositis secondary to cancer therapy: MASCC/ISOO Mucositis Guidelines. Cancer 2014;120:1453–61.

7. Sharma R, Tobin P, Clarke SJ. Management of chemotherapy-induced nausea, vomiting, oral mucositis, and diarrhoea. Lancet Oncol 2005; 6:93–102.

8. Saif MM, Farid SF, Khaleel SA, Sabry NA, El-Sayed MH. Hepatoprotective Efficacy of Ursodeoxycholic Acid in Pediatrics Acute Lymphoblastic Leukemia. Pediatr Hematol Oncol 2012; 29:627–32.

9. Wong RKS, Bensadoun R-J, Boers-Doets CB, Bryce J, Chan A, Epstein JB, et al. Clinical practice guidelines for the prevention and treatment of acute and late radiation reactions from the MASCC Skin Toxicity Study Group. Support Care Cancer 2013; 21:2933–48.

10. Dave PS, Patel BM, Patel H, Mankad MH. Obstructive Uropathy in Gynecologic Malignancy and Value of Percutaneous Nephrostomy. GCMC J Med Sci 2015;4:114-9.

11. Vadhan-Raj S. Management of chemotherapy-induced thrombocytopenia: current status of thrombopoietic agents. Semin Hematol 2009; 46 (Suppl 2):S26–32.

12. Schiffer CA, Bohlke K, Delaney M, Hume H, Magdalinski AJ, McCullough JJ, et al. Platelet Transfusion for Patients With Cancer: American Society of Clinical Oncology Clinical Practice Guideline Update. J Clin Oncol 2017;36:283–99.

13. Subenthiran S, Choon TC, Cheong KC, Thayan R, Teck MB, Muniandy PK, et al. *Carica papaya* Leaves Juice Significantly Accelerates the Rate of Increase in Platelet Count among Patients with Dengue Fever and Dengue Haemorrhagic Fever. Evid Based Complement Alternat Med 2013;2013: 616737.

Genetics of Gynecologic Cancers

Poonam Sachdeva, Amee Prapanna

Introduction

In the past two decades, cancer research has undergone dramatic changes following the identification of cellular oncogenes and subsequent recognition that cancer is largely a genetic disease. The basic genetics and pathogenesis of gynecological cancers like cervical, ovarian and endometrial cancers has been a topic of ongoing research. This has lead to the development of alternative therapeutic strategies for these cancers. This chapter throws light on the genetic framework of various gynecological cancers.

Q1. What are the characteristics of cancer cells?

There are several essential properties that cancer cells share like:

- Self sufficiency in growth signals
- Insensitivity to any antigrowth signals
- Apoptosis evasion
- Replicative potential that is limitless
- Sustained angiogenesis
- Tissue invasion and metastasis
- Development of any kind of genomic instability
- Growing independently of growth factor support
- Escape from any kind of anti-tumor immune responses

Combination of these properties that are normally under tight genetic control cause the development of malignancy. Cancer develops as a result of mutation of one or more genes in a cell. Under normal circumstances the body is usually able to cope up and correct these errors. However, if any error causes a defect in the ability of a cell to repair DNA damage then mutations can accumulate and the control of cell proliferation, apoptosis and cell to cell contact will be lost thus facilitating carcinogenesis.[1]

Q2. What is Knudson's hypothesis?

Knudson's hypothesis is the two-hit genetic model for hereditary and sporadic cancer development. In hereditary cancers, the first hit is present in the genome of every cell. Only one additional hit is necessary, therefore, to disrupt the correct function of the second cancer gene allele.[2]

In contrast sporadic cancers develop in cells without hereditary mutation in the cancer predisposing alleles. In this case both hits must occur in a single somatic cell to disrupt both cancer gene alleles.

Genetic mutations can be acquired or germline. Acquired mutations can occur from genetic damage that is gained during everyday life from exposure to any carcinogen such as the human papillomavirus (HPV), alcohol, tobacco, or ultraviolet radiation and are the commonest cause of cancer. Sporadic tumors occur because of acquired mutations. Of all cancers, around 5–10% are inherited, commonly in an autosomal dominant fashion. They generally arise because of highly penetrant genetic mutations. These mutations are commonly known as 'germline' and are the cause of 'cancer syndromes'. Of these over

200 have so far been described.[3] There is a multifactorial interaction between low penetrant genes and environmental factors in another 10–15% of cancers which are often referred to as 'familial'.

The study of cancer syndromes has improved the way these cancers are managed and has also improved our understanding of sporadic cancers.

Q3. What is hereditary cancer?

Cancers are mainly caused by spontaneous somatic mutations. A small percentage of cancers arise on a heritable genomic background. About 12% of ovarian and 5% of endometrial cancers are considered to be hereditary.[4]

Germ line mutations require additional mutations at one or more loci for tumorigenesis to occur. These mutations occur via different mechanisms for example, via environmental factors such as ionising radiation or mutations of stability genes. (Table 28.1)

Characteristics of hereditary cancer include:
- diagnosis at an early age
- family history of cancer, usually of a specific cancer syndrome, in two or more relatives.

Q4. What are the various cancer causing mechanisms?

The Fanconi anemia (FA)—BRCA pathway is the key to repair double stranded DNA breaks, through homologous recombinations (HR). When HR is deficient double stranded DNA breaks are repaired via non-homologous joining ends. This is a much more error prone mechanism. Biallelic mutations of the FA BRCA genes lead to the very rare autosomal recessive disorder, i.e. Fanconi anaemia which is characterized clinically by childhood

Table 28.1: Hereditary cancer syndromes		
Hereditary syndrome	*Gene mutation (gynecologic tumors)*	*Tumor phenotype*
Hereditary nonpolyposis colorectal cancer (HNPCC)/LYNCH syndrome	MLH1, MSH2, MSH3, MSH6, PMS2	Cancer of endometrium and ovary
Hereditary breast and ovarian cancer	BRCA1, BRCA2	Cancer of breast, ovary and fallopian tubes
Li-Fraumeni syndrome	TP53, CHEK2	Breast cancer
Cowden syndrome, Bannayan-Zonana syndrome	PTEN	Breast cancer, endometrial cancer
Multiple endocrine neoplasia Type I	Menin	Ovarian carcinoid
Multiple endocrine neoplasia Type II	RET	Ovarian carcinoid
Peutz-Jeghers syndrome	STK11	Ovarian sex cord tumor with annular tubules (SCTAT)

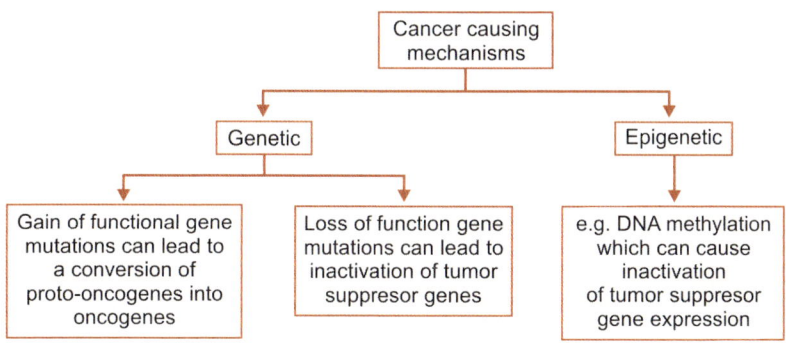

Fig. 28.1: Cancer causing mechanisms

aplastic anaemia increased risk of hematological and other malignancies.[5] The cause of hereditary breast and ovarian cancer are monoallelic mutations. The FA-BRCA pathway has been implicated in breast cancer with many of its genes displaying moderate penetrance in familial diseases. Until recently, most hereditary breast and ovarian cancers were attributed to BRCA 1 and BRCA 2 mutations with the other FA-BRCA genes being associated with breast cancer only. Now there is evidence of other HR repair genes specific to ovarian cancer as well.

Q5. What are cancer susceptibility genes?

Cancer susceptibility genes are divided into gatekeepers and caretaker genes. Gatekeeper genes control cellular proliferation and are divided into oncogenes and tumor suppressor genes. Gatekeepers prevent development of tumors by inhibiting growth or promoting cell death, e.g. p53 and retinoblastoma gene.[4]

Oncogenes stimulate cell growth and proliferation whereas tumor suppressor genes reduce the rate of cell proliferation or induce apoptosis.

Caretaker genes also preserve the integrity of genome and are involved in DNA repair as well (stability genes). The inactivation of caretaker genes increases the likelihood of persistent mutations in gatekeeper genes and other cancer related genes, e.g. DNA Mismatch repair genes like MLH1, MSH2 and MSH6[4] (Table 28.2).

Q6. What are genetic aberrations?

They are genomic alterations such as gene amplification, point mutations and deletions or rearrangements. They are identified in premalignant, malignant and benign neoplasms. (Table 28.3)

Q7. What are the factors that trigger neoplasia?

- Increased age
- Environmental factors
- Smoking
- Radiation
- Immune function
- Diet

CERVICAL CANCER

Q8. What is the etiopathology of cervical carcinogenesis?

Specific types of human papilloma viruses are the principal etiologic agents for both cervical

Table 28.2: Cancer susceptibility genes
Oncogenes
• Family of genes that result from gain of function mutations of their normal counterparts, proto-oncogenes.   • Proto-oncogenes stimulate proliferation in a controlled context. Activation of oncogenes can lead to stimulation of cell proliferation and development of a malignant phenotype.   • For example, ras genes- c-H(Harvey)-ras, c-K(Kirsten)-ras and N(Neuroblastoma)-ras
Tumor Suppresor Genes
• They are involved in development of most cancers.   • They are inactivated in a two step process in which both copies of tumor suppresor genes are mutated or inactivated by epigenetic mechanisms like methylation.   • For example, p53
Stability Genes
• The main function of stability genes is the preservation of correct DNA sequence during DNA replication (caretaker function).   • The inactivation of stability genes leads to a higher mutation rate in all genes. Mutations in oncogenes and tumor suppressor genes lead to cancer.   • Both alleles of stability genes must be inactivated to cause loss of function.   • For example, mismatch repair genes, nuclear-type excision repair genes, and base excision repair genes.

Table 28.3: Genetic aberrations

Amplification

- Amplification refers to an increase in copy number of a gene. Proto-oncogene amplification is a relatively common event in malignancies of female genital tract.
- E.g. HER2/neu proto-oncogene interacts with a variety of cellular proteins that increase cell proliferation. Overexpression of HER2/neu was demonstrated in about 30% of breast cancers, 20% of advanced ovarian cancers and 50% of endometrial cancers.
- High tissue expression of HER2/neu is associated with a decreased overall survival, especially in patients with endometrial cancer.

Point Mutations

- Point mutations cause a change in the codon sequence at the base pair level- it may or may not disrupt the function of a gene product.
- For example, ras gene family-oncogene encoded proteins that disrupt the intracellular signal transduction system following point mutations.
- The most common genetic mutation described in solid tumors is point mutation of p53 gene. {These mutations occur at preferential 'hotspots'. When DNA damage occurs p53 can arrest cell cycle progression to allow the DNA to be repaired or undergo apoptosis. The lack of normal p53 results in loss of control of cell proliferation with ineffecient DNA repair and genetic instability.} Mutations of p53 occur in 50% of advanced ovarian cancer and 30–40% of endometrial cancers but are uncoommon in cervical cancers.
- Point mutations in BRCA1 and BRCA2 genes can predispose to the development of breast and ovarian cancer. BRCA proteins are involved in DNA repair. If DNA is damaged, e.g. by ionising radiation or chemotherapy, the BRCA 2 protein binds to RAD51 which is central for the repair of double stranded breaks via homologous recombination and BRCA 1 mediates the repair by BRCA 1 associated surveillance complex (BASC).
- The prevalence of BRCA 1 and 2 mutation in general population in USA is 1:250. Specific founder mutation, e.g. two BRCA 1(185delAG and 5382insC) and one BRCA 2 mutation (6174delT) are found in 2.5% of Ashkenazi Jews of Central and Eastern European descent.

Deletions and Rearrangements

- They reflect gross changes in DNA template that may result in synthesis of markedly altered protein product.
- Commonly reported in leukemias, lymphomas and mesenchymal tumors.
- For example, Philadelphia chromosome in chronic myeloid leukemia is a result of reciprocal translocation between chromosome 9 and chromosome 22.

cancers and its precursors. HPV types 16, 18, 31, 35, 39, 45, 51, 56, 58 have high oncogenic risk. Types 16 and 18 are clinically most important. The high oncogenic risk HPV types produce two oncoproteins designated E-6 and E-7, which interact with endogenous cell cycle regulatory proteins, including p53 and Rb. The interaction of virally derived and endogenous cellular proteins converges in deregulation of cell cycle progression and appears to be critical for development of cervical cancer. Integration of HPV DNA into host genome also appears to play a role in tumor progression. Integration of HPV DNA frequently disrupts the E2 open reading frames, resulting in overexpression of

E6 and E7 oncoproteins and possibly causing genomic instability.[6]

However, because HPV infection is not sufficient for cervical carcinogenesis, attention has been focused on molecular cofactors important to this process. Various kinds of alterations in oncogenes and tumor suppressor genes may play a role in carcinogenesis of cervical cancer.

Q9. How does HPV cause cervical cancer?

HPV is a critical factor for oncogenesis as it produces two oncogenic proteins E6 and E7. E6 protein binds p53 resulting in loss of its tumor suppressor activity in cells. Normally, p53 induced G1 growth arrest presumably allows the cell to repair the damage to its DNA and to maintain genomic integrity.[6]

E7 protein binds to the retinoblastoma (Rb) protein. In normal cells not infected with a high-oncogenic risk HPV, the hypophosphory-lated forms of Rb protein forms complexes with transcription factors of the E2F family. These complexes negatively regulate the cell growth by repressing transcription of E2F-dependent genes. If the E2F-Rb complexes dissociate, free E2F becomes available. Free E2F stimulates the transcription of E2F dependent genes and allows DNA replication.[7]

In benign precursor lesions, viral DNA is maintained in a free, extrachromosomal, circular form termed as episome. In cervical cancer, the HPV genome is integrated into host genome.[8] Since there is a long latency between occurrence of HPV infection and development of cervical cancer, it is likely that other factors or intracellular alterations are involved in cervical carcinogenesis.

Q10. What are the genes involved in cervical cancer?

Tumor Suppressor Genes in Cervical Cancer

Loss of heterozygosity in invasive cervical cancers has been observed predominantly on chromosome 3, 5 and 11 and less frequently on chromosomes 1, 4, 6, 10,17, 18, and X. Specific chromosomal segments are lost during carcinogenesis, and these can be used to identify potential tumor suppressor gene. Data from several studies indicate the presence of several tumor suppressor genes on chromosome 3 (3p13-21.3) and chromosome 5 and 11 at 5 pp 15.1-15.2 and 11q22-24.[9–12]

In general, more than 90% of squamous cell cervical cancers contain HPV DNA, and p53

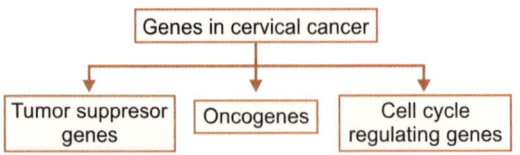

mutations are rarely seen. p53 mutations appear to be more common in HPV-negative cancers , although HPV-negative cancers that do not contain p53 mutations exist. This suggests that loss of function of p53 or Rb by binding with E6 and E7 protein is the key mechanism in cervical carcinogenesis. Studies have shown that HPV negative tumors have a worse prognosis.[13]

Oncogenes in Cervical Cancer

Rearrangements, amplifications or over-expression of c-myc proto-oncogene are found in cervical cancers. c-myc amplification is related to early relapse and is superior as a prognostic factor for nodal status. Over-expression of c-erbB2 is associated with poor prognosis and when there is increased expression of Ha-ras there is resistance to radiation.[14]

Alterations in other Cell Cycle Regulating Genes

Bcl-1 (cyclin D1) is capable of binding to Rb protein, and is over expressed and amplified in the majority of cervical cancer cell lines. Bcl-2 overexpression was not found to relate to HPV status and was more likely to be seen in CIN 3 rather than low grade dysplasias; thus, its expression may be an early event in malignant transformation.[15]

OVARIAN CANCER

Q11. What are the tumor suppressor genes in ovarian cancer?

Many studies of loss of heterozygosity in ovarian cancer have found a high frequency of allelic deletion (>33%) for seven chromosome arms—6p, 6q, 13q,17p, 17q, 18q and Xp. Among them the most important allelic loss area in ovarian cancer is p53 locus of 17p. p53 mutation has been reported in epithelial ovarian cancer and borderline ovarian tumors.[16]

Functional wild-type p53 has been shown to be required for sensitivity to a variety of chemotherapeutic drugs and radiation, playing a crucial role in the pathway of apoptosis. p53 mutation of one allele predisposes the cell to the loss of wild-type p53 function, which has been shown in ovarian cancer cells to lead to the development of cisplatin resistance.

Nearly 90% of the ovarian cancers that express p53 mutations. In ovarian cancers the overexpressed or mutant p53, which is seen in 50% of advanced cases, is associated with high grade and poor survival, but not with clinical chemoresponsiveness.[17]

The important role of p53 in regulation of cellular proliferation has led to speculation that gene therapy, designed to reintroduce wild type p53 genes into cancer cells that have mutant p53 genes, might be successful in suppressing tumor growth.[18]

Role of BRCA1 and BRCA2: Mutations of BRCA1 and BRCA2 can account for many of the familial cases of breast-ovarian cancer syndrome and site-specific ovarian cancers, but not for the sporadic ovarian cancers. In sporadic ovarian cancers frequent allelic losses that included the BRCA1 region of chromosome 17q were demonstrated.[19]

Vandamme, et al. have identified two deletion units in the region 11p13 and 11p15.5.[20] These regions correspond to the location of WT-1 and WT-2 genes, raising the possibility that the same genes could be involved in ovarian carcinogenesis. In chromosome 6, allelic losses were found on both p and q arms. Especially 6q 24–27 has been reported to have frequent loss of heterozygosity at the estrogen receptor gene locus which has been strongly suggested as one of the putative tumor suppressor gene.[21]

Q12. What are the various oncogenes involved in ovarian cancer?

Amplification of c-myc proto-oncogene has been reported in approximately one-third of advanced stage epithelial ovarian neoplasms.[22] This gene encodes a DNA binding protein that is exhibited in increased amounts in dividing cells and has a role in cellular proliferation.

The c-fms proto-oncogene encodes the receptor for colony stimulation factor (CSF) and has a role in autocrine and paracrine secretion of Interleukin 1 (IL1), IL6 and tumor necrosis factor (TNF) during ovarian carcinogenesis. CSF is elevated in 70% of ovarian cancer patients.[23]

The c-erbB protooncogene encodes the transmembrane receptor for epidermal growth factor (EGF). The EGF receptor is expressed by most advanced stage ovarian cancers and EGFR positive tumors have worse prognosis than EGFR negative tumors.[24]

The HER-2/neu or erbB2 oncogene is related to erbB oncogene and its over-expression was found in 30% of ovarian cancers and was associated with poor prognosis.[25]

The Ha-ras gene over expression or mutation results in alteration in cell growth leading to ovarian cancer. The Ki-rasgene mutations are reported in 30% of ovarian cancer patients and significantly high in mucinous adenoma of ovary.[26]

Q13. What are the molecules involved in adhesion and invasion?

Metastasis is the most life threatening aspect of cancer. The loss of normal adhesive functions and gain of new adhesive functions are crucial in this metastatic cascade.

The cell adhesion molecule CD44 is expressed when ovarian cancer cells are attached to peritoneal mesothelium but such expression is lost when the cells are found in ascitic fluid. Overexpression of CD44R1 variant increases the potency of metastasis and is associated with poor prognosis.[27]

ENDOMETRIAL CANCER

Q14. What causes endometrial cancer?

Endometrial cancer is a hormone dependent tumor. Aromatase cytochrome p450 is part of complex mechanism responsible for conversion of C19 steroids to estrogen. Its expression is increased in endometrial cancers. There is also overexpression of c-myc gene and p53, the latter is associated with poor prognosis.

Q15. What are the tumor suppressor genes in endometrial cancer?

In endometrial cancers most chromosomes contain regions of sustained allelic loss.[28] Chromosome 17p contains the p53 gene which when mutated or deleted plays an important role in transition to carcinoma from atypical hyperplasia.

Q16. What are the oncogenes in endometrial cancer?

Ki-ras point mutations have a role in development of atypical endometrial hyperplasias and endometrial carcinomas. The Ki-ras mutation may be an early oncogenic event in endometrial cancer.[29]

Over-expression of HER-2/neu was associated with advanced stage, deep myometrial invasion and poor survival in endometrial cancers.

Recently, another new chromosomal region which has putative tumor suppressor gene for endometrial cancer has been identified in chromosome 10q25-26.

CLINICAL IMPLICATION

Q17. What is the clinical impact of knowing the molecular biology of cancer?

Two decades ago, cancer research was dramatically changed by identification of cellular oncogenes and subsequent recognition that cancer is largely a genetic disease. This advance shifted the focus from carcinogenesis and mutagens to oncogenes and tumor suppressor genes. This has lead to development of alternative therapeutic strategies for cancer treatment including gene therapy. Gene Therapy (also called human gene transfer) is the therapeutic delivery of nucleic acid into patient's cells as a drug to treat the disease.[30] Gene therapy uses virus as vectors to insert new gene into the genome of a cell and the new gene makes a functional protein to treat that disease.

Prognosis of a cancer can be given and the risk of developing cancer can also be calculated with the help of molecular biology.

This has lead to early screening and identification of cancer in high risk population.

 Key Points

- Cancer develops when one or more genes in a cell are mutated and the DNA repair mechanism fails to correct the damage.
- Hereditary cancers are specific cancer syndromes that run in families and present at earlier age.
- There are various cancer susceptibility genes like oncogenes, tumor suppressor genes and stability genes, genetic aberration of which leads to cancers.
- Main cause of cervical cancer is HPV virus (type 16,18) which affects p53 and Rb gene through E6 and E7 proteins and incorporation of viral DNA in host genome.
- In ovarian cancer, most important allelic loss area is p53 locus of 17p. p53 mutation has been reported in epithelial ovarian cancer and borderline ovarian tumors. Mutations of BRCA1 and BRCA2 can account for many of the familial cases of breast-ovarian cancer syndrome and site-specific ovarian cancers, but not for the sporadic ovarian cancers.
- Mutations in p53, Ki-ras and over-expression of HER-2/neu and of Aromatase cytochrome p450 is seen in many endometrial cancer.
- Better understanding of genetics of gynecological cancers has led to development of gene therapy for treatment of cancer, screening, prognosis and better calculation of risk of developing cancer.

REFERENCES

1. Negrini S, Gorgoulis VG, Halazonetis TD. Genomic instability-an evolving hallmark of cancer. Nat Rev Mol Cell Biol 2010;11:220–8.
2. Knudson AG Jr. Mutation and cancer: statistical study of retinoblastoma. ProcNatlAcadSci U S A. 1971;68:820–3.
3. Nagy R, Sweet K, Eng C. Highly penetrant hereditary cancer syndromes. Oncogene 2004; 23:6445–70.
4. Berek and Novak's Gynecology. 15th Edition; Lippincott Williams and Wilkins, 2012.
5. Taniguchi T, D' Andrea AD. Molecular pathogenesis of Fanconianemia : recent progress. Blood 2006;107:4223–33.
6. Vogelstein B, KinzlerK. The multistep nature of cancer. Trends Genet 1993;9:138–41.

7. ChellappanS, KraousVB, Kroger B, Munger K, HowleyPM, Phelps WC, et al. Adenovirus ElA, simianvirus 40 tumor antigen, and human papilloma virus E7 protein share the capacity to disrupt the interaction between the transcription factorE2F and the retinoblastoma gene product. Proc Natl AcadSci USA 1992;89:4549–53.

8. Cullen AP, Reid R, Campion M, LorinczAT. Analysis of the physical state of different human papilloma virus DNAs in intraepithelial and invasive cervical neoplasia. J Virol 1991;65:606-12.

9. Jones MH, Nakamura YH. Deletion mapping of chromosome 3p in female genital tract malignancies using micro satellite polymorphisms. Oncogene 1992;7:1631–4.

10. Kohno T, TakayamaH, Hamaguchi M, Takano H, Yamaguchi N, TsudaH. Deletion mapping on chromosome 3p in human uterine and cervical cancer. Oncogene 1993;8:1825–32.

11. Mitra AB, MurtyVV, PratapM, LuthraUK. Allelotypeanalysis of cervical carcinoma. Cancer Res 1994;54:4481–7.

12. Hampton GM, Penny LA, Baergen RN, Larson A, Brewer C, Liao S et al. Loss of heterozygosity in cervical carcinoma: subchromosomal localization of a putative tumoro suppressor gene to chromosome llq22-q24. Proc Natl AcadSci USA 1994; 91:6953–7.

13. IkenbergH, SauerbreiW, Schottmuller U, Spitz C, PfleidererA. Human papilloma virus DNA in cervical carcinoma. Correlation with clinical data and influence on prognosis. Int J Cancer 1994; 59:322–6.

14. Bourhis J, Le MG, BarroisM, GerbauletA, Jeanne D, Duvillard P, et al. Prognostic value of c-myc proto-oncogene overexpression of NIH3T3 cells to ionizing radiation. Science 1988;239:645–7.

15. SaegusaM, Takano Y, HashimuraM, Shoji Y, OkayasuI. The possible role of bcl-2 expression in the progression of tumors of the uterine cervix. Cancer 1995;76:2297–303.

16. Berchuck A, Kohler MF, Marks JR, Wiseman R, Boyd J, BastRC. Thep 53 tumor suppressor gene frequently is altered in gynecologiccancers. AmJ Obstet Gynecol 1994;170:246–52.

17. Brown R, Clugston C, Burns P, EdlinA, Vasey P, VojtesekB, et al. Increased accumulation of p53 protein in cisplatin-resistant ovarian cell lines. IntJ Cancer 1993;55:678–84.

18. Fujiwara T, Grimm EA, MukhopadhyayT, CaiDW, SchaubLB, Roth JA. Cancer Res 1993;53: 4129–33.

19. Takahashi H, BehbakhtK, McGovern PE, Chiu HC, Couch FJ, Weber BL. Mutation analysis of the BRCAIgene in ovarian cancers. A retroviral wild-type p53 expression vector penetrates human lung cancer spheroids and inhibits growth by inducing apoptosis. Cancer Res. 1993;53:4129–33.

20. Vandamme B, Lissens W, AmfoK, DeSutterP, BourgainC, VamosE et al. Deletion of chromosome llp13-ll p15.5 sequences in invasive human ovarian cancer is a subclonal progression factor. Cancer Res 1992;52:6646–52.

21. Foulkes WD, Ragoussis J, Stamp GW, Allan GJ, TrowsdaleJ. Frequent loss of heterozygosity on chromosome 6 in human ovarian carcinoma. Br J Cancer 1993;67:551–9.

22. Sasano H, NaguraH, Silverberg SG. Immunolocalization of c-mycconcoprotein in mucinous and serous adenocarcinomas of the ovary. Human Pathol 1992;23:491–5.

23. Chow SN, ChienCH, Chen CT. Molecular biology of human ovarian cancer. Int Surg 1996;81:152-7.

24. ScambiaG, CatozziL, Panici PB, FerrandinaG, CoronettaF, BarozziR, et al. Expression of ras oncogene p21 protein in normal and neoplastic ovarian tissues: Correlation with histopathologic features and receptors for estrogen, progesterone, and epidermal growth factor. AmJ Obstet Gynecol 1993;168:71–8.

25. BerchuckA, KamelA, Whitaker R. etal. Overexpression of HER-2/neuis associated with poor survival in advanced epithelial ovarian cancer. Cancer Res 1990;50:4087–91.

26. McGrath J, Capon D, GoeddeD, Levinson A. Comparative biochemical properties of normal and activated human rasp21 protein. Nature 1984; 310:644–55

27. Naor D, Sionov RV, Ish-Shalom D. CD44: structure, function, and association with the malignant process. Adv Cancer Res. 1997;71:241–319.

28. Fujino T, Risinger JI, Collins NK, Liu FS, Nishii H, Takahashi H, et al. Allelotype of endometrial carcinoma. Cancer Res 1994;54:4294–8.

29. Jeyarajah A, Oram D, Jacobs I. Molecular events in endometrial carcinogenesis. Int J Gynecol Cancer 1996;6:425–38.

30. Kaji EH, Leiden JM. Gene and Stem Cell Therapies. JAMA 2001;285:545–50.

Prevention of Gynecologic Cancers

Niharika Dhiman, Swati Rai

Gynecologic cancers have a major impact on women's health and affect their quality of life. There are various methods that can prevent Gynecologic cancers, however, these are often not implemented due to lack of awareness and resources.

The various levels of prevention are described in Table 29.1.

CERVICAL CANCER

Cervical cancer is one of the most common cancers among Indian women. Globally 5, 28, 000 new cases are diagnosed every year and 2, 66, 000 deaths occur. 83% of these cases burden the developing countries among which the highest incidence rates are in Latin America,

Table 29.1: Levels of prevention	
Primordial	**Defined as prevention of emergence/development of risk factors before they have appeared** Purest form of prevention Target population—general population. Approach—individual and mass education.
Primary	**Defined as intervention taken prior to the onset of disease.** Risk factors are present in population. It acts in pre-pathogenesis phase of disease. Target population—susceptible individuals. Goal: To prevent the disease by reducing the risk factors. WHO has recommended the following strategies: – Population/mass strategy – High risk strategy Example: life style modification, medication.
Secondary	**Defined as intervention that arrest the progress of disease at an early stage and thereby prevent complication.** Risk factors are present. Disease process has started. Target population—asymptomatic. Goal: To arrest the disease process at an early stage Intervention: Early diagnosis /screening tests Health programs started by government act at this level
Tertiary	**Defined as intervention at the stage when the disease process has started and advanced beyond early stages.** Target population—symptomatic individuals It is done in late pathogenesis phase Intervention: Disability limitation and rehabilitation

sub-Saharan Africa and South East Asia accounting for 15% of all cancers.[1]

The rate of cervical cancer varies widely and is inversely proportional to effectiveness and implementation of prevention programs. In developed countries due to extensive screening programs cervical cancer has become a relatively uncommon disease.

I. Primary Prevention

The goal is to prevent the disease by reducing the modifiable risk factors. (Table 29.2)

It has been now proven, that there is a strong causal association between human papilloma virus (HPV) infection of cervix and cervical cancer. This offers a unique opportunity for prevention of cancer at primary level by intervening in the natural history of the disease.

i. **Education:** It plays an important role in prevention in prevention by spreading awareness, promoting safe sexual practices and imparting knowledge regarding the screening methods available for cervical cancer. Barrier method (male condom) when used 100% of the time reduce the risk of HPV infection to 70% as compared to women whose partner used it less than 5% of the time.

Table 29.2: Risk factors for cervical cancer

Modifiable	Non-modifiable
Low socioeconomic status	Genetic predisposition
Low education level	Older age
Early age at first coitus	Racial factors
Early age at first pregnancy	
Multiple sexual partners	
Multiparity	
Long term use of oral contraceptives	
History of sexually transmitted infections	
History of genital warts	
Cigarette smoking	
Immunosuppression	
HIV infection	
Lack of routine cytological screening	
Diet low in folates, carotene, vitamin C	

ii. **HPV vaccination:** It has been proven now that HPV infection precedes the development of cervical cancer by a number of decades and persistent HPV infection is necessary for the development and progression of precancerous lesions of cervix to a higher grade or even frank malignancy. The lifetime risk of acquiring a genital HPV infection is nearly 80% and the probability of transmission per active intercourse is 40%.[3]

In a study by Munoz et al[3] pooled data from 11 case control studies involving 1918 women with histologically confirmed squamous cell carcinoma found that 15 HPV types were classified as high risk types (16, 18, 31, 33, 39, 45, 51, 52, 56, 58, 59, 68, 73 and 82) and considered carcinogenic. A meta-analysis confirmed high prevalence of HPV in cervical cancers worldwide with HPV 16 (51%) and HPV 18 (16.2%) being most common. HPV 16 type was more prevalent in squamous cell carcinomas and HPV 18 type more prevalent in adenocarcinoma.

Papilloma viruses are double-stranded DNA viruses that infect squamous or mucosal epithelia. They consist of non-enveloped capsid containing major structural protein L1 and minor structural protein L2. In episomal state in host cell, the HPV genome expresses proteins coded by E1, E2, E6 and E7 regions. During infection HPV remains in episomal state but in cancer it integrates with host genome leading to upregulation of E6 and E7 genes and their proteins. These oncoproteins cause oncogenic transformation of infected cells. Many animal and human studies of papilloma virus infection have provided good evidence that neutralizing antibodies to viral capsid proteins L1 and L2 can block new infections with HPV. This forms the basis for prophylactic vaccines, in which empty viral capsids called VLPs (virus like particles) are synthesized from microbial and cellular expression systems.[4]

Two HPV vaccines are currently in market: Cervarix and Gardasil. Both are FDA approved not requiring a booster dose. The protection against HPV 16 and 18 post vaccination have lasted for 5 years with Gardasil and more than 6 years with Cervarix (Table 29. 3).[5]

According to Indian Academy of Pediatrics Advisory Committee on Vaccines and Immunization the dosage schedule is:[6]

Routine vaccination
- Minimum age: 9 years
- 9–14 years: 2 doses 6 months apart (0, 6)
- >15 years and immunocompromised individuals: 3 dose schedule
- Dose: 0.5 mL intramuscular either in deltoid muscle/anterolateral thigh.

Catch-up vaccination
- Administer the vaccine series to girls and women at age 13 through 45 years if not previously vaccinated.
- Either HPV2/4 .

Side effects: The most common adverse effects are local reactions like pain in 83%, swelling with erythema in 25% and fever in 4%. No serious vaccine related adverse effect has been reported till date. It is contraindicated in people with a history of immediate hypersensitivity to yeast or any other vaccine component. The vaccine should be administered in sitting or lying down position and the person should be observed for 15 minutes post vaccination for syncope. The vaccine is contraindicated during pregnancy (category B) but can be given during lactation or after MTP.[5]

Efficacy: Phase III trials of HPV vaccines were used to demonstrate efficacy in preventing incident vaccine-related HPV infection and the pre-neoplastic lesions caused by it. The Future I and Future II trials, evaluated HPV4, and PATRICIA and the COSTA RICA HPV vaccine trial evaluated HPV2. The efficacy was 95% (HPV4) and 100%(HPV2) respectively. As per the data available, the results of the modeling predict that anti-HPV 16 and anti-HPV 18 antibody levels will gradually decrease, but will remain several folds higher as compared with natural infection for at least 20 years postvaccination.[7–10]

II. Secondary Prevention

The core of secondary prevention is screening tests. These are simple, rapidly applied tests to detect unrecognized disease among apparently healthy individuals. They diagnose precancerous lesions at early stages. Methods for screening precancerous disease:
- DVI (direct visual inspection)
- VIA (visual inspection after application of acetic acid)
- VILI (visual inspection after application of Lugol's iodine)
- Cytology based:
  a. Conventional
  b. Liquid based—Thin Prep (Hologic), Sure Path(BD), QIA sure Methylation Test

Table 29.3: Types of HPV vaccines		
Name	*Gardasil*	*Cervarix*
Manufacture	Merck and Co.	Glaxo Smith Kline
Age group	9–26 years	9–26 years
Type	Recombinant vaccination	Recombinant vaccination
Also known as	HPV4, qHPV	HPV2, bHPV
Protection against	HPV6,11,16,18 (Quadrivalent)	HPV 16, 18 (Bivalent)
VLP dose	L1 dose 20/40/40/20 µg	L1 dose 20/20 µg
Adjuvant	225 µg aluminum hydroxyphosphate sulfate (ASO4)	500 µg aluminum hydroxide, 50 µg 3-O-deacylated-4-monophosphoryl lipid A (MPLA) Alum
Produced in	Saccharomyces cerevisiae (baker's yeast) expressing L1	Trichoplusiani (Hi 5) insect cell line infected with L1 recombinant baculovirus 0, 1, 6 months
3 dose schedule	0, 2, 6 months	

(Qiagen) Topoisomerase IIA (TOP2A) and MCM2 (BD)

- HPV DNA testing
- Speculoscopy
- Polar probes
- Colposcopy
- Cervicography
- Microcolpohysteroscopy
- CARE HPV—latest test for developing countries, result is available within 2.5 hours.
- Newer development—biomarkers used as surrogate markers for cervical dysplasia- E6/7m RNA, L1 capsid protein, Ki-67, p16INK4a :CINtec (Roche), CINtec PLUS (p16INK4a + Ki-67)

III. Tertiary Prevention

The WHO guidelines for screening and treatment of precancerous lesions for cervical cancer (2013) recommend **"screen-and-treat"** strategies according to the resources available (Table 29.4).[11]

Screening tests recommendations: HPV (cutoff level ≥1.0 pg/mL), cytology (cut-off level ASCUS+, atypical squamous cells of undetermined significance), and VIA.

Screen-and-treat recommendations: Cryotherapy is the first-choice for treatment provided entire transformation zone (TZ) and lesion is visible, the lesion does not cover >75% of the ectocervix and is not extending into the endocervical canal. If the patient is not eligible for cryotherapy then Loop electrosurgical excision procedure (LEEP) is the alternative option.[11]

Case 1

A 28-year-old lady who has been sexually active for 3 years was diagnosed as HIV positive and was referred from ART clinic for cervical cancer screening.

Q1. What would you do for her?

Follow the **"Screen and treat"** approach

Screen her with HPV testing/cytology. If test is negative rescreen every 2–3 years. HPV vaccination 3 doses after counseling her regarding the reduced efficacy in this age group.

If testing is positive perform VIA to rule out any large lesion or suspected cancer and to assess for eligibility for cryotherapy.

Treat by using cryotherapy, if not eligible for cryotherapy treat with LLETZ. Perform posttreatment screening at one year to ensure effectiveness of treatment.

Case 2

A 48-year-old lady presents to the gynecology outpatient clinic for a routine check-up following an abdominal hysterectomy done in another hospital 2 years back.

Q1. Does she require screening for cervical cancer?

Take appropriate history to know the indication for hysterectomy, whether done for benign

Type of resource setting	Screening method	Age to start screening	Interval of screening	Treatment method	Single visit treatment approach
Good resource setting	HPV testing (preferred) Co-testing (HPV+ Cytology) or Cytology or VIA	Cytology-25 years HPV-30 years	Cytology-3 years Co-testing/ HPV-5 years	LEEP Cryotherapy Conization Thermal coagulation	See and Treat
Restricted resource setting	VIA	30 years	3 years	Cryotherapy LEEP Conization Thermal coagulation	Screen and treat or See, screen and treat

Table 29.4: Treatment approach according to the resource settings[11]

or malignant condition, type of hysterectomy (total or subtotal) and ask for documents of the surgery. Examine her to see for presence or absence of cervix.

- If total hysterectomy was done for a benign condition she does not require any further screening.
- If previous history or records of CIN— screen with HPV at 6 and 18 months.
- If history or records are inconclusive— screening is at the discretion of the treating clinician.

ENDOMETRIAL CANCER

Endometrial cancer (EC) is the most common gynecologic cancer in developed countries. There are two distinct histological types of endometrial cancer—Type I/endometroid (estrogen dependent) and Type II/non-endometroid (non-estrogen dependent). Most of the preventive and proposed screening methods help in detecting Type I endometrial carcinoma.

I. Primary Prevention

In the year 2015 in USA alone, 50,000 new cases of endometrial carcinoma and >10,000 related deaths were reported. The various risk factors associated with endometrial carcinoma are enlisted in Table 29.5.[12]

A. Lifestyle modification

i. *Obesity and physical activity:* Obese women have 2.4 to 4.5 times risk of being diagnosed with EC as compared to normal weight women.[13]

ii. *Exercise:* In a large prospective cohort study, the women who did high intensity exercise had a 35% reduced risk of EC as compared to those who do not perform any vigorous activity.[13] Daily walking or physical activity in otherwise sedentary women also reduces the risk.[13]

iii. *Diet:* In Women's Health Initiative study done on 84000 postmenopausal women who were randomized to a low fat diet rich in fruits, vegetables and grains showed no difference after an average follow up of 8 years.[14] Increased glycemic load in the diet increases the risk of EC.

iv. *Coffee, tea, alcohol and other beverages:* A meta-analysis of 13 cohort studies found a dose response relationship and an overall reduced risk of EC with coffee consumption (RR=0.80). Similar reductions have been noted with consumption of green tea. A meta-analysis of six cohort and 14 case control studies found no association of alcohol with EC.[15]

v. *Smoking:* Decreases the risk of EC probably due to anti-estrogenic effect, but due to known side effects of smoking it cannot be recommended. In a meta-analysis of ten cohort studies, the risk was reduced by 19%.

B. Surgical prevention

A meta-analysis of three cohort studies reported a reduction of 60% in risk of EC after bariatric surgery compared to obese controls who did not have surgery (RR = 0.4).

Table 29.5: Risk factors associated with endometrial cancer	
Modifiable (relative risk)	*Non-modifiable (relative risk)*
Long-term use of unopposed estrogen therapy (4–8)	Early menarche <12 years (3)
Tamoxifen therapy (2–3)	Late menopause >52 years (2–3)
Obesity	Atypical endometrial hyperplasia (8–29)
• BMI 30–34 kg/m^2–1.7	
• BMI 35–39 kg/m^2–4.3	
• BMI >40 kg/m^2–6.4	
Nulliparity (3)	HNPCC syndrome (20)
Diabetes, hypertension, thyroid and gallstone disease (3)	Polycystic ovarian disease

C. Chemoprevention

i. *Oral contraceptive pills:* Progestin containing contraceptive pill have anti-estrogen effect on the endometrium and decrease the EC risk. A meta-analysis of 36 case-control studies showed a 31% risk reduction in women who had ever used OCPs compared to non-users (RR = 0.69; 99% CI 0.66–0.73).[16] The effect persisted for 30 years even after cessation of use.

ii. *Other contraceptives:* One large case-control study found that injectable progestin (DMPA) is protective against EC with effects lasting up to 8 years (RR = 0.21, 95% CI 0.06–0.79)[17]. For MIRENA, a pooled analysis of four cohort and 14 case-control studies found a 31% reduction rate, with stronger effects with longer use.[18]

iii. *Hormone replacement therapy (HRT):* There is strong evidence that estrogen-only HRT increases the risk of EC in women with an intact uterus whereas, combined usage with progestin reduces the risk.

iv. *Other chemo protection:* A meta-analysis of nine case-control studies of non-steroidal anti-inflammatory drugs (NSAID) usage in obese women found reduction in risk (RR = 0.72).[19] Oral hypoglycemic agents like metformin have anti-proliferative effect on hyperplastic and cancerous endometrium in vitro. However, the results are conflicting and inconclusive.

v. *Breast-feeding:* A recent meta-analysis found that breast-feeding reduces the risk of EC by 33%. For each one month duration of breast feeding, risk of EC was reduced by 2%.

III. Secondary Prevention

Universal screening of asymptomatic/low risk women by endometrial sampling or by any blood or radiological tests is not recommended and none of the methods have been found to be sufficiently sensitive or specific. However, screening is justified in high risk women (postmenopausal on exogenous estrogen therapy without progestin, family history of HNPCC and premenopausal women with anovulatory cycles, e.g. polycystic ovarian disease). In menopausal and premenopausal women a cutoff of 3 mm for endometrial thickness on transvaginal sonography requires endometrial sampling.

Case 3

A 26-year-old lady has a family history of colorectal cancer in her mother which was diagnosed at 48 years of age and endometrial cancer in her sister diagnosed at 35 years of age. She presents to the gynecology outpatient clinic seeking advice for her risk of developing the cancers.

Q1. How will you counsel and screen her?

The family history is suggestive of Lynch syndrome (HNPPC) in her first-degree relatives. Prepare a pedigree chart. Counsel her regarding the benefits and drawbacks of genetic testing.

Surveillance for cancer

- Endometrial—annual screening with transvaginal sonography (TVS)/endometrial cytology; prompt evaluation in case of abnormal uterine bleeding.
- Ovarian—Ca-125 annually
- Colon—colonoscopy every 1–2 years

A prophylactic hysterectomy with salpingectomy can be offered once family is complete.

OVARIAN CANCER

I. Primary Prevention

A. Life style modification

i. *Weight loss and physical activity:* A meta-analysis of 47 studies reported a 12% increased risk of epithelial ovarian cancer (EOC) for obese women (BMI >30kg/m^2).[20]

ii. *Diet:* Two meta-analysis of cohort and case-control studies reported 11–16% risk reduction with daily vegetable consumption.[21]

iii. *Coffee, tea, alcohol and other beverages:* Unproven benefit in EOC.

iv. *Smoking:* A meta-analysis of 51 studies found an increased risk of mucinous EOC (RR =1.79), with a dose response relationship, hence, smoking cessation should be recommended for all women.[22]

v. *Breast-feeding:* A meta-analysis of five cohort studies reported a 24% reduction in EOC risk.[23]

B. Surgical prevention

In most recent meta-analysis it was found that tubal ligation decreased the risk of EOC by up to 30%. The Society for Gynecologic Oncology recommends salpingectomy after childbearing is complete during elective pelvic surgeries.[24] Those at high genetic risk (BRCA-1 carrier, HNPCC) are advised to undergo to undergo bilateral salpingo-oophorectomy at age 35 or after completion of child bearing, that decreases their risk of EOC by 80%.

C. Chemoprevention

Only oral contraceptive pill among all the contraceptives plays a protective role in EOC. In a large meta-analysis 27% risk reduction in EOC was found and the benefit persisted for 30 years after use.

II. Secondary Prevention

There is no established role of screening with TVS, Ca-125 or any other modality in early detection of ovarian cancer in low risk population. The role of proteomic patterns by using surface-enhanced laser desorption ionization time-of-flight (SELDI-TOF) and the measurement of plasma DNA levels and allelic imbalance by digital single nucleotide polymorphism (SNP) analysis is still under evaluation.

Case 4

A 25-year-old lady married for 2 years, whose elder sister has been diagnosed with breast carcinoma at 32 years of age and tested positive for BRCA mutation, seeks your advice regarding genetic testing and her chances of having affected children.

Q1.   What would you advise her?

This is a case of hereditary breast and/or ovarian cancer syndrome (HBOS) in the first-degree relative hence the criterion for genetic testing is met. Full pedigree analysis is done. A pre-test and post-test counseling is to be done. If found positive for BRCA mutation management has to be done as follows:

- Self-breast examination —monthly
- Clinical breast examination—six monthly
- Breast mammography/MRI—annually
- TVS and CA-125—six monthly
- Reproductive concerns—advise about prenatal diagnosis using preimplantation genetic testing (PGD) and artificial reproductive techniques with discussion about their benefits, risks and limitations.
- Option of risk reducing bilateral mastectomy can be offered.
- After completion of child bearing, risk reducing salpingiooprectomy at 35–40 years can be offered.

VAGINAL AND VULVAL CANCER

The relationship between the malignancies of cervix, vagina and vulva and HPV infection has long been established. Hence, vaccination against HPV plays preventive role for these cancers also. Various measures should be implemented for reducing the risk of STI. Quitting cigarette plays a protective role against both vaginal and vulval cancer.

Key Points

- Most of the risk factors associated with gynecological malignancies can be modified by following simple lifestyle changes.
- Routine screening and HPV vaccination can significantly bring down the incidence of cervical cancer.
- The approach to screening for cervical cancer has to be done according to the resources available.
- There is still no effective screening method available for early detection of endometrial and ovarian malignancy.

REFERENCES

1. Frisch M. Human Papillomavirus associated cancers in patients with HIV and AIDS. J Natl Cancer Inst 2000;92:1500–10.

2. Walboomers JM, Jacobs MV, Manos MM,Bosch FX, Kummer JA, Shah KV, et al. Human papilloma virus is necessary cause of invasive cervical cancer worldwide. J Pathol 1999;189:12–19.

3. Munoz N, Bosch FX, de Sanjose S, Herrero R, Castellsagué X, Shah KV et al. Epidemiologic classification of human papillomavirus types associated with cervical cancer. N Engl J Med 2003;348:518–27.

4. Kirnbauer R, Booy F, Cheng N, Lowy DR, Schiller JT. Papilloma virus L1 major capsid protein self-assembles into virus-like-particles that are highly immunogenic. Proc Natl Acad Sci USA 1992; 89:12180–84.

5. Markowitz LE, Dunne EF, Saraiya M, Lawson HW, Chesson H, Unger ER; Centers for Disease Control and Prevention (CDC); Advisory Committee on Immunization Practices (ACIP). Quadrivalent Human Papillomavirus Vaccine: Recommendations of the Advisory Committee on Immunization Practices (ACIP). MMWR Recomm Rep 2007; 56:1–24.

6. Vashishtha VM, Choudhury P, Kalra A,Bose A, Thacker N, Yewale VN. Indian Academy of Pediatrics (IAP) recommended immunization schedule for children aged 0 through 18 years India, 2014 and updates on immunization.Indian Pediatr 2014;51:785–800.

7. Garland SM, Hernandez-Avila M, Wheeler CM, Perez G, Harper DM, Leodolter S. Quadrivalent vaccine against human papillomavirus to prevent anogenital diseases. N Engl J Med 2007;356: 1928–43.

8. Future II Study Group Quadrivalent vaccine against human papillomavirus to prevent high-grade cervical lesions. N Engl J Med 2007;356: 1915–27.

9. Paavonen J, Jenkins D, Bosch FX, Naud P, Salmerón J, Wheeler CM, et al. Efficacy of a prophylactic adjuvanted bivalent L1 virus-like-particle vaccine against infection with human papillomavirus types 16 and 18 in young women: an interim analysis of a phase III double-blind, randomised controlled trial. Lancet 2007; 369:2161–70.

10. Herrero R, Hildesheim A, Rodríguez AC, Wacholder S, Bratti C, Solomon D, et al. Rationale and design of a community-based double-blind randomized clinical trial of an HPV 16 and 18 vaccine in Guanacaste, Costa Rica. Vaccine 2008; 26:4795–4808.

11. WHO Guidelines for Screening and Treatment of Precancerous Lesions for Cervical Cancer Prevention.Geneva: World Health Organization; 2013. ISBN-13: 978-92-4-154869-4.

12. Brinton LA, Felix AS, McMeekin DS,Creasman WT, Sherman ME, Mutch D, et al. Etiologic Heterogeneity in Endometrial Cancer: Evidence from a Gynecologic Oncology Group Trial. Gynecol Oncol 2013;129:277–84.

13. Du M, Kraft P, Eliassen AH, Hankinson SE, De Vivo I. Physical activity and risk of endometrial adenocarcinoma in the Nurses Health Study. Int J Cancer 2014;134:2707–16.

14. Filomeno M, Bosetti C, Bidoli E, Levi F, Serraino D, Montella M, et al. Mediterranean diet and risk of endometrial cancer: a pooled analysis of three Italian case control studies. Br J Cancer 2015; 112:1816–21.

15. Sun Q, Xu L, Zhou B, Wang Y, Jing Y, Wang B. Alcohol consumption and the risk of endometrial cancer: a meta-analysis. Asia Pac J Clin Nutr 2011; 20:125–33.

16. Collaborative Group on Epidemiological Studies on Endometrial Cancer and oral contraceptives: an individual participant meta-analysis of 27, 276 women with endometrial cancer from 36 epi-demiological studies. Lancet Oncol 2015;16:1061–1070.

17. DMPA and risk of endometrial cancer. The WHO Collaborative study of Neoplasia and Steroid Contraceptives. Int J Cancer 1991;49:186–190.

18. Felix AS, Gaudet MM, La Vecchia C, Nagle CM, Shu XO, Weiderpass E,et al. Intrauterine devices and endometrial cancer risk: a pooled analysis of the Epidemiology of Endometrial Cancer Consortium. Int J Cancer 2015;136:E410–422.

19. Neill AS, Nagle CM, Protani MM, Obermair A, Spurdle AB, Webb PM; Australian National Endometrial Cancer Study Group. Aspirin, nonsteroidal anti-inflammatory drugs, paraceta-mol and risk of endometrial cancer: a case-control study, systematic review and meta-analysis. Int J. Cancer 2013;132:1146–55.

20. Kotsopoulos J, Baer HJ, Tworoger SS. Anthropo-metric measurement and risk of epithelial ovarian cancer: results from the nurses' health study. Obesity 2010;18:1625–1631.

21. Hu J, Hu Y, Zheng S. Intake of cruciferous vegetables is associated with reduced risk of ovarian cancer: a meta-analysis. Asia Pac J Clin Nutr 2015;24:101–109.

22. Faber MT, Kjaer SK, Dehlendorff C, Chang-Claude J, Andersen KK, Høgdall E, et al. Cigarette smoking and risk of ovarian cancer: a pooled analysis of 21 case-control studies. Cancer Causes Control 2013;24:989–1004.

23. Crane TE, Alberts DS, Thompson CA, Basen-Engquist K, Thomson CA. Dietary intake and ovarian cancer risk: a systematic review. Cancer Epidemiol Biomarkers Prev 2014;23:255–73.

24. Walker JL, Powell CB, Chen LM, Carter J, Bae Jump VL, Parker LP, et al. Society of Gynecologic Oncology recommendations for the prevention of ovarian cancer. Cancer 2015;121: 2108–20.

30 | Urinary Incontinence in Women: Approach to Diagnosis and Management

Nikhil Khattar, Hemlata Garg, Rubee Khattar

"Any unintentional/involuntary loss of urine is incontinence"

Workup of a woman complaining of urinary incontinence (UI) is often perceived to be a difficult task due to lack of understanding of physiology of micturition and pathophysiology of various forms of incontinence. The major types of UI are stress, urge and overflow incontinence.[1] A careful history of complaints of the woman helps in making a diagnosis.

History

A. When does the leak occur? Is it at all times or conditional?

This question segregates incontinence due to complete sphincteric loss (highest degree of intrinsic sphincter deficiency) and fistulas from urge or stress urinary incontinence.

1. *If it is only during stress:* With stress one means conditions of sudden rise in intra-abdominal pressure like cough, sneeze, laugh or giggle, lifting of weight. Generally a leak on single cough indicates severe stress urinary incontinence (SUI), whereas the same after a series of cough is a milder SUI. Similarly, a leak on laugh indicates severity. An underlying chronic respiratory condition leading to cough makes a minor incontinence a severely debilitating condition.

2. *If only during urge:* Urgency is an intense desire to pass urine because of "fear of leaking" and if it actually leaks during that urge then it is urge incontinence. It is usually a manifestation of involuntary detrusor contractions during the storage phase of micturition cycle. This can either be because of some underlying inflammation (urinary tract infection, stone in bladder, vaginitis), neurogenic condition or idiopathic.

3. *If continuous:* Then the primary differentiation to be made is between a urethral and an extraurethral incontinence (which can be checked during examination).

   Extraurethral UI is a manifestation of genito-urinary fistulae – vesicovaginal fistula (VVF) or ureterovaginal fistula (UVF). In UVF and small VVFs the patient also intermittently voids spontaneously.

   Urethral If the leak is urethral, intrinsic sphincteric defect (ISD) or overflow incontinence are the two main possibilities that are differentiated by presence of an empty or a full bladder.

4. *Mixed urinary incontinence:* Stress and urge urinary incontinence can co-exist. Usually either of the two will be predominant.

5. *Enuresis:* Refers to complete loss of urine. It occurs as a complete evacuation of urine and is different from incontinence. Nocturnal enuresis occurs only during sleep. Daytime enuresis can be a manifestation of complete lack of awareness of surroundings due to neurological or psychological conditions.

B. Quantification and impact on quality of life.

Whether any pads are used and if so how many? Does the incontinence restrict any social area of life? Any precipitating factors?

Examination

1. Smell of urine is unmistakable, and wet pads or underclothing points towards the severity and so does any feature of local dermatitis.
2. Pooling of urine in vagina on per speculum examination is confirmation of extra-uretheral incontinence.
3. A percussable bladder should point towards overflow incontinence (can also be confirmed by ultrasonography in obese patients).
4. Presence of concomitant pelvic organ prolapse/or hypermobile urethera can be seen.
5. Demonstration of UI on cough or Valsalva maneuver confirms SUI.
6. Basic neurological examination should include checking for anal tone, anal reflex.

This chapter will deal with only the urethral forms of incontinence and their management. Genitourinary fistulae are covered in another chapter of the book.

Overflow Incontinence

It is very important for any physician dealing with UI to identify this form of incontinence as this is the only form of UI that can lead to serious complications like renal damage or severe infections leading to sepsis.

It is also called as "paradoxical incontinence" as the underlying cause is bladder outlet obstruction and still the patient is leaking. The hallmark of this form of UI is a continuous dripping of urine in a patient who may be otherwise spontaneously voiding. The presence of a distended bladder can be appreciated by percussion, bimanual examination or by presence of high postvoid residual urine on ultrasonography (USG) or catheterization. In such a scenario, presence of bilateral hydronephrosis may suggest an obstructive uropathy. The determination of detrusor leak point pressure (DLPP) is important in urodynamic study (UDS) in such cases to predict or monitor the efficacy of treatment. High DLPP increases the risk of upper urinary tract deterioration and renal failure.

Stress Urinary Incontinence

The proximal female urethra is above the pelvic diaphragm and hence is an abdominal organ. Any increased abdominal pressure is equally transmitted to both the bladder and the proximal urethra, in effect, nullifying the pressures and maintaining the continence. This proximal part slips below the pelvic diaphragm in conditions of prolapse or hypermobile urethra leading to unequal pressure causing genuine stress incontinence. All colposuspension procedures are based on this earlier concept and fix the urethra to correct the hypermobility.

As the understanding of continence mechanisms evolved, the focus came on the posterior support provided by urethral fascia ligaments that act as a hammock to support the urethra (De Lancey's hammock hypothesis). The success of sling surgeries (i.e. tension-free mid urethral slings) depends on restoring this hammock rather than correcting the hypermobility.

Apart from the supports of the urethra and the intra-abdominal portion, which are the passive mechanisms of continence, the urethra itself has its **sphincteric muscles**, which provide the active continence.

On closure during the filling phase, the urethral mucosa is thrown into folds. Because of rich submucosal vascularity and hormonal influence the mucosal glands secrete mucus that forms a plug to seal the urethra. This **"mucosal seal"** is an important adjunct to sphincteric and fascial mechanisms of continence in women. During the postmenopausal phase this support decreases and along with weakening pelvic floor muscles becomes an important contributory factor to incontinence.

Evaluation of SUI

Clinical demonstration of SUI requires examining the patient with a full bladder. Very often, urge incontinence accompanies the stress incontinence. This mixed urinary incontinence usually has a predominant component, which can be judged on detailed history. Differentiating the hypermobility component from pure or intrinsic sphincteric deficiency (ISD) is an important aspect of SUI evaluation. The traditional Q tip test or simply observing for the downward rotational motion of urethra on Valsalva maneuver is indicative of hypermobility. Tension free slings act best for hypermobile urethra.

ISD is associated with severe stress incontinence. If it is not total (gravity) incontinence, the demonstration of ISD requires a urodynamic study. An abdominal or Valsalva leak point pressure of <90 cm H_2O is suggestive of a component of ISD, whereas <60 cm H_2O is diagnostic. Autologous pubovaginal slings are indicated for such severe incontinence.

Treatment Strategies for Stress Urinary Incontinence

Conservative Management

Pelvic floor muscle therapy (PFMT) regimens that focus on repeated contraction of pelvic floor muscle unit as a whole is helpful for lower grades of SUI especially when it is associated with urethral hypermobility or pelvic organ prolapse. These exercises are best explained by keeping a finger in the rectum or vagina and asking the patient to give a "squeeze" over it. Biofeedback mechanisms also focus on doing the PFMT in the correct manner by giving a visual feedback of their efforts of pelvic floor contraction.

Vaginal laser therapy with CO_2 laser focuses on superficial bursts of energy in subvaginal tissue to induce generation of more collagen to strengthen the supports. Present evidence suggests it to be of possible benefit in low grade SUI.

The main issue with all conservative options is the low longevity of response with these measures.

Mechanical: Soft plugs made of silicon are commercially available and can be useful for women who either do not want surgery or are not fit for it.

Surgery for SUI

The choice of best surgical method for SUI is an evolving issue. Available options are:
A. Retropubic suspension procedures
B. Autologous facial slings (Rectus fascia/fascia lata)
C. Synthetic slings
   - Tension free slings (Retropubic sling-TVT/transobturator sling—TOT)
   - Single incision sling
D. Adjustable slings

A. Retropubic suspension procedures

Suspension procedures aim to correct the hypermobility of the urethra and bladder neck and reinstate the sagging bladder neck with the vaginal tissue to fix supports.[2]

Burch Colposuspension: This is the standard retropubic surgical method for correcting SUI.
- In this procedure, the retropubic exposure of the anterolateral fornices of vagina is done aided by a finger in the vagina.
- Vagina on either side is fixed to the Cooper ligament (ileopectineal part of the inguinal ligament) with three interrupted sutures thereby reinstating it to supposedly normal position.
- The sutures are tied loose so that two fingers can be inserted between the vaginal wall and the lateral pelvic wall.
- The cure rates are in the range of 85–90%.
- Voiding dysfunction lasting 2–3 weeks is seen in approximately 10–15% of patients. Voiding dysfunction persisting beyond four weeks is seen in less than 5%. Occasionally there is a need to revise the procedure if obstruction does not resolve. There is a slight long-term risk of vault and posterior vaginal wall prolapse.

Other modifications are paravaginal repair and vaginal obturator shelf procedure, which essentially achieve the same restoration by fixing the paravaginal tissue to the obturator internus fascia. The urethrovesical angle formed is slightly different in each. The long-term results are also slightly different.

B. Autologous fascial slings[3]

Use of rectus fascia as sling is more common than fascia lata.

- Using a pfannenstiel incision a 8 × 1.5–2 cm transverse strip of the rectus sheath is taken and a 1–0 prolene suture is taken on both the ends and left long so that the sling is hung on the string.
- The bladder is kept drained with a Foley's catheter.
- A longitudinal or inverted U-shaped vaginal incision is used to dissect the mid and proximal urethra till the bladder neck. After raising adequate flap, ischiopubic rami are felt on each side. Endopelvic fascia is pierced with a Metzenbaum scissors pointing to the ipsilateral shoulder, and the long suture on the sling is fed from the retrobubic space. This brings along the rectus fascia strip in the vaginal incision.
- The same procedure is repeated on the other side but this time taking the long suture from the vaginal side to the retropubic area. Both the long ends are then tied over the closed rectus thereby providing the suspension to the bladder neck or even compression to the urethra if so desired.
- A cystoscopy is mandatory to rule out any inadvertent bladder injury.
- Success rates range from 70–97%. The procedure gives excellent outcomes in recurrent SUI. Being autologous material, it is the procedure of choice when stress incontinence surgery is combined with a urethral reconstructive procedure. It is also the treatment of choice for ISD. The urethra requires compression for restoring continence in such cases.
- Transient voiding dysfunction, postoperative retention and bladder outlet obstruction (<5%) and de novo urgency are important complications. Occasionally such complications may require sling incision and complete take down.
- Pubovaginal slings have a higher rate of success but slightly more morbidity than Burch's colposuspension.

C. Synthetic Slings

Midurethral synthetic slings: These are tension-free loose slings made of polypropylene that are placed behind the mid urethra. These induce fibrosis to provide a board like rigidity and allow the urethra to be apposed during transient increases in intra abdominal pressure. These are the easiest to place and can be performed as daycare procedures.

Retropubic mid urethral slings/tension-free vaginal tape (TVT):

- It is inserted in almost the same fashion as a pubovaginal sling but the level of dissection is not the bladder neck.
- There is no tension on the sling as the ends are not tied and are left loose after tensioning the sling with a gap of a surgical instrument (e.g. tip of scissors or an artery forceps) between the sling and the mid urethra.
- This procedure is slowly loosing popularity because as compared to trans obturator tape, it has slightly more complications like intraoperative bladder injury and vascular injury.
- The sling is indicated when there is a component of ISD along with urethral hypermobility.

Trans obturator midurethral slings:

- These can be either 'outside in' or 'inside out'.
- In either case, a curved needle is used to create a passage of sling track from medial thigh just below the adductor longus insertion at the level of clitoris to the vaginal incision at the level of mid urethra though the obturator internus fascia. Piercing of the obturator internus fascia is the most crucial step so that the sling lies deep to the ischiopubic ramus.
- Thus, it provides a sling track that is less angulated compared to the retropubic sling and gives a more physiologic hammock behind the urethra.
- Being more physiological, it is associated with less chances of bladder perforations, postoperative voiding dysfunction or *dnovo* urgency, while maintaining equivalent cure rates to other surgical procedures.

- As the track is very close to the obturator nerve, a higher incidence of thigh and groin pain is noted which is often transient but at times has mandated sling removal.
- Studies reporting outcomes >5 years after the procedure report cure rates of 70–95% in short term (mean 83–84%) that eventually settle to 61–64% by 5 years.[4,5]

Urgency Incontinence (Overactive Bladder)

Clinical Presentation

A woman presenting with episodes of uncontrollable urge often leading to incontinence is likely to have an overactive bladder (OAB) and urge incontinence. Usually there are no accompanying problems in voiding.

Such women will have a normal urine examination and culture and the uroflowmetry will be normal with insignificant residual urine. A voiding diary will reveal frequent voids throughout day and night (usually more than 8 in a day) and unpredictable episodes of incontinence.

It is important to rule out any causes that are causing irritation to the bladder like urinary tract infection (UTI), stone, outlet obstruction, adjacent organ inflammation like vaginitis, prolapse and neurogenic causes. If these causes have been ruled out, the diagnosis would be idiopathic overactive bladder (OAB).

Definition

The International Continence Society (ICS) defines OAB as "urinary urgency, usually accompanied by frequency and nocturia, with or without urgency incontinence, in the absence of urinary tract infection or other obvious pathology".[1]

The diagnosis is usually clinical and urgency is pivotal to the diagnosis.

OAB is a quality of life problem and affects a person's social and work life. The nocturia affects sleep and thus productivity at work apart from sexual life.

Pathophysiology and Etiology

The sensation of filling is conveyed to the cortex via two types of afferent fibers mediating the micturition reflex—(a) myelinated A-delta fiber and (b) unmyelinated C-fiber. A-delta fibers respond to passive bladder distension and active detrusor contraction, thus conveying information about active bladder filling, whereas unmyelinated fibers respond to chemical irritation of bladder mucosa.[6,7]

Storage Phase

During the storage phase of the bladder—with increasing bladder volume the detrusor is kept relaxed and the sphincters activity is slowly increased (the "guarding reflex"). Beta-3 adrenergic receptors help increase the sphincteric tone and keep the detrusor relaxed. The suprapontine micturition center is in a state of inhibition during entire filling.

Voiding Phase

The voiding phase receives command from cortex, which first switches off the sympathetic activity to relax the guarding reflex and then the pontine micturition center discharges a strong parasympathetic impulse that causes detrusor contraction to evacuate the urine.

The voiding phase is parasympathetic dominated after all sympathetic activity is switched off leading to pelvic floor and sphincter relaxation followed by a strong cholinergic discharge causing detrusor contraction.

Detrusor over activity (DO) and OAB might arise in circumstances in which the afferent activity is inappropriately high for any given degree of bladder distension.

Etiology of OAB is complex and poorly understood[7,8]

1. **Neurogenic hypothesis:** When the balance of inhibitory and stimulatory afferent impulses to the bladder is tilted to stimulatory bursts, OAB ensues. DO arises from generalized, nerve-mediated excitation of the detrusor muscle. Normally the bladder control is modulated in an inhibitory fashion

by the cerebral cortex. Damage to the brain can induce DO by reducing supra-pontine inhibition. Damage to axonal pathways in the spinal cord allows the expression of primitive spinal bladder reflexes.[9]

2. **Myogenic hypothesis:** Some detrusor muscle fibers attain autonomic behavior and increased phasic activity occurs. Overactive detrusor contractions result from a combination of increased spontaneous excitation within smooth muscle of the bladder and enhanced propagation of this activity to affect an excessive proportion of the bladder wall.[10]

Risk Factors for OAB

Bladder inflammation, chronic bladder outlet obstruction, central nervous system disorders, diabetes mellitus, pregnancy, vaginal delivery, postmenopausal status and old age (risk increases with age), the commonest cause being idiopathic.

Any patient coming to gynecology outpatient clinic with the symptoms of urgency, urge incontinence, frequency with or without nocturia should be evaluated properly because OAB is a diagnosis of exclusion.

Clinical Evaluation

History

- Presence or absence of symptoms, their severity and effect on quality of life for each of the symptoms including urgency, frequency and incontinence should be elicited.
- Voiding symptoms like poor flow, urethral pain, interrupted urinary stream and feeling of incomplete evacuation should also be assessed and if present, a uroflowmetry should be obtained to rule out voiding dysfunction.
- Drug history of medications that can exacerbate the symptoms of OAB like intake of diuretics and alpha agonist should be taken.
- Medical condition, e.g. closed-angle glaucoma and cognitive impairment can limit treatment options.

Physical Examination

- A thorough abdominal, per vaginal and per rectal examination should be undertaken.
- Conditions like pelvic organ prolapse with or without cystocele should be looked for, as this could be the cause of frequency or urgency.
- For women with an atrophic vagina and symptoms of OAB, estrogen deficiency may contribute to their symptoms.
- Clinical evaluation should exclude other possible causes of urgency and frequency of micturition like:

  Urological causes: UTI, bladder tumor, bladder stone, urethral diverticulum, small capacity bladder, interstitial cystitis, radiation cystitis.

  Gynecological causes: Cystocele, previous pelvic surgery, pelvic mass (fibroids).

  Medical causes: Upper motor neuron lesion (cerebrovascular stroke, Parkinson's disease), impaired renal function, congestive heart failure, diabetes mellitus, diabetes insipidus.
- Post-micturition residual urine estimation can be performed to rule out overflow incontinence or incomplete bladder emptying, which can cause symptoms of OAB.

Frequency volume charts or bladder diaries are a useful adjunct to assist history.

- Generally a three-day diary is maintained.
- The patient should be asked to record the quantity of fluid intake and urine output and record all her voids with time.
- Any leakage of urine and number and degree of soakage of pads is noted.

The diaries are superior to patient recall and help clinician to rule out excessive fluid intake and polyuria as diagnosis. A voiding diary can provide patients with insights into those behaviors that need modification to decrease the urinary frequency.

Urodynamic evaluation: Conservative management and oral pharmacotherapy are commonly prescribed without a urodynamic diagnosis.

Clinical evaluation with urodynamics is indicated when conservative and drug therapy fail to manage OAB adequately or in complicated cases of OAB or before invasive surgery.

The main urodynamic finding associated with OAB is presence of uninhibited detrusor contractions or urodynamic DO along with increased filling sensation or leak in the filing phase.

Failure to demonstrate DO on urodynamic study does not rule out its existence. It is well known that up to 50% of women with urge incontinence do not demonstrate detrusor contractions on urodynamic study and in fact, are able to suppress the motor activity in test conditions.[11]

Treatment

1. **Noninvasive treatment**
   a. Behavioral therapy
   b. Pharmacotherapy—oral medication (anticholinergic or beta 3 agonist).
   c. Combined behavioral and pharmacologic therapy.
   d. Estrogen for postmenopausal women.
2. **Minimally invasive treatments:**
   a. Botulinum a-toxin.
   b. Neuromodulation (post tibial nerve, sacral nerve stimulation).
   c. Interruption of innervation (central sub-arachnoid block or sacral Rhizotomy, peripheral motor and/or sensory block).
3. **Invasive treatments:**
   a. Augmentation cystoplasty.
   b. Urinary diversion.

1. Noninvasive Treatment

a. *Behavioral modifications:* This includes
   • *Lifestyle modification* like decrease in weight, avoidance of smoking, decreased consumption of tea, coffee and spicy food.
   • Avoidance of diuretics before bedtime.
   • *Timed (scheduled) voiding:* Incontinent patients should be advised to follow a voiding schedule based on trigger of time rather than wait for urge (timed voiding).

The time can be initially started with an interval of 2 hours and gradually increased. This will allow emptying before the surge in afferent sensations resulting in an uninhibited detrusor contraction.

Bladder can be slowly retrained by gradually increasing the voiding interval. This can be assisted with pharmacotherapy and pelvic floor exercises. Patient should be asked to suppress the intense urge and wait for it to calm down, and to walk to toilet rather than rush for it (any uninhibited detrusor contraction generally comes down to baseline in a while). Bladder training requires a motivated patient with sufficient cognitive function.

• *Pelvic floor training* (Kegel exercises) consists of intermittent voluntary maximal contraction of pelvic floor muscles. Each contraction is held for 6–8 seconds followed by brief period of relaxation. A common regimen is set of 10 contractions three times per day. Continence improves after 6–2 weeks of exercise. Contraction of pelvic floor muscle is best done when lying down, but can be done during different activities such as sitting or when talking on telephone.

b. *Pharmacotherapy:* The commonly used drugs used to manage urge incontinence are anticholinergics and beta agonists (Table 30.1)
   • *Anticholinergic agents:* Generally a first line option for OAB. Most physicians regard a trial of 6–12 weeks as reasonable. Studies have found discontinuation rates of 43–83% in first 30 days of treatment, commonly because of side effects like dry mouth and constipation. Tendency to cause retention especially in patients with high residual urine and blurring of vision in patients with narrow angle glaucoma should be kept in mind. Regular follow up is necessary for monitoring treatment, side effects and adherence to treatment.

Drugs	Dosage	Side effects	Contraindications	Special precautions
MIRABEGRON α3 agonist	25–50 mg/OD	Cardiovascular, hypertension	Severe uncontrolled hypertension, hypersensitivity	Hepatic, renal disorder, recipient of CYP2D6 substrate
SOLIFENACIN anticholinergic	5–10 mg/OD	Constipation, xerostomia	Narrow angle glaucoma, gastric retenion	Hepatic, renal disease, dementia, delirium, pregnancy, lactation
TOLTERODINE anticholinergic	1–2 mg/BD	Xerostomia, headache, constipation	Narrow angle glaucoma, gastric retention	Hepatic, renal disease, CYP3A4 inhibitor, pregnancy lactation
DARIFENACIN anticholinergic	20 mg/BD	Constipation, headache, UTI	Narrow angle glaucoma, hypersensitivity, Urinary retention	Narrow angle glaucoma, hypersensitivity, Urinary retention
TROSPIUM anticholinergic	7.5–15 mg/OD	Xerostomia, headache, constipation	Narrow angle glaucoma, hypersensitivity, Urinary retention	Narrow angle glaucoma, hypersensitivity, Urinary retention

Table 30.1: Commonly used drugs for overactive bladder

- *Beta-adrenergic agonist:* Only available option for use is Mirabegron. The onset of action is slower than anticholinergics but side effects like dry mouth, risk of retention and constipation are not known with this class of drug.

c. *Combined behavioral and pharmacologic therapy*

d. *Estrogen for postmenopausal women:* Local estrogen therapy is the most beneficial route in treatment of OAB due to direct effect on reversal of vaginal atrophy.

2. Minimally Invasive Treatments

a. *Intravesical therapy with botulinium toxin* is a useful second line strategy after failure of initial pharmacotherapy. It acts by inhibiting detrusor contraction by inhibiting release of acetylcholine at neuromuscular junction. It is invasive and requires a visit to the operation theatre and has a risk of temporary retention requiring clean intermittent self-catheterization. The effect of the drug is reversible and wanes off in 6–9 months and the injection has to be repeated.

b. *Sacral neuromodulation (Interstism) and posterior tibial electrical nerve stimulation (P-TENS):* Modifies voiding reflex by electric stimulation of S3 afferent nerve. Stimulation of the sacral roots has effectively suppressed the hyperactivity of the detrusor muscle. Indicated in patients who fail or cannot tolerate conservative treatment because of side effects. The treatment is costly and available only at specialized centers.

3. Surgery for Urge Incontinence

Surgery is the last resort for patients failing all other less invasive therapies.

Types of surgery:
- Augmentation enterocystoplasty (using bowel as a detubularised patch to increase bladder capacity).
- Auto augmentation (taking off the bladder muscle from the bladder mucosa to allow a low pressure expansion).
- Urinary diversion as ileal conduit—done rarely.

Results of augmentation cystoplasty—most patients become dry. However, 10–40% require clean intermittent self catheterization for emptying as the detubularised intestine does not produce a synchronous contraction to facilitate emptying.

Failure rates of autoaugmentation are more due to limited increase in bladder capacity.

💡 Key Points

- Urinary incontinence is a distressing symptom that requires thorough evaluation.
- The common types are stress and urge incontinence.
- History, examination and investigations involving urodynamic studies and uroflowmetry help in identifying different types of incontinence.
- Initial management involves behavioral modification, pelvic floor exercises and correction of any underlying cause.
- Pharmacotherapy with specific drugs helps alleviate symptoms however the side effects may be a limiting factor for their use.
- Surgery is used for patients not responsive to non-invasive measures.

REFERENCES

1. Haylen BT, de Ridder D, Freeman RM, Swift SE, Berghmans B, Lee J, et al; International Urogynecological Association; International Continence Society. An International Urogynecological Association (IUGA)/International Continence Society (ICS) joint report on the terminology for female pelvic floor dysfunction. Neurourol Urodyn 2010;29:4-20.

2. Retropubic Suspension Surgery for Incontinence in Women. In: Wein AJ, Kavoussi LR, Partin AW, Peters CA, eds. Campbell-Walsh Urology. 11th ed. Elsevier 2016;1918–1938.

3. Slings: Autologous, Biologic, Synthetic, and Midurethral, In: Wein AJ, Kavoussi LR, Partin AW, Peters CA, eds. Campbell-Walsh Urology. 11th ed. Elsevier 2016;1987–2038.

4. Gomelsky A. Midurethral sling: is there an optimal choice? Curr Opin Urol 2016;26:295–301.

5. Leone Roberti Maggiore U, FinazziAgrò E, Soligo M, Li Marzi V, Digesu A, Serati M. Long-term outcomes of TOT and TVT procedures for the treatment of female stress urinary incontinence: a systematic review and meta-analysis. Int Urogynecol J 2017;28:1119–1130.

6. Physiology and Pharmacology of the Bladder and Urethra. In: Wein AJ, Kavoussi LR, Partin AW, Peters CA (eds). Campbell-Walsh Urology. 11th ed. Elsevier 2016;1631–1684.

7. Badlani GH, Davila GW, Michel MC, Rosette JJ MCH (eds). Continence: Current Concepts and Treatment Strategies. Springer, 2009.

8. Overactive Bladder. In: Wein AJ, Kavoussi LR, Partin AW, Peters CA (eds) Campbell-Walsh Urology. 11th ed. Elsevier 2016;1796–1806.

9. de Groat WC. A neurologic basis for the overactive bladder. Urology 1997;50(6A Suppl):36–52.

10. Brading AF. A myogenic basis for the overactive bladder. Urology 1997;50(6A Suppl):57–67.

11. Hashim H, Abrams P. Is the bladder a reliable witness for predicting detrusor overactivity? J Urol 2006;175:191–4.

31 | Genitourinary Fistulas

Karishma Bhatia, Devender Kumar

A fistula is an abnormal passage or communication that leads from one hollow organ to another. The close anatomical relation of lower urinary tract to vagina and uterus makes the reproductive tract susceptible to fistula formation during complicated childbirth and gynecological surgery (Fig. 31.1).

These acquired tracts between two viscus cause physical, social as well as emotional suffering to the patient. Continuous dribbling of urine or fecal matter (recto-vaginal fistula) into the vagina leads to recurrent infections, lower self-esteem, abandonment and/or divorce sometimes. The global incidence is 1 in 100,000 cases but in developing countries it is 1–3 in 1000 cases.[1] Majority (approx. 90%) of these are caused by neglected or operative deliveries in developing countries and radiotherapy or gynecological surgeries in developed countries.[2]

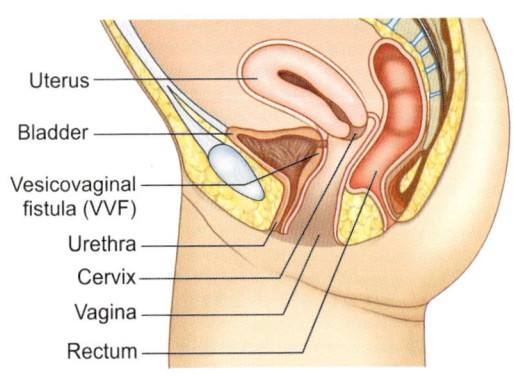

Uterus ——

Bladder ——

Vesicovaginal ——
fistula (VVF)

Urethra ——

Cervix ——

Vagina ——

Rectum ——

Fig. 31.1: Vesicovaginal fistula

Prevention and early diagnosis followed by appropriate treatment are the important aspects of management of genitourinary fistulae.

Case 1

Mrs X, 19-year-old girl had her first child at home, delivery conducted by Dai. Labour lasted for three days. She delivered a stillborn baby. Ten days later, she had complaints of dribbling of urine. She ignored it and then developed rashes in her perineum. Now she has come to the OPD.

Q1. What history does one need to illicit?

A detailed history should be obtained in patients presenting with urinary incontinence.
1. History related to delivery is obtained.
   a. Duration of labor, place and time of birth
   b. Whether it was conducted by skilled or unskilled birth attendant.
   c. Was there any manipulation or instrumentation?
2. Information about the baby—if the baby cried or not, weight of the baby.
3. Any history of excessive bleeding, fever after delivery.
4. History of urinary complaints/leakage:
   a. Was there any difficulty in passing urine?
   b. Did she pass urine voluntarily after delivery or there was any need of catheterization?
   c. When did involuntary passage of urine begin?

d. Does the leak occur on coughing, straining, conditions associated with increased abdominal pressure (stress incontinence)

5. Is there history of irresistible desire to pass urine associated with incontinence (urge incontinence)
   a. Amount of urine leak
   b. Whether it is continuous or intermittent
   c. If it is dependent on patient s position
   d. Does patient void transurethral as well
   e. History of any systemic illnesses

6. Sometimes patients may give history of foot drop which can result from neurological damage secondary to compression of sciatic nerve due to cephalo-pelvic disproportion or obstruction.

Q2. What are the important points in examination?

A complete general physical examination, height, weight, BMI of the patient should be calculated. Genitourinary fistulas are more common in women with short stature, young age, poor nutritional status, low socio-economic status and deliveries conducted at home by dais or unattended deliveries.

Per abdomen examination: Look for any organomegaly, any scar marks.

Local examination: Note any rashes, excoriation of perineal skin which can result due to acidic pH of urine and its continuous dribbling from the vagina on the perineum.

Cough test for urinary incontinence: With bladder full patient is made to lie down and asked to cough while the examiner looks for urinary leak through the urethral meatus and also from the vagina when a fistula is suspected.

Per speculum examination: On per speculum examination one needs to look for any defect, its size and location, surrounding mucosa and its edges. Look for any inflammation, induration, edema, fibrosis and leakage of urine.

In this patient findings were

Patient is of short stature (height 136 cm) BMI is 17.5, her vitals were stable.

Per abdomen: Soft, no guarding , tenderness, no organomegaly seen.

Local examination: Rashes and itching marks seen on perineum.

Per speculum examination: Defect seen on anterior vaginal wall about 3 × 4 cm in size, about 3 cm from the Introitus. Surrounding vaginal mucosa is fibrosed.

Q3. Where are obstetric fistulas commonly located? What is the pathogenesis of obstetric fistulas?

Obstetric fistulas are generally large and are located distally in the vagina. They involve large portions of the bladder neck (trigonal

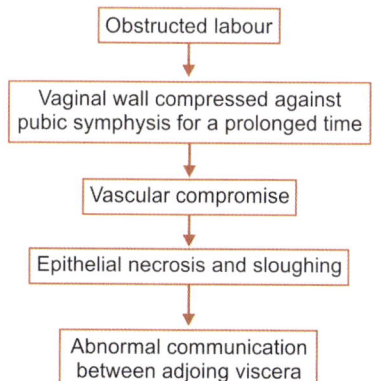

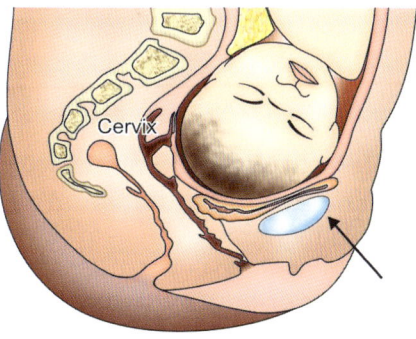

Fig. 31.2: Pathophysiology of obstetric fistula (compression of bladder against pubic bone marked with arrow point)

area) and proximal urethra sometimes. This is explained by the mechanism of formation of such fistulas. In cases with CPD or obstructed labor, the bladder neck is compressed against pubic bone by fetal head. It causes ischemic injury which may lead to sloughing of tissue after 3–5 days depending upon insult.

In developing countries like India, fistulas mostly result from obstetric causes (90%).[2] This is due to the large numbers of unattended deliveries, younger age at childbirth, lower socioeconomic status, small pelvis due to malnutrition, rickets, etc.

Obstructed labor injury complex includes urethral loss, stress incontinence, hydro-ureteronephrosis, renal failure, rectovaginal fistula, renal atresia and sphincter incontinence, cervical destruction, amenorrhea, pelvic inflammatory disease, secondary infertility, vaginal stenosis, osteitis pubis and foot drop.[3]

Q4. What is the approach to management for this patient ?

Obstetric fistulas are difficult to manage due to extensive tissue necrosis. Patient should be catheterised using foley's catheter and worked up. Repair of obstetric fistulas should be delayed by about 3 months to allow for tissue healing. Also meanwhile serial urine cultures are sent to ensure that urine is sterile at the time of surgery. Three consecutive cultures should be negative before surgery.

Patient should be encouraged to take high protein diet, good nutrition needs to be provided. Any anemia should be corrected with oral or intravenous iron or blood donation. Patient should be counselled as emotional support is also of extreme importance in such cases.

Q5. Could fistula in this patient be prevented?

Patients with obstructed labor should be catheterized for a minimum of 21 days to allow for bladder drainage and prevent its distention. This aids in healing of the epithelium thus preventing fistula formation. If it occurs and is small then catheter should be left for up to 6 weeks. Adequate diet and water intake needs to be ensured.

Q6. What are the principles of surgical repair of fistula?

Principles of surgical repair: These principles were given by Marion Sims in the mid 19th century and are followed till present day.[4]

1. The tissue should not have any edema or infection at the time of repair
2. All scar tissue should be excised and margins should be freshened.
3. Tension free closure of the defect by wide mobilization of the tissues.
4. Minimal use of cautery and atraumatic handling of tissues.
5. Excellent hemostasis to be achieved using fine suture material.
6. Good post operative bladder drainage until healing is achieved. To achieve this dual drainage of urine is ensured via a suprapubic as well as a transurethral Foleys catheter.
7. In the 20th century, the use of transplanted blood supply from the bulbocavernosus muscle, gracilis muscle, vestibular fat pad, omentum was also advocated. This provides an additional external blood supply which promotes healing of the fistula. This is especially helpful in fistulas developing secondary to radiation.

Q7. What are different approaches to fistula repair? How to go about fistula repair for this patient ?

There are two approaches for fistula repair-abdominal and vaginal (Table 31.1). There are

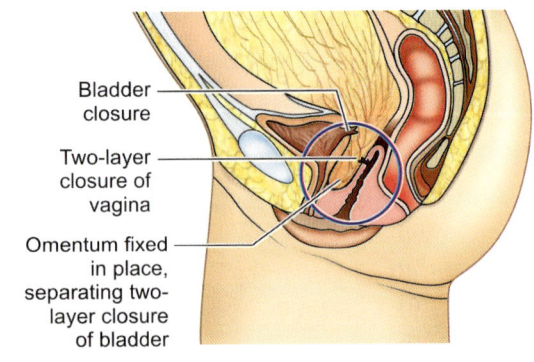

Bladder closure

Two-layer closure of vagina

Omentum fixed in place, separating two-layer closure of bladder

Fig. 31.3: Placement of omental flap using abdominal approach

Table 31.1: Abdominal vs vaginal approach for fistula repair		
	Abdominal	*Vaginal*
Incision	Abdominal	Vaginal
Timing of repair	Delayed	Maybe be done immediately if no infection
Exposure limitation	Fistula low on the trigone or low on the bladder neck is difficult to expose abdominally	Fistula at vaginal cuff is difficult to expose vaginally
Sexual function	No change in vaginal length	Vaginal shortening may occur
Flaps used	Omentum (Fig. 31.3), peritoneal flap, rectus abdominis flap	Labial fat pad (martius flap), peritoneal flap, gluteal skin or gracilis myocutaneous flap.
Relative indications	Large fistula, located high in a deep narrow vagina, radiation fistulae, failed vaginal approach, small bladder needing augmentation, need for ureteral reimplantation	Uncomplicated fistulae, low fistulae

relative indications for both but the single most important factor is the surgeon's experience. Approach needs to be individualized.

Q8. What are the advantages of vaginal approach over abdominal?

- Avoidance of laparotomy
- Short operative time
- Brief hospital stay
- Minimal blood loss
- Anti-incontinence, prolapse surgeries can also be performed
- Local grafts-martius, peritoneal can be used.

Q9. What are the various techniques of fistula repair?

1. Vaginal
   - *Vaginal flap or flap splitting technique:* 3-layer closure without flap, four layer with flap.
   - *Latzko technique:* Margins of fistula are dissected for 1 to 2 cm circumferentially and then approximated. Results in vaginal shortening.

   Complications: Vaginal shortening, stenosis Most important complication of fistula is recurrence.

2. *Abdominal:* Suprapubic extraperitoneal or intraperitoneal approach.

Case 2

A 42-year-old lady got operated for fibroid uterus, it was a 24 week size uterus. She was catheterised and Foley's catheter was removed on day 2 of surgery. On the 4th postoperative day she developed urinary leakage. It was less on lying down and increased when she stands.

Q1. What is the differential diagnosis of postoperative urinary leakage?

The differential diagnosis of urinary incontinence post operatively:
- Urogenital fistula
- Stress incontinence
- Urge incontinence
- Overflow incontinence

Q2. What are the causes of fistula formation?

Various obstetric conditions that can result in fistula formation are:
- Prolonged or obstructed labor (discussed in detail above)
- Caesarean section especially repeat caesarean section.
- Caesarean hysterectomy
- Cervical cerclage
- Placenta percreta
- Operative vaginal delivery

In developed countries fistulas result from complications of surgery and radiation therapy for cancers. Gynecological procedures resulting in fistula formation are:

- Hysterectomy especially radical hysterectomies for cancers
- Myomectomy
- Bursch colposuspension
- Mid urethral sling surgery

These result from extensive and blunt dissection between the bladder and the uterus, unrecognized bladder laceration, inappropriate stitch placement, or devascularization in the tissue planes.

Rate of bladder injury during abdominal hysterectomy is 0.5 to 1%.[5] VVF is more common after abdominal hysterectomy compared to vaginal approach. Post hysterectomy VVFs are thought to result most commonly from an incidental unrecognized iatrogenic cystotomy near the vaginal cuff. Other mechanisms for post hysterectomy VVF include tissue necrosis from cautery, a suture placed through both the bladder and vaginal wall during closure of the vaginal cuff, or suture ligation in an attempt to control pelvic bleeding. Tissue ischemia and resulting necrosis promotes fibrosis and induration, resulting in an epithelial lining of the tract and development of a fistula tract.[6]

Fistula can also form due to malignancy, irradiation or occur congenitally.

Q3. What are the different types of fistulas?

Genital fistulas can be classified in various ways:

1. *Based on location* (Fig. 31.4)
   - Vesicovaginal
   - Urethrovaginal
   - Vesicouterine
   - Vesicocervical
   - Ureterovaginal
   - Ureterouterine

Combination fistulas: Vesicoureterovaginal, vesicoureterouterine, vesicovaginorectal.

2. Based on size
   - Small <2 cm
   - Medium 2–3 cm
   - Large 4–5 cm
   - Extensive >6 cm

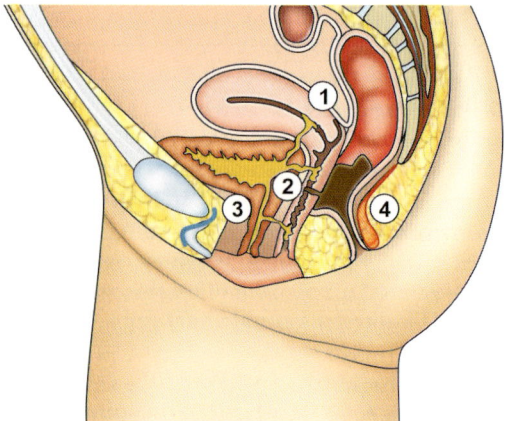

Fig. 31.4: Various fistulae locations (1. Vesicouterine, 2. Vesicovaginal, 3. Uretherovaginal, 4. Recto-vaginal)

3. Simple and complicated

Simple	Complicated
Less than 2 to 3 cm	Greater than 3 cm
Near the cuff (supratrigonal)	Distant from cuff/ trigonal involvement
No history of radiation or malignancy	Pelvic malignancy is present/prior radiation therapy
Vaginal length is normal	Vaginal length shortened

Q4. How can one prevent gynecological fistulas?

Primary prevention: Bladder is catheterized to ensure it is empty and not distended during surgery. Bladder is adequately mobilized to access the vaginal cuff. Blunt dissection should not be done especially in cases with prior surgeries as the vesicovaginal space may be scarred. Retractors for the bladder should be held carefully. If hysterectomy is performed for benign lesions then, cruciate incision should be given on isthmic area of uterus and pubocervical, pubovesical fascia should be pushed along with bladder. Avoid involving fascia during vaginal cuff suturing.

Secondary prevention involves timely detection and repair of any bladder injury if it occurs and ensuring a watertight closure of bladder. Uninterrupted postoperative bladder drainage should be achieved.[7] The American

Association for the Surgery of Trauma (AAST) grade of the bladder trauma is the strongest predictor of subsequent VVF formation. Higher the grade more is the likelihood of fistula formation. A grade V bladder injury implies injury to the trigone. The proximity of the injury to the vaginal cuff increases VVF formation because the site of the bladder injury comes in direct contact with the healing cuff.[8]

Q5. How would you manage a bladder injury detected intraoperatively?

If bladder is injured intraoperatively, cystoscopy should be performed to identify the injury, its size as well as proximity to the ureters and the bladder trigone.

Routine use of cystoscopy during hysterectomy is controversial.

Before repair of injury, bladder is catheterized with transurethral Foley's catheter.

a. If bladder injury is close to ureter, ureteral catheterization is recommended.

b. Vesicovaginal space should be sufficiently dissected to allow tension free closure.

c. The urothelial/lamina propria layer is closed with interrupted or continuous 2–0 or 3–0 sutures.

d. A second layer is put using interrupted sutures in a staggered fashion.

e. A third layer of peritoneum is put using delayed absorbable 3–0 suture in interrupted fashion.

For repairing a cystotomy at the trigonal area, a transverse closure is preferred. Vertical closure would produce ureteral obstruction as ureteral orifices are drawn toward each other. Ureteral catheters should be considered in repair of a cystotomy involving the ureteric orifices.

Patient has height of 160 cm, BMI of 29, vitals are stable, passed flatus and stool, vitals are stable, on local examination, there is no bleeding and perineum is normal.

On a gentle per speculum examination a tiny hole is seen at the apex of vagina through which urine is coming out and pooling on the speculum.

Q6. What are the various tests used to confirm site of fistula?

A simple speculum examination sometimes does not help know the exact type of fistula. For this we can use the *three swab* test (Fig. 31.5).

Using a speculum three swabs are put into the vagina-upper (next to cervix), middle and lower (at introitus). Using a catheter the bladder is filled with methylene blue dye. Then the patient is asked to walk for about half an hour and the swabs are removed.

Double dye test confirms a ureterovaginal fistula. Patient is given oral phenazopyridine or pyridium 200 mg three times a day. If upper swab is stained orange it confirms ureterovaginal fistula.

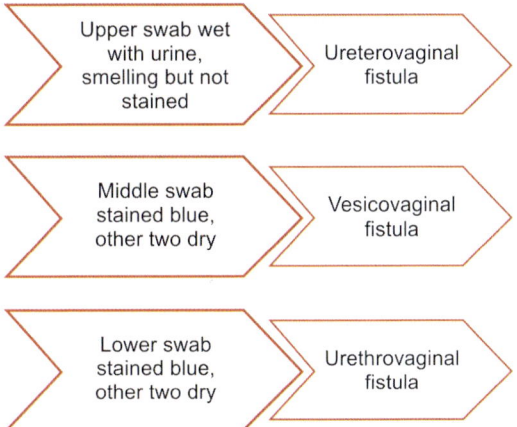

Fig. 31.5: Three swab test to locate fistula and its interpretation

Three swab test

These tests were performed for this patient and the middle swab stained blue, others were dry implying that it is a vesicovaginal fistula.

Q7. What is the role of cystoscopy? What is the role of ureteral catheterization?

Cystoscopy helps in localizing the fistula in relation to the ureteric orifices.

Ureteroscopy and ureteral catheterization has been used in the management of ureterovaginal fistula.[9] It is helpful where the fistula is small and there is ureteric continuity. A guide wire is passed retrograde and a double J (DJ)

stent is inserted. This is left for 4 to 6 weeks allow to healing of the ureter. A one year follow up with intravenous urography is done to look for any late stenosis occurring due to peri-ureteric fibrosis.

Q8. What further investigations are indicated in a post surgical VVF?

As up to 12 % of post surgical VVFs are found to be associated with a ureteral injury or ureterovaginal fistula, upper urinary tract evaluation should be done prior to repair using intravenous urography (IVU) or computed tomography (CT) urography.[10]

Q9. How will this patient be managed?

Management of the fistula depends on various factors which are

- Size
- Location
- Simple or complicated
- Time of presentation—early is less than 3 weeks, >3 weeks—late presentation.

Since this patient has a small simple fistula we should first attempt conservative management.

Non-surgical management: A trial of conservative management should be offered especially for patients with fistula small in size, i.e. less than 0.5 cm and certainly <1 cm. Patient is catheterized for 4 to 6 weeks. In 1985, Zimmern concluded that if the fistula's catheter decreases in size in 30 days it may completely heal by leaving Foley's for another 2 to 3 weeks.[11] Good nutrition is provided, anemia if present should be corrected.

Conservative surgical management: VVF repair can be done with

- Fibrin glue
- Cystoscopic laser treatment
- Autologous platelet rich plasma with interposition of platelet rich fibrin

Surgical repair: Obstetric fistulas repair is attempted only after 3 months. In this period patient is kept catheterized to prevent exposure of the epithelial surfaces to urine. Small fistulas may heal with prolonged catheterization. Three successive urine cultures should be negative. However in patients with post hysterectomy fistulas detected soon after surgery one can go for a repair straight away after ensuring urine is not infected.

Q10. What is classical presentation of a vesicouterine fistula?

Patient reports:

a. Cyclical hematuria, i.e. menouria
b. Amenorrhea—if fistula is located above the cervix menstrual blood may be redirected into the bladder.
c. Urinary incontinence
   This is known as YOUSSEF syndrome.

The most common cause of a vesicouterine fistula is lower segment caesarean section. Non surgical management can be done by inducing involution of uterus hormonally and maintaining bladder drainage. Surgical management is individualized and depends on need for future fertility. If family is complete hysterectomy with bladder repair is done.

Case 3

Mrs X is 55-year-old, she developed carcinoma cervix stage 2b, 8 years ago for which she received chemoradiation. Now she is complaining of urinary leakage since the past 3 months which is continuous in nature.

Q1. What is the differential diagnosis?

We need to take a comprehensive history and examine the patient. It can be due to urinary incontinence or fistula formation. Fistula secondary to radiation may present even after decades as it occurs as a result of fibrosis and devascularization of tissue.

Q2. Is a biopsy indicated?

Yes a biopsy should be done as the fistula may represent a recurrence of the malignancy.

Q3. What is the approach to management?

Repair should be performed after a minimum of 6 months of cancer treatment, as tissue needs more time to heal. Also one should consider using grafts as they provide vascularity essential for healing and recovery.

 Key Points

- Majority of genitourinary fistulas are caused by neglected or operative deliveries in developing countries and radiotherapy or gynecological surgeries in developed countries.
- Prevention and early diagnosis followed by appropriate treatment is the key to manage genitourinary fistulae.
- Obstetric fistulas are generally repaired after 3 months, post surgical fistulas may be repaired immediately if diagnosed intraoperatively whereas post radiation fistulas should only be repaired after about 6 months of completion of treatment.
- Repair of genitourinary fistulas is done based on the principles described by Marion Sims removal of necrotic tissue, tension free closure, excellent hemostasis and maintenance of good post-operative bladder drainage.

REFERENCES

1. Hilton P, Ward A. Epidemiological and surgical aspects of urogenital fistulae: a review of 25 years experience in south-east Nigeria. Int Urogynaecol J Pelvic Floor Dysfunct 1998;9:189–94.

2. Nawaz H, Khan M, Tareen FM, et al. Retrospective study of 213 cases of female urogenital fistulae at the department of urology & transplantation civil hospital Quetta, Pakistan. J Pak Med Assoc 2010;60:28–32.

3. Arrowsmith SD. Genitourinary reconstruction in obstetric fistulae J Urol 1994;152:403–6.

4. Sims JM. On the treatment of vesicovaginal fistula.1852. Int Urogynaecol J Pelvic Floor Dysfunct 1998;9;236–48.

5. Keettel WC, Sehring FG, deProsse CA, et al. Surgical management of urethrovaginal and vesicovaginal stulae. Am J Obstet Gynecol 1978; 131:425–31.

6. Kursh ED, Morse RM, Resnick MI, et al. Prevention of the development of a vesicovaginal stula. Surg Gynecol Obstet 1988;166:409–12.

7. Hutch JA, Noll LE. Prevention of vesicovaginal stulae. Obstet Gynecol 1970;35:924–7.

8. Duong TH, Taylor DP, Meeks GR. A multicenter study of vesicovaginal stula following incidental cystotomy during benign hysterectomies. Int Urogynecol J 2011;22:975–9.

9. Koonings P, Huffman JL, Schlaerth JB. Ureteroscopy: A new aspect in the management of postoperative uretero-vaginal fistulae. Obstet Gynecol 1992; 80:548–9.

10. Goodwin WE, Scardino PT. Vesicovaginal and ureterovaginal fistulae: a summary of 25 years of experience. J Urol 1980;123:370–4.

11. Genitourinary fistulas: vaginal approach for repair of vesicovaginal fistulas. Clin Obstet Gynaecol 1985;12:403–13.

Section

VI

General

- Contraception
- Care of a Survivor of Sexual Violence: Clinical and Medicolegal Aspects

Rachna Sharma, Sneha Sharma

Approximately 4.2 crore couples have an unmet need for contraception. Presently, the spacing options are limited to only condom, intrauterine contraceptive device (IUCD) and oral pills which contribute to 5.9, 1.9 and 4.2% share of contraceptive use respectively. So there is a need for contraceptive counseling in every eligible couple. Here we will discuss different case scenarios and contraceptive choices available for that particular case.

Case 1

A 28-year-old G2P1L1 at 38 weeks gestation delivers a live baby of weight 3 kg with normal APGAR and is breastfeeding. Patient wants contraceptive advice. She is not willing for IUCD insertion.

Q1. What are the options available to her?

The options available to her are:

a. Oral pills
   - Progestogen-only pills (POP)
   - Centchroman
b. Lactational amenorrhea method

Q2. What are POPs? How are they used and when is the earliest time when breast feeding women can start taking them?

Women can start POPs immediately after giving birth whereas COCs should be started six months postpartum. They can be started in breastfeeding women earlier than 6 weeks as they do not affect quality and quantity of milk and infant growth.[1–3]

Progestin only pills also called as "mini pills" contain low doses of synthetic hormone progestin and are to be taken continuously every day[4,5] Women can start using POPs anytime, if it is certain that she is not pregnant. There is no need for backup, if started within 5 days of start of cycle whereas backup method should be used for the first two days of taking pill if started anytime after 5th day of menstrual cycle. All pills in the pack are of same color and are active pills containing hormone. One pill should be taken every day and at the same time.

Q3. What are the side effects of POPs?

The side effects include irregular bleeding, headache, breast tenderness, nausea, dizziness and ovarian cysts.[6,7]

Q4. How are missed pills managed?

If she misses a pill or if she takes pill 3 or more hours late then she should take a pill as soon as possible, other pills are continued as usual. Backup method to be used for next 2 days or emergency contraceptive pill can be taken if she had sexual intercourse in preceding 72 hours.

If she has severe vomiting and vomits within 2 hours of taking the pill, another pill from the pack should be taken as early as possible and rest of the scheduled pack continued, but if vomiting continues, a backup method should be used.

Q5. What is the efficacy of POPs?

In the first year of use, documented failure rates range from 1.1 to 9.6 per 100 women.[8]

Q6. What are Centchroman pills?

Centchroman (ormeloxifene) is a non steroidal, non hormonal selective estrogen receptor modulator (SERM) oral contraceptive pill.

Q7. When to start and how to use centchroman?

For initiation, first pill is to be taken on first day of period and the second pill three days later. This pattern is to be repeated for the first 3 months. From fourth month, the pill is to be taken once a week on the first pill day and should be continued on the weekly schedule.

In case of missed pill it should be taken as soon as possible. If pill is missed by 1 or 2 days but lesser than 7 days normal schedule is continued and backup method is used till the next period starts but if pill is missed by more than 7 days, pills should be started all over again like new user.

Q8. What are the side effects of ormeloxifene?

It can cause delayed periods in some users as well as scanty periods in some, usually in first 3 months which is not harmful and rather helpful for anaemic woman.

Q9. In which conditions should ormeloxifene not be given?

- Polycystic ovarian syndrome
- Recent history of jaundice or liver disease
- Severe allergic state
- Cervical dysplasia
- Chronic illness like tuberculosis

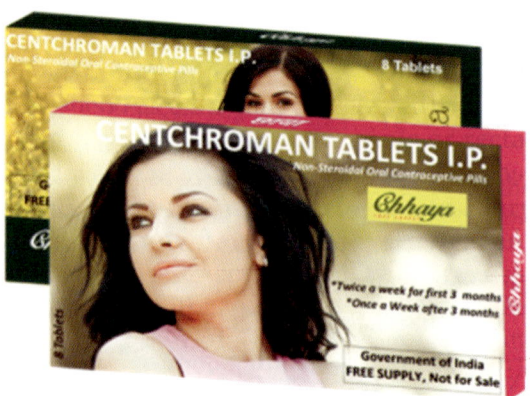

Case 2

A 21-year-old woman P1L1 came to OPD as she had unprotected intercourse 36 hours ago, and also 4 days before that and is worried about pregnancy. Her last menstrual period started 14 days ago and she bleeds for 4 days every 28 days.

Q1. What are the contraceptive options available for her?

- Emergency Contraceptive Pills (ECPs)
- IUCD

Q2. What are emergency contraceptive pills?

ECPs are also known as "morning after pills". The government supplies it by the name "Ezy" pill. It contains only one 1.5 mg tablet of progestin levonorgestrel.[9,10] It is used to prevent pregnancy after unprotected sexual intercourse. It does not disrupt existing pregnancy.

Q3. How should she use ECPs?

Pill is to be taken immediately after unprotected intercourse preferably within 12 hours or as soon as possible within 72 hours.

Case 3

A 25-year-old primigravida with term pregnancy comes with labor pains and delivers a live baby.

Q1. What contraceptive advice should be given to her?

She can be advised to have any of the following contraceptives:

a. Postpartum IUCD
   - Cu T 380 A—for 10 years.
   - Cu T 375 (Multiload)—for 5 years.
b. Depot medroxy progesterone acetate (DMPA) after 6 weeks.
   - ANTARA—in government institutes.
   - KHUSHI—in non-government set-up.
c. Progestogen-only pills (POPs) after 6 weeks
d. Follow lactation amenorrhea method

INTRAUTERINE CONTRACEPTIVE DEVICE

Mechanism of action: Copper IUCDs release copper ions which cause:

- Biochemical and morphologic impact on the endometrium
- Alterations in cervical mucus and endometrial secretions
- Production of cytokine peptides known to be cytotoxic to the endometrium.[11]

Postpartum IUCD

Postpartum IUCD (PPIUCD) can be inserted immediately after delivery of placenta in which case it is called post-placental IUCD insertion.

A written and informed consent from patient alone is sufficient for PPIUCD insertion after counseling her (husband's consent is not required). Consent should ideally be taken before delivery preferably in antenatal period but can be taken at the time of delivery in case patient is not willing before and changes her mind after delivery or if she is an unbooked patient.

For a woman who wants birth spacing between two children, the best option is Cu T 375 or Multiload as it is for five years and can be removed whenever she wants to conceive or at the completion of 5 years.

A woman who has completed her family is an ideal candidate for sterilization but if she is not willing, Cu T 380 A can be inserted as postpartum IUCD as it is effective for 10 years. After ten years if she has not attained menopause, Cu T 380 A can be removed and either reinserted or if patient is willing she can be counseled for permanent sterilization.

If a non-willing woman becomes willing for IUCD insertion, it can be inserted in the next 48 hours post-delivery provided the health care provider is experienced and internal os can be easily negotiated. It can only be inserted in patients who have had a vaginal delivery and not in post-caesarean cases.

Interval IUCD

- It is inserted after 6 weeks postpartum.
- IUCD insertion is not done between 48 hours after delivery to 6 weeks postpartum.

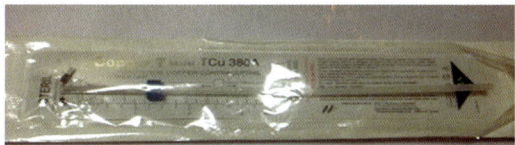

Lactational Amenorrhea Method (LAM)

For use of lactational amenorrhea as contraceptive three criteria have to be met

- She should have amenorrhea
- She should be exclusively breastfeeding
- Child should be less than 6 months old.

Efficacy of Lactation Amenorrhea Method is 0.7 per 100 women at 6 month postpartum.

Case 4

A woman G4P2L2A1 at 11 weeks gestation with history of MTP pill intake with bleeding per vagina comes to gynae casualty in shock with severe anemia. She was admitted, retained products of conception were removed and three unit packed cells were transfused.

Q1. Before discharge what contraceptive advice is given to her??

If a patient has taken MTP pills and presents with complications such as sepsis or anemia, the complications should be managed and after completing the abortion process medically or surgically, contraception should be given immediately.

Post abortal woman who has not completed her family, can be offered the following methods:

a. Contraceptives that can be started on the day misoprostol is given are:
- Combined oral contraceptives (COCs)
- Progesterone-only pills (POPs)
- DMPA and NET-EN
- Medroxy progesterone acetate—ANT ARA, available in government institutes
- Implants

Combined oral contraceptives

- Polyphasic pills—deliver different amount of estrogen and progestins. Aim is to alter steroid levels to achieve lesser metabolic effects, minimize breakthrough bleeding and amenorrhea, while efficacy is maintained.
- Monophasic pills—deliver same amount of estrogen and progestin each day. These pills are used to prevent pregnancy and to regulate cycles in PCOS patients.

b. Copper/levonorgestrel (LNG) IUCD can be inserted after ensuring that abortion is complete.

c. After 2nd trimester abortion provider should be skilled in copper IUCD and LNG IUD insertion and it should not be used in post abortion cases with sepsis.

Post-abortion Woman who has Completed her Family

Sterilization can be offered.

Woman who has Completed her Family and is Seeking an Abortion

- Medical termination of pregnancy and sterilization should be done at the same time.
- Two types of sterilization can be done depending on the facility and skill of the service provider.
  1. Mini-laparotomy
  2. Laparoscopic ligation

1. **Mini-laparotomy**
   - It is the most common method in developing countries.
   - Suprapubic incision is given.
   - Pomeroy's tubal ligation is most commonly done.
   - It is simple and safe.

2. **Laparoscopic ligation**
   - Permits direct visualization and manipulation of the abdominal and pelvic organs.
   - Its advantages are short hospital stay, less discomfort, small scar, and sexual activity need not be restricted.

- Surgeon inspects the pelvic and abdominal organs for abnormalities.
- The disadvantages include the cost, fragile equipment, special training is required and the risks of inadvertent bowel or vessel injury.

Case 5

A 24-year-old woman six weeks postpartum brings her baby for immunization. She is breastfeeding the child and she wants to know regarding contraception options available for her. Discuss whether OCPs are right choice for her or not?

Oral contraceptive pills interfere with breastfeeding so they should not be used in women less then 6 months postpartum.

Options available for her are:

- POPs
- Inj. DMPA
- Centchroman
- IUCD

Q1. What is DMPA?

Inj. DMPA is an aqueous suspension of Pregnane 17 Alpha hydroxyl progesterone—a derivative of progestin medroxy progesterone acetate for depot injection. DMPA is a progestogen only injectable given intramuscular every three months. One dose comprises of one vial of 150 mg, aqueous suspension of DMPA.

Q2. When should she start DMPA injection?

- Can be started within 7 days of menstrual cycle.[12,13]
- Can be started anytime after 7 days of menstrual cycle—with need of backup method for 7 days after injection.
- For breastfeeding women—wait till 6 weeks postpartum and then start DMPA.
- Immediate postpartum in non breast feeding women and post-abortion.

Effectiveness depends on time of injection, regularity, injection technique, post injection care. With perfect use failure rate of 0.3% is noted.

Q3. What is the mechanism of action of DMPA?

- Inhibits ovulation by suppressing midcycle peaks of LH and FSH[14]
- Thickening of cervical mucus—due to depletion of estrogen
- Thinning of endometrial lining—due to high progesterone and depleted estrogen

Q4. What are its limitations?

- Does not protect against sexually transmitted diseases
- Action cannot be stopped immediately
- It has to be repeated every 3 months to achieve desired contraception
- Return of fertility takes 7–10 months from the date of last injection[15]
- It causes changes in the menstrual cycle and bleeding
- Osteoporosis/osteopenia

Q5. What category of patients is DMPA best suited for?

- Breastfeeding women
- As a long term contraception
- Women with iron deficiency anemia

- Women with endometriosis, benign breast disease, ovarian cysts, dysmenorrhea
- Provides protection against endometrial cancer, PID and depression.[16]
- It reduces sickle cell crisis in patients with sickle cell anemia.[17]

Q 6. What are MEC categories?[18]

It refers to medical eligibility criteria

MEC 1: Method can be used without restriction

MEC 2: Advantages of method generally outweigh risks

MEC 3: Method usually not recommended unless other more appropriate methods are not available or not acceptable

MEC 4: Method not to be used

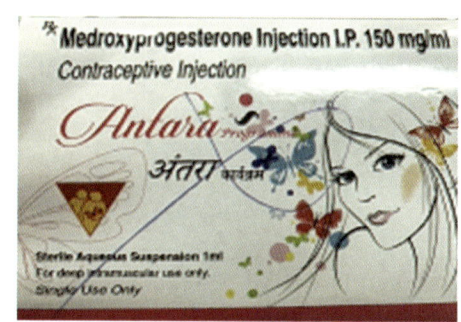

Condition	Qualifier for condition	Contraceptive methods				
		COC	POP	Inj DMPA	IUCD	LNG-IUD
Lactation	<48 hours postpartum	4	2	3	1	2
	>48 hours to <6 weeks postpartum	4	2	3	3	3
	6 weeks–6 months postpartum	3	1	1	1	1
Hypertension	<160/100	3	1	2	1	1
	>=160/100	4	2	3	1	2
HIV	NRTIs	1	1	1	2	2
	NNRTIs	1	1	1	2	2
	Ritonavir boosted protease inhibitors	3	3	3	2	2
Tuberculosis	Pulmonary	3	3	1	1	1
	Abdominal	3	3	1	4	4
Heart disease	Uncomplicated	4	2	3	1	2
	Complicated	4	2	2	2	2
Epilepsy	On anticonvulsants	3	3	1	1	1
DVT	History of DVT, on anticoagulant	4	2	2	1	2
	Acute DVT	4	3	3	1	3
Diabetes Mellitus	History of GDM	2	2	2	1	2
	Without vascular disease	2	2	2	1	2
	With end organ damage or >20 years duration	4	2	3, 4	1	2

Case 6

A 35-year-old G4P2L2A1 at 35 weeks gestation with imminent eclampsia is admitted from casualty, her BP is 170/110 and urine albumin is 2+, MgSO$_4$ is started and labor induction is done. She delivers vaginally. What contraceptive advice should be given to her postpartum?
- Patient should be counselled for PPIUCD.
- Centchroman/POPs after 6 weeks
- Sterilization

Case 7

A 25-year-old G2P1L1 with rheumatic heart disease-severe MS, moderate MR, and moderate PAH delivers a live baby vaginally at 38 weeks. What are the contraceptive options available for her?
a. Valvular heart disease (complicated)
- POP
- DMPA
- Copper IUD
- LNG IUD
- Implant

Prophylactic antibiotics should be given for copper IUD and LNG IUD. Thread should be cut short to prevent infections.

b. Stroke, ischemic heart disease, multiple risk factors
- Copper IUCD
- LNG IUD
- POP
- Implant

NEWER METHODS OF CONTRACEPTION

- Contraceptive patch—known as ortho-Evra has an area of 20 cm^2. It contains 750 µg ethinyl estradiol and 6.0 mg of norelgestromin and delivers 20 µg ethinyl estradiol and 150 µg norelgestromin.
- Patch is applied once weekly for 3 weeks on the same day, but not on the same site followed by a week without use of the patch. Failure rate is <1%.
- Transdermal spray—progesterone only spray (nestrone) with metered dose of 1.2 mg per day. It avoids first pass metabolism and is applied to the skin daily for 3 months.
- Vaginal ring—available as Nuva Ring vaginal steroid contraceptive is a flexible, soft, transparent ring. The Nuva Ring releases 15 µg ethinyl estradiol and 120 µg Etonogestrel per day. Failure rate is less than one percent.[19]
- Vaginal gel—it contains glyminox 1%, applied 15 minutes before intercourse and has microbicidal along with spermicidal effect. Failure rate is 1.2–1.5%.

 Key Points

- COCs should not be given to breastfeeding women till 6 months postpartum.
- POPs are safe for breastfeeding women and can be started earlier than 6 weeks postpartum.
- Apart from prolongation of menstrual cycle centchroman is not known to cause any side effects.
- Emergency contraceptive pills should be taken within 72 hours of unprotected intercourse; they do not disrupt an existing pregnancy.
- Inj DMPA can be started any time after it is certain that woman is not pregnant. Return of fertility takes 7–10 months from the date of last injection.

REFERENCES

1. Tankeyoon M, Dusitsin N, Chalapati S, Koetsawang S, Saibiang S, Sas M, et al. Effects of hormonal contraceptives on milk volume and infant growth. WHO Special Programme of Research, Development and Research Training in Human Reproduction Task force on oral contraceptives. Contraception 1984;30:505–22.
2. Progestogen-only contraceptives during lactation: I. Infant growth. World Health Organization Task force for Epidemiological Research on Reproductive Health; Special Programme of Research, Development and Research Training in Human Reproduction. Contraception 1994;50:35–53.
3. Progestogen-only contraceptives during lactation: II. Infant development. World Health Organization, Task Force for Epidemiological Research on Reproductive Health; Special Programme of Research, Development, and Research Training in Human Reproduction. Contraception 1994;50:55–68.

4. Chi I. The safety and efficacy issues of progestin-only oral contraceptives an epidemiologic perspective. Contraception 1993;47:1–21.

5. McCann MF, Potter LS. Progestin-only oral contraception: a comprehensive review. Contraception 1994; 50: S1–195.

6. Vessey M, Metcalfe A, Wells C, McPherson K, Westhoff C, Yeates D. Ovarian neoplasms, functional ovarian cysts, and oral contraceptives. Br Med J 1987;294:1518–20.

7. Tayob Y, Adams J, Jacobs HS, Guillebaud J. Ultrasound demonstration of increased frequency of functional ovarian cysts in women using progestogen-only oral contraception. Br J Obstet Gynaecol 1985;92:1003–9.

8. Trussell J, Kost K. Contraceptive failure in the United States: a critical review of the literature. Stud Fam Plann 1987;18:237–83.

9. Von Hertzen H, Piaggio G, Ding J, Chen J, Song S, Bartfai G, et al. WHO Research Group on Post-Ovulatory Methods of Fertility Regulation, Low dose mifepristone and two regimens of levonorgestrel for emergency contraception: a WHO multicentre randomised trial. Lancet 2002; 360:1803–10.

10. Arowojoulu AO, Okewole IA, Adekunie AO. Comparative evaluation of the effectiveness and safety of two regimens of levonorgestrel for emergency contraception in Nigerians. Contraception 2002;66:269–73.

11. Nyman T, Strengell L, Rutanen EM. Effect of intrauterine contraceptive devices on cytokine messenger ribonucleic acid expression in the human endometrium. Fertil Steril 1995;63:773–8.

12. Siriwongse T, Snidvongs W, Tantayaporn P, Leepipatpaiboon S. Effect of depo-medroxyprogesterone acetate on serum progesterone levels when administered on various cycle days. Contraception 1982;26:487–93.

13. Petta CA, Faundes A, Dunson TR, Ramos M, DeLucio M, Faundes D, et al. Timing of onset of contraceptive effectiveness in Depo-Provera users: Part I. Changes in cervical mucus. Fertil Steril 1998;69:252–7.

14. Mishell Jr DR. Effect of 6 methyl-17-hydroxyprogesterone on urinary excretion of luteinizing hormone. Am J Obstet Gynecol 1967;99:86–90.

15. Said S, Omar K, Koetsawang S, Kiriwat O, Srisatayapan Y, Kazi A, et al. A multicentred phase III comparative clinical trial of depot-medroxyprogesterone acetate given three-monthly at doses of 100 mg or 150 mg: 1. Contraceptive efficacy and side effects. World Health Organization Task Force on Long-Acting Systemic Agents for Fertility Regulation. Special Programme of Research, Development and Research Training in Human Reproduction. Contraception 1986;34:223–35.

16. Multinational comparative clinical trial of long-acting injectable contraceptives: norethisterone enanthate given in two dosage regimens and depot-medroxyprogesterone acetate. Final report. Contraception 1983;28:1–20.

17. Reference Manual for injectable contraceptive (DMPA) Family Planning Division Ministry of Health and Family Welfare Government of India, March 2016.

18. Medical Eligibility Criteria (MEC) Wheel for Contraceptive Use. Family Planning Division Ministry of Health and Family Welfare Government of India, 2015.

19. Roumen FJ. Review of the combined contraceptive vaginal ring, Nuva Ring. Ther Clin Risk Manag 2008;4:441–51.

Care of a Survivor of Sexual Violence: Clinical and Medicolegal Aspects

Bidhisha Singha

Sexual violence is defined " as any sexual act, attempt to obtain a sexual act, unwanted sexual comments/advances and acts to traffic, or otherwise directed against a person's sexuality, using coercion, threats of harm, or physical force, by any person regardless of relationship to the victim in any setting, including but not limited to home and work (WHO, 2003).[1] Sexual violence is a global public health problem which leads to negative consequences on physical and mental health of a person.

Numerous studies have been done both globally and in India which reveal a high prevalence of sexual violence. In 2009, a meta-analysis was done which analyzed 65 studies over 22 countries, reported that Africa had highest prevalence of child sexual abuse (34.4%); 7.9% males and 19.7% females have faced sexual abuse below the age of 18 years; Europe, America, and Asia had prevalence rate of 9.2%, 10.1%, and 23.9%, respectively.[2]

A National study was conducted by Ministry of Child Development on Child Abuse (2007), it showed that across 13 states, 53% children faced some forms of sexual abuse and 22% were subjected to severe form of sexual abuse. Andhra Pradesh, Assam, Bihar, Delhi showed the highest number of child sexual abuse.[3] Most of the perpetrators are well known rather than strangers.

Health professionals play an important role in responding to survivors, providing medical treatment, psychological support, collecting evidences and good documentation of the findings.

Q1. What is POCSO ACT? What are the relevant acts and rules for medical professionals?

- POCSO stands for Protection of Children From Sexual Offences Act, which is a special law, came into effect from 14th November, 2012.[4]
- Protects children from sexual assault (penetrative/non penetrative), sexual harassment and pornography. The act also strengthens legal provision, integrates child friendly procedures for reporting, recording and investigation, provision of special courts.
- Any person below the age of eighteen years is considered a child.
- Any form of sexual offence is considered to be punishable by law.
- Any sexual offence committed by any person of authority, position of trust, e.g army personnel, teacher, police officer, doctor or any staff of hospital, etc. is considered as "Aggravated sexual assault".
- Mandatory reporting of any sexual offence, failure to do so is a punishable offence (imprisonment for six months and/fine).
- Medical examination of a female child should be conducted by a female doctor, in presence of parent/guardian/any person whom the child trust and in absence, a female has to be appointed by the hospital.
- Emergency medical care to be provided (both government and private hospitals), free of cost, even without a legal requisition.

Q2. What is the definition of rape?

- Rape is defined as per Criminal Law Amendment Act, 2013.[1]
- May be penetrative or non-penetrative.
- Penetrative sexual violence is penetration of vagina, anus, urethra or mouth to any extent by penis/object/any part of the body or manipulates any part of body to cause penetration or applies his mouth to the penis/vagina/anus/urethra.
- Non-penetrative sexual violence includes touching, fondling, stalking, etc.
- A sexual act need not be a complete penetration but also includes a minimal passage of glans between the vulva with or without rupture of hymen or with or without emission of semen.

Case 1

A 23-year-old woman comes to casualty on her own with history of sexual violance.

Q1. Should the doctor go ahead with the examination and treatment? Who should examine the survivor?

- A survivor can come directly to a doctor. Even without a police requisition/magisterial order the doctor can go ahead with the examination and treatment.[1]
- A survivor should be immediately attended to as it is considered to be a medico-legal emergency (Supreme Court Directives, 2000), within 15 minutes of arrival.[5]
- Health provider should be nonjudgemental, empathetic and establish rapport with the survivor. Health provider has to explain the survivor in simple manner the procedure and details of the whole process of reporting, medical examination, forensic evidence collection. Informed consent should be recorded before proceeding for any examination.
- Mandatory reporting to be done, MLC (medicolegal case) to be made.
- If survivor refuses police information, it should be explained that hospital is bound by law to report. However, she has a right not to lodge a FIR.
- Survivor has a right to treatment and it is free of cost. Both private as well as Government institutions are obligated to provide treatment. Denial of treatment is an offence under law (imprisonment of one year/fine/both).
- Any Registered medical practitioner (government or private sector) can examine a survivor (Gynecologist not mandatory). A male doctor can also examine in presence of a female attendant. Female doctor has to examine a girl survivor (POCSO Act), if less than 18 years of age.

Case 2

A 11-year-old girl gives history of sexual violence. She has been brought to the hospital by police. Her parents had accompanied her.

Q1. Whose informed consent/refusal should be sought and for what purposes?

In this case consent has to be taken from her parents, as she is less than 12 years of age.[1]

- Minimum age for giving consent for examination is 12 years (sections 89 and 90 of IPC).
- If below 12 years, parents/guardians can give consent.
- If parents are not available, consent from a panel of doctors from the institution is to be taken for the best interest of the survivor.
- In case of mentally challenged survivor, consent can be taken from parents/guardians. In absence of parents/guardians, consent can be taken from a panel of doctors from the hospital/Child Welfare Committee.
- In case of life threatening situation, doctors can initiate treatment even without consent.

Informed consent/refusal should be taken for:

- Medical examination that is required for treatment
- Medico-legal examination (involves examination of mouth, breast, vagina, anus and rectum)

- Sample collection for treatment and forensic evidence collection
- Information to police

Refusal for any of the above should be documented. Survivor can refuse at any step and her decision is to be respected.

Consent form has to be signed by:
- Survivor/parents/guardian (as appropriate)
- Examining doctor
- Witness (major, disinterested person).

Case 3

A 23-year-old woman, a victim of sexual voilence was brought to hospital by police.

Q1. What are the important points to be kept while taking history?

Detailed history taking is important as history will guide us regarding treatment, and evidence to be collected.[1]
- History should be recorded verbatim.
- History narrated by whom should be recorded (in case of children, history can be elicited with the help of dolls/body charts).
- Sexual violence history should be taken in details
  - date/time/place
  - number (if more than one assailant)
  - name of the perpetrator if revealed, should be countersigned by the informant
  - history of any physical violence suffered and in which part of body
  - history of any verbal threats/use of any objects or weapons/any restraints/use of drugs or alcohol. In case of use of any objects history of any use of lubricants to be elicited.
  - any injury marks left on the assailants body
  - history regarding attempted/complete penetration of vagina, anus and mouth by penis/objects/fingers to be recorded. History regarding other sexual acts also to be elicited.

  - history regarding emission of semen and on which part of the body or use of condom
  - history of post assault activities, e.g bathing, douching, changing clothes, etc. should be taken
- Menstrual history—date of last menstrual period (LMP) is to be recorded, whether the survivor was menstruating at the time of assault needs to be documented (if yes, second examination is to be done later).
- Details of clothing worn at the time of sexual violence should be enquired.
- Previous significant medical or surgical history.

Case 4

An 18-year-old girl was brought to casualty with history of sexual violence. The survivor gives detailed history of peno-vaginal penetration by her neighbour, verbal threats and physical assault.

Q1. What are the important points to be noted during examination of a survivor?[1]

A thorough examination of the survivor is done as detailed below:
- General examination—any signs and symptoms of any intoxication, state of pupils, condition of the clothes worn.
- Examination of injuries on the body:
  - to be examined carefully from head to toe for any injuries, e.g. contusions, lacerations, abrasions.
  - Injuries to be marked on body charts
  - description of injuries in details, e.g. site, shape, dimensions, color
- Presence of any stains on the body to be documented
- Local examination of external genitalia:
  - for any stains, injuries
  - in case pubic hair has been removed, it should be mentioned
  - vulva should be examined in a systemic manner

- per speculum and per vaginal examination to be done in this case *only if indicated*, e.g. bleeding per vagina. Speculum to be lubricated with sterile warm water.
- old injuries of hymen should not be documented. Recent findings should be documented (e.g. bruise, bleeding, tear, etc.)
- Local examination of anus and rectum/oral cavity—for any stains, injuries bleeding, discharge, tenderness to be documented.
- Systemic examination

Case 5

A 15-year-old girl gives history of sexual assault (peno-vaginal penetration with condom) two days back. She had taken bath after the assault. She gives history of being hit by a stick in the thigh. On detailed examination a bluish discoloured area was noted on the right thigh of 3 × 3 cm, probably caused by a blunt object. No other injuries noted on genital examination.

Q1. What medical evidence should be collected during examination of the survivor?

Ask about the clothes worn at the time of assault. If changed or washed it should be documented. Clothes have to be collected by the police.

As her examination revealed a bruise on the right thigh, same finding to be documented on the body charts.

The swabs have to be collected for forensic evidence as the girl has reported after 48 hours.

History of vaginal penetration with condom—two vaginal swabs are collected for evidence of lubricant.

- Evidence collection depends on the type of assault, post assault activities and the time when the survivor has approached after the assault.[1]
- After 96 hours of assault, forensic evidence is unlikely to be found, so swabs to be taken after relevant history. Evidences on the clothing can be collected even after 96 hours

- If the clothing is present, careful documentation of any tears/stains to be mentioned. It should be packed in such a manner that the stain part does not come in contact with the unstained part. All clothes are packed separately in paper bags.
- Nail clippings and nail scrapings to be taken if there is history of struggle during sexual violence or if the survivor gives history of scratching.
- Scalp hair to be combed when there is a history of struggle.
- Blood and urine samples to be taken in case of history of drug/alcohol intoxication, any history of unconsciousness or any sign or symptoms of intoxication.
- Any debris found on the body should be collected.
- Oral swab to be collected from behind the last molars, if history relevant of oral penetration.
- In case of presence of matted pubic hair, it should be cut/removed and packed after drying.
- While taking swabs from dried stains, it should be kept in mind that the swab should be just moistened with only distilled water, properly *air dried* before packing. Swabs should be taken only which are relevant, e.g. vaginal swab should not be collected when only history of oral penetration is given. Number of swabs collected from which site and for what evidence should be mentioned. Number written on the envelope should be in consonance with the numbers written in Forensic lab form (Table 33.1).

Q2. What will be the Provisional Opinion of the above mentioned case? When should the final opinion be given?

The provisional and final opinion in this case are:

Provisional Opinion

A 15-year-old girl has presented 48 hours after assault. She has reported peno-vaginal penetration (penetrative sexual assault) with physical assault. There is history of taking bath

History of sexual violence	Type of swab(s)	Purpose	Any other points to consider?
Peno-vaginal	Vaginal	• Semen/sperm detection • Lubricant • DNA	• Whether ejaculation occurred inside vagina or outside • Use of condom
	Body	• Semen/sperm detection • Saliva (in case of sucking/licking)	• If ejaculation occurred outside
Peno-anal	Anal	• Semen/sperm detection • Lubricant • DNA • Fecal matter	• Whether ejaculation occurred inside anus or outside • Use of condom
	Body	• Semen/sperm detection • Saliva (in case of sucking/licking)	• If ejaculation occurred outside
Peno-oral	Oral	• Semen/sperm detection • DNA • Saliva	• Whether ejaculation occurred inside mouth or outside • Use of condom
	Body	• Semen/sperm detection • Saliva (in case of sucking/licking)	• If ejaculation occurred outside
Use of objects	Swab of the orifice (anal, vaginal, oral)	• Lubricant	• Detection of lubricant used if any
Use of body parts (fingering)	Swab of the orifice (anal, vaginal, oral)	• Lubricant	• Detection of lubricant used if any
Masturbation	Swab of the orifice or body part	• Semen/sperm detection • DNA • Lubricant	• Whether ejaculation occurred or not • If ejaculated in orifice or body parts

Table 33.1: Type of swabs collected for forensic analysis*

*Table from Ministry of Health and Family Welfare guidelines and protocols.

after the assault. On examination a bluish discoloured area of 3 × 3 cm noted in the right thigh, probably caused by a blunt object. No genital injuries are noted which may be due to use of lubricated condom. There are no signs of use of force however vaginal penetration cannot be ruled out. Vaginal swab for presence of lubricant has been sent.

• Provisional opinion is to be formed immediately after detailed medical examination of the survivor on the basis of history and findings.[1] It should also mention after what time the survivor has reported for examination, any history of post assault activities. WHO states that only in 33% cases of sexual violence, injuries are found.[6,7] It should be always borne in mind that absence of findings does not disprove or prove forceful penetrative intercourse.[8–11] Probable reasons for absence of findings should be documented. Mention the samples collected for forensic evidence.

Wherever there is a history of sexual violence and even, if no trace evidence/ injuries are detected during examination— it should always be mentioned that sexual violence cannot be ruled out.

- **Final opinion:** It is given after collection of the reports of forensic analysis and laboratory investigations.

Case 6

An 18-year-old girl brought by police with history of penetrative sexual violence (peno-vaginal) by 3–4 person with physical assault with knife 8 hours back. On taking her menstrual history her LMP was two weeks back. On examination there was a 2 cm superficial incised wound on the right thigh and a vaginal tear of around 3 cm in the posterior fornix was noted.

Q1. How will you manage the case? When should the survivor be called for follow up?

- First and foremost first aid should be given.
- Injection Tetanus Toxoid is to be given.
- Evidence collection and treatment should be done simultaneously.
- The wound in the thigh should be cleaned with antiseptic solution.
- Patient should be taken to operation theatre for surgical management of the vaginal tear.
- Swabs to be collected prior to cleaning and surgical draping.
- Emergency contraception to be given.
- HBsAG immunoglobulin to be given.
- Antibiotics for sexually transmitted disease should also be started.
- Post exposure prophylaxis (PEP) for HIV to be given to her considering her high risk; after explaining the risk, benefits and side-effects of antiretroviral therapy (ART). The drug should be started with her consent and proper counselling.
- Psychological counselling is very important.
- Blood sample should be sent for HIV/ VDRL/HBsAG.

- After her discharge, the survivor is asked to follow up for another medical examination after 3 weeks or earlier if she misses her periods.

Treatment Guidelines[1]

Sexually transmitted infection (STI)

- If clinical signs are suggestive of STI—collect swabs and start PEP.
- In absence of clinical signs—wait for lab results. In settings where lab investigations are not available, start PEP.

  In non-pregnant women—Azithromycin 1 gm stat or Doxycycline 100 mg bd/ Metronidazole 400 mg for 7 days.

  In pregnant women—Amoxycillin/Azi-thromycin with Metronidazole. Metronida-zole is to be avoided in first trimester.

Hepatitis B

- Administer 0.06 ml/kg HB immuno-globulin immediately (within 72 hours).
- WHO recommendation—HBsAG vaccina-tion without HB immunoglobulin should be offered.[12,13]

Emergency contraception

- Should be given preferably within 72 hours, can be given up to 5 days.
- Can be given to girls who are in the begin-ning stages of puberty (Tanner stage 2 and 3) premenarche.[12]

  Levonorgestrel—two tablets of 0.75 mg or single dose of 1.5 mg. Repeat the dose if there is history of vomiting within 3 hours of taking the tablets.

  OR

  Mala-D—two tablets stat and repeat after 12 hours.

Laceration

- Clean the wound/tetanus toxoid/surgical treatment if required

PEP for HIV

- Within 72 hours after assessing HIV risk, proper counselling of risks/benefits/side effects of the drug. ART should be started after obtaining consent.[12,13]

Psychological Care

Guidelines for follow-up

- Re-examination after 2 days to note any development of bruises or other injuries, thereafter at 3 and 6 weeks.
- Test for pregnancy
- Repeat test for STI after the incubation period.
- To assess for psychological sequel and send for psychological support.

Case 7

A 23-year-old lady was brought by parents to the hospital as she was found drowsy. She had gone out with her friends at night. Patient complained of discomfort in the genital area. She only remembers taking a soft drink with one of her friends.

Q1. What are the probable drugs causing such symptoms?

Drugs are being used to incapacitate the victims for rape/sexual assault. These drugs are known as "Date Rape Drugs/Predator drugs". These drugs are odourless, colourless and tasteless. Commonly used drugs are Rohypnol, Gamma hydroxybutyric acid, Ketamine, which makes the victim confused, physically helpless, causes antegrade amnesia and are fast metabolized in the body. For detection of these drugs, blood and urine samples should be tested within 72 hours.[14]

Case 8

A 5-year-old girl child was brought to the casualty by her parents. The child was found by her brother who saw the neighbour undressing the child and touching her breast and genitals. The child is not allowing any examination.

Q1. How would you proceed for examination?

- First and foremost—physical examination should not cause any trauma[15–17]
  - Use clinical judgement

- Address the child's fear and anxieties, explain each step, and protect privacy.
- Provide utmost comfort or care, e.g., examining on the mother's lap or when mother is lying with her on the couch.
- Examination can be deferred or abandoned.
- Never force any examination if there are no reported symptoms or injuries.
- Child should not be held or restrained during examination (except for infants or very young toddlers).
- Sedation or general anaesthesia (GA) to be considered if child refuses examination and conditions requires medical attention, such as bleeding or suspect foreign body. Conscious sedation can be given if examination and evidence collection are necessary and child is not able to co-operate.
- Speculum examination to be done under general anesthesia in pre-pubertal girls (if indicated).

Case 9

A 13-year-old girl came to the outpatient clinic with her mother and she is 9 weeks pregnant. History of repeated sexual assault by her cousin brother was revealed.

Q1. What should the doctor do regarding MTP, collection of sample?

- Pregnancy is to be terminated as per MTP Rules.[1]
- Consent of her mother should be taken as it is an invasive procedure (as per law section 87 IPC girl of 18 years and above can give consent for invasive procedures). In case her mother refuses, consent can be taken from a panel of doctors of the hospital or Child Welfare Committee (CWC).
- The police has to be informed, as the products of conceptus have to be collected and sent to forensic lab as evidence.
- Products of conception are to be only rinsed in normal saline and not to be completely soaked in saline. Immediately hand the samples to the police along with the DNA kit.

Flowchart showing the management of sexual violence survivors[1]

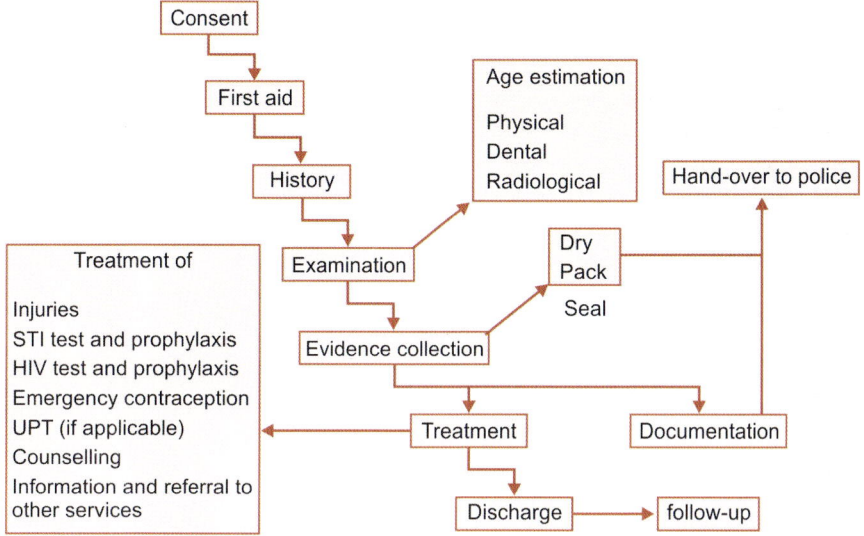

- Sample should be transported by the police in ice-box, temperature should always be maintained at around 4°C (2 to 8°).
- In case the police fail to collect the sample, written intimation should be sent to the police station In-Charge, stating that the hospital will not be responsible if there is degradation of sample leading to loss of evidence.

Key Points

- Care of a survivor of sexual violence needs to be given in a sensitive non judgemental manner.
- It is mandatory to register as a medicolegal case with the police.
- Informed consent should be taken for examination. If refused it should also be documented.
- Careful history taking and thorough examination should be done.
- Per speculum and per vaginal examination are done only if indicated as in vaginal bleeding.
- Medical evidence as detailed in the chapter should be collected meticulously and handed over to the police for forensic analysis.
- The survivor should be given proper medical care including protection against sexually transmitted infections, emergency contraception and psychological counseling.
- Provisional opinion should be drafted carefully and correctly. Final opinion is given after collection of forensic analysis reports.

REFERENCES

1. Guidelines and Protocols, Medicolegal care for survivors/victims of Sexual Violence. Ministry of Health and Family Welfare, Government of India. Available at *https://mohfw.gov.in/reports/guidelines- and-protocols-medico-legal-care-survivors-victims-sexual-violence*
2. Singh MM, Parsekar SS, Nair SN. An epidemiological overview of child sexual abuse. J Family Med Prim Care 2014;3:430–5.
3. Study on Child abuse: India 2007, Ministry of Women and Child Development, Government of India. Available at *https://www.childline india.org.in/pdf/MWCD-Child-Abuse-Report.pdf*
4. The Protection of Children from Sexual Offences Act, 2012. Available at http://indiacode.nic.in/amendmentacts 2012.
5. Comprehensive Standard Operating Procedure for "One Stop Centre in Delhi". Delhi State Legal Services Authority, New Delhi.
6. Bowyer L, Dalton ME. Female victims of rape and their genital injuries. Br J Obstet Gynaecol 1997; 104:617–20.
7. *http://www.who.int/violence_injury_prevention_/_publications/violence/med_leg_guidelines/en/*
8. Tjaden PG, Thoennes N. Full report of the prevalence, incidence, and consequences of violence against women. Research report. Findings from the National Violence Against Women Survey. Washington DC: National

Institute of Justice and Centers for Disease Control and prevention 2000.

9. Strengthening the medico-legal response to sexual violence. WHO publication. November 2015.

10. McLean I, Roberts SA, White C, Paul S. Female genital injuries resulting from consensual and non-consensual vaginal intercourse. Forensic Sci Int 2011;204:27–33.

11. Zilkens RR, Smith DA, Phillips MA, Mukhtar SA, Semmens JB, Kelly MC. Genital and anal injuries: A cross-sectional Australian study of 1266 women alleging recent sexual assault. Forensic Sci Int 2017; 275:195–202.

12. Responding to children and adolescents who have been sexually abused, WHO Clinical Guidelines, 2017.

13. Responding to intimate partner violence and sexual violence against women, WHO clinical and policy guidelines, 2013, *http://www.who.int, reproductivehealth/publications/violence*

14. Pal R, Teotia AK. Date rape drugs and their forensic analysis: An update. Int J of Medical Toxicology and Legal Medicine 2010;12:36–47.

15. Model Guidelines under Section 39 of The Protection of Children from Sexual Offences Act,2012.Ministry of Women and Child Development 2013.

16. Child Sexual Abuse: Prevention and Response 2015, Information for Health Care Professionals UNICEF.

17. Child Sexual Abuse: Prevention and Response 2012, Information booklet for doctors and health care professionals, UNICEF.